Perspectives in Public Health

Edited by

Siân Griffiths and David J Hunter

Foreword by

The Minister of State for Public Health

Radcliffe Medical Press

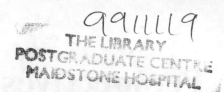
©1999 Siân Griffiths and David J Hunter

Radcliffe Medical Press Ltd
18 Marcham Road, Abingdon, Oxon OX14 1AA

British Library Cataloguing in Publication Data

A catalogue record for this book is available from the British Library.

ISBN 1 85775 209 0

Typeset by Advance Typesetting Ltd, Oxfordshire
Printed and bound by the Alden Press, Oxford

Contents

Foreword   vi

List of contributors   x

1   Introduction   1
Siân Griffiths and David J Hunter

2   Public health policies   11
David J Hunter

Part 1   Posing the problems: case studies in public health

3   Past and present public health in Liverpool   23
John Ashton

4   Tackling inequalities in health: public policy action   34
Michaela Benzeval

5   Food as a public health issue   47
Tim Lang

6   Transport   59
Gary McGrogan

7   Why should public health include housing?   66
Geoff Matthews

8   Domestic violence   85
Siobhan McCartney

9   Tobacco control: a losing battle?   95
Donald Reid

10   Children and young people   107
Aidan Macfarlane

11   Occupational health   115
Kit Harling

12   **Population ageing**   121
      John Grimley Evans

13   **Genetics**   131
      Ron Zimmern

Part 2   Meeting the challenges: practice perspectives

14   **Multidisciplinary public health in practice**   143
      Ros Levenson, Nikki Joule and Jill Russell

15   **Public health practice in health authorities**   159
      Tony Jewell

16   **Annual public health reports**   171
      Anne Davies

17   **Primary care perspectives**   179
      David Colin-Thomé

18   **Public health and local government**   192
      Tony Elson

19   **Environmental health perspectives**   198
      Graham Jukes

20   **Public health and health promotion**   203
      Charlotte Black

21   **The practice of public health medicine: past, present, future** 214
      June Crown

22   **Public health and clinical practice**   223
      Nicholas Hicks

23   **Public health nursing**   235
      Ron De Witt and Jackie Carnell

24   **Public health scientists**   250
      Janet Baker

25   **The socially constructed dilemmas of academic public health** 261
      John Gabbay

Part 3   Facing the future

26   Futures I   271
Walter Holland and Susie Stewart

27   Futures II   281
Kenneth Calman

28   Futures III   289
Lord Hunt of King's Heath

29   Postscript/signposts   295
Siân Griffiths and David J Hunter

Index   297

Foreword

In the year in which the NHS celebrates its fiftieth anniversary, it may appear facile to write that society has changed since 1948, but there are still occasional voices of dissent about the need for change, so it is worth repeating it. Britain today is a much more diverse and less deferential country than it was in the 1940s and 1950s. In the post-war spirit of national collective action, from a country that had pulled together and sustained itself through a harrowing war, mass solutions for a mass population were the obvious response. Big governments did big things for a passive population. The tendency was towards 'a one size fits all' and 'any colour so long as it is black' model of provision.

Just as the global economy has diversified that approach to production, so too have society, culture and public expectations become more sophisticated. So just as we are seeking to modernise our health service – through our commitments on waiting lists and through intiatives such as *NHS Direct* – we must also seek a third way of promoting and protecting the public health of the country – a way that recognises the realities of the present rather than the habits of the past. The Green Paper, *Our Healthier Nation*, was our first step in setting out what that new public health might look like.

In doing so we also had to recognise that the pattern of disease and death in England has changed dramatically since the 1948 Act. The combination of truly national and free health service with new vaccines meant that tuberculosis, polio and measles were soon no longer the awesome killers that they had been. Medical technology, new treatments and new ways of diagnosing illness helped to tackle old problems. New drugs allowed some people with mental health problems to leave the Victorian watertower hospitals and return to the community. The Lunacy Act gave way to the Mental Health Act.

Life expectancy improved. Diet improved. The number of people who smoked began to fall. As some of these challenges were met, new challenges arose or longstanding ones became more apparent. Above all, inequalities in health have persisted and in some cases widened. Life expectancy at birth for a baby boy has been estimated to be about 5 years less in children of manual and unskilled workers than in those of professional and managerial workers. Children born to parents of unskilled workers are five times as likely to suffer accidental death than the children of professional workers. The district with the worst infant mortality rate in England has a rate more than three times as high as that of the best.

Such inequalities are unacceptable, which is why we set out our aim in *Our Healthier Nation* to improve the health of the worst off in society and to narrow the health gap. The Independent Inquiry into Inequalities in Health reported recently to Government on its conclusions following a review of the evidence for the most effective action we can take to reduce health inequalities. The report will inform the development of the White Paper which will set out our definitive strategy for improving the health of the people of England.

The third way is also about realism in what can be achieved. Health inequalities have persisted throughout the century, only narrowing at times of war. They have widened in many cases, particularly over the past two decades. So we need to be quite clear that, although there may be some quick wins, the overall task is a difficult one and a long-term one. In the past the difficulty of the challenge meant that government ignored or denied it. Inequalities were euphemistically and deceptively referred to as 'variations' and explained away as statistical artefacts or the fault of those who suffered most from them. This Government will not shy away from the task. Health inequality is unacceptable in a civilised society and we must bend our efforts to a long-term haul to reduce them.

Another key challenge that has become apparent as life expectancy increases, is that although we are living longer, too many of those additional years are spent in poor health and dependence. In 1994, for example, life expectancy at birth for a baby girl was almost 80 years, but over 17 of those years could be expected to be years of illness. Good health is not just about how long people live. It is also about quality of life and how well people are during their extra years, so that they can enjoy the dignity and independence that we take for granted when we are well.

If we meet the targets proposed in *Our Healthier Nation* then we will be saving at least 15 000 preventable deaths each year – and when I write 'we' I do not mean 'we, the Government', I mean 'we, the country'. *Our Healthier Nation* sets out a third way for public health between top-down, nanny state planning and individual victim blaming. The Government rejects the old notion that the state can somehow organise the country in such a way as to ensure that people become healthier automatically through no effort on their own part. Equally, it is unsustainable to say that all ill health is all the fault of the person who suffers it. Health is not about blame. It is about opportunity and responsibility.

The national contracts for health set out a third way. Individuals on their own can find it hard to make a difference, but with help from friends and families, and support, when it is needed, from local and community agencies, they can make real changes. Those local agencies need central government to provide leadership and put in place the national building blocks and support. Without individuals, families and communities working together, government achievements will be limited. Without government playing its full part, as we found in the past, communities and individuals will struggle to make a real difference.

To help bring the nation together in a concerted and co-ordinated drive for better and more equitable health, we have proposed a national contract for better health. It sets out our mutual responsibilities for improving health in the areas where we can make most progress towards our overall aims of reducing the number of early deaths, increasing the length of our healthy lives and tackling inequalities in health.

The government role is an explicitly wide one in the national contracts. The Government is firmly committed to tackling inequalities in health, through the concerted efforts of everyone who can play a part. The New Deal, our education reforms, the national minimum wage, the Capital Receipts initiative and our commitment to strategic policies on transport and the environment – together with Health Action Zones, Education Action Zones, and Employment Action Zones – these policies form a critical mass that can finally begin to tackle inequalities in health. Problems that have grown up and worsened over decades will not be solved overnight. Our establishment of the Independent Inquiry into Inequalities in Health was a clear sign of our commitment on this front.

So the new public health is about partnership and mutual responsibility at all levels of society and between all levels of society – individual, community and national. It is as much about wider socio-economic and environmental policies as it is about those policies that fall within the portfolio of the Department of Health. We now need to think very carefully about how we flesh out a new – and critical – dimension: psycho-social health.

When ill-defined, it is an approach that is all too easy to hold up to mockery, particularly when politicians start to write about feelings and emotional well being. However, there is no doubt that it is a very serious and important factor. Too much stress makes you ill. Our ability to cope with stress affects our health. The quality of relationships in society – at home, at work, in the street – is incredibly influential on our health. Socially cohesive societies, where people trust each other, respect each other and are able to say what they feel, are more likely to be healthy societies. Societies where people walk the streets in fear of each other, mutually suspicious and closing off their feelings are neither happy nor healthy places to be. How people feel – their well being – is an excellent predictor of their physical health.

So we cannot approach public health merely on medical and material foundations. We need to have the self-confidence and maturity to recognise that the way we handle our relationships with each other is a key component of health. We need to start learning the practical business of building and sustaining well being – nurturing and strengthening the factors that seem to protect some individuals from the worst effects of multiple deprivation.

We are only beginning to understand the pathways and connections between the psychological and physiological, but there are already policies we can point to which will help to bolster the psychological resilience and emotional self-confidence of society. Pre-school education will be a vital part of that. So too will be the quality of relationships that the very young have with their parents. Educational achievement, at whatever age, helps to protect against poor health. The sure start, parenting and nurturing programmes and measures to reduce crime, and fear of crime, will also be important.

Action against social exclusion and social isolation will be a vital component of that work. Disabling poor health is socially excluding, preventing people from playing a full part in social and economic life. Nowadays, a lot is talked about social exclusion, and quite rightly, but we should never forget that premature death is the ultimate social exclusion.

Unemployment, low educational attainment, poor housing and a degraded environment are central both to health inequality and to social exclusion. The Government has signalled its clear intention to make headway on these issues. The public health agenda is a major driver in this effort.

In moving forward from the NHS's fiftieth anniversary and developing the new public health, it is worth reminding ourselves from time to time about the founding principles that underpin it and who better to quote in this year than Nye Bevan?

The preventive health services of modern society fight the battle over a wider front and therefore less dramatically than is the case with personal medicine. Yet the victories won by preventive medicine are much the most important for mankind. This is not so only because it is obviously preferable to prevent suffering rather than alleviate it. Preventive medicine, which is merely another way of saying collective action, builds up a system of social habits that constitute an indispensable part of what we mean by civilisation.

I hope that readers of this volume will find the stimuli of debate, discussion, and innovation a spur to further concerted action in this vital arena of public policy.

Rt Hon. Tessa Jowell
Minister of State for Public Health
January 1999

List of contributors

Professor John Ashton
Regional Director of Public Health
NHS Executive, North West Region

Janet Baker
Assistant Director of Public Health
NHS Executive, West Midlands

Charlotte Black
Executive Director
Cambridge and Huntingdon Health
  Authority

Michaela Benzeval
Senior Research Fellow
The London School of Economics and
  Political Science

Sir Kenneth Calman
Vice-Chancellor and Warden
University of Durham
Former Chief Medical Officer

Jackie Carnell
Chief Executive
Community Practitioner & Health Visitors
  Association

David Colin-Thomé
General Practitioner
Cheshire

June Crown
Director, South East Institute of Public
  Health
Past President, Faculty of Public Health
  Medicine

Anne Davies
Freelance Policy Analyst

Ron De Witt
Chief Executive, Leeds Health Authority
Chairman, English National Board
  for Nursing, Midwifery and Health
  Visiting

Tony Elson
Chief Executive
Kirklees Metropolitan Council

Professor John Gabbay
Professor of Public Health
Wessex Institute for Health Research,
  University of Southampton

Siân Griffiths
Director of Public Health and Health
  Policy
Oxfordshire Health Authority

Professor Sir John Grimley Evans
Professor of Clinical Gerontology
University of Oxford

Kit Harling
Consultant Occupational Physician
Bristol Royal Infirmary
President, Faculty of Occupational
  Medicine

Nicholas Hicks
Consultant Public Health Physician
Oxfordshire Health Authority

Professor Walter Holland
Visiting Professor
LSE Health, London School of Economics
Past President, Faculty of Public Health
    Medicine

Lord Hunt of King's Heath
Former Chief Executive
NHS Confederation

Professor David J Hunter
Professor of Health Policy and
    Management
Nuffield Institute for Health
University of Leeds

Tony Jewell
Director of Public Health and
    Health Policy
North West Anglia Health Authority

Nikki Joule
Independent Policy and Research
    Consultant

Graham Jukes
Director of Professional Services
Chartered Institute of Environmental
    Health

Professor Tim Lang
Professor of Food Policy
Thames Valley University

Ros Levenson
Independent Policy and Training
    Consultant
Visiting Fellow, King's Fund

Siobhan McCartney
Research and Development Officer
Greater Glasgow Health Board

Gary McGrogan
Head of Environment and Regulatory
    Services
Sheffield City Council

Aidan Macfarlane
Public Health Consultant
Oxfordshire Health Authority

Geoff Matthews
Policy Officer (Housing)
Local Government Association

Donald Reid
Chief Executive
Association for Public Health

Jill Russell
Honorary Research Fellow
Royal Free and University College
    Medical School, University College,
    London

Susie Stewart
Research Manager
Department of Public Health, University
    of Glasgow

Ron Zimmern
Director of the Public Health Genetics
    Unit
Cambridge and Huntingdon Health
    Authority

For our long suffering families

Jessica, Allie, Sam and Ian

and

Jacqui, Eve and Miles

CHAPTER ONE

Introduction

Siân Griffiths and David J Hunter

Public health has become more topical since the election of the Labour Government in 1997, particularly with the appointment of the first Minister for Public Health, who has spelt out her vision for public health in the Foreword. But one of the problems with public health is that it can be everything – the air we breathe, the food we eat, our water, housing, health behaviours and also our health services. As such it also risks being nothing – merely a diffuse and confusing collection of ideas that are not seen to deliver any concrete product. It was just this 'everywhere but nowhere' tension which prompted us to collect together contemporary perspectives in public health in the UK. We have invited public health practitioners from a variety of backgrounds to give their views on important themes in public health today. Our aim has been to reflect the practice of public health. A snapshot of public health in its 150th year, we look at the past, present and future. An exploration of the historical perspective is followed by case studies of important issues such as food, tobacco and inequalities. Practitioners of public health have developed the theme of current practice and the final chapters reflect on possible future scenarios. We hope that readers will learn from the diverse perspectives something about the scope, passion, problems and future of public health.

In the 150 years since the Public Health Act was passed in Britain the context and challenges facing public health may have changed but the basic principles have remained the same. The Government has signalled the importance of redirecting the focus of the NHS from ill health and health services, to a broader view which recognises not only positive health but the impact of environmental and social factors on people's health. To quote *Modernising Health and Social Services*:

> *The Government recognises the complex causes of ill health and the part that economic and social factors have to play. It also recognises the fundamental inequalities in health; that the worst off in our society are more ill and die earlier.*[1]

The same document recognises that 'public health has been relatively neglected', whilst the recent Health Improvement Programme guidance highlights the shared responsibility for health between local authorities, health authorities and their partners.[2]

This modern face of public health needs to be set within the context of historical development. Since 1848, public health has moved through many phases and incarnations, assimilating scientific developments which have made it possible to practise population healthcare as well as to create healthier environments.

To some extent, progress in public health can be monitored by the rise, and fall, of the Medical Officer of Health (MOH). The establishment of the office of MOH was the symbolic recognition of the importance of public health – and its disestablishment indicative of the breadth of its responsibilities which are not containable within the medical model. George Bernard Shaw, writing the preface to his play *The Doctor's Dilemma* gives an important insight into the role of the MOH at the turn of the century.[3] He describes the MOH as follows:

> *He has a safe, dignified, responsible independent position based wholly on the public health ... his position depends, not on the number of people who are ill ... but on the number who are well. He is judged, as all doctors and treatments should be judged, by the vital statistics of his district.*

Shaw recognised that public health had a broader role than merely involving doctors, and spelt out his vision that:

> *the MOH as we know him is only the beginning of that army of Public Hygiene which will presently take the place in general interest and honour now occupied by our military and naval forces. It is silly that an Englishman should be more afraid of a German soldier than of a British disease germ, and should clamour for more barracks in the same newspaper that protests against more school clinics and cry out that if the state fights disease it makes us paupers.*

The reaction against the imposition of a hygienic orthodoxy by both media and the profession is not dissimilar to the present-day reaction to the nanny state. It is arguable whether Shaw's vision has been achieved. Recognising the scale of the task in taking on board the importance of collective as well as individual action, he proffered some advice in the conclusion of his treatise for both the public and the profession. He recommended to the public that they should:

> *take the utmost care to get well born and well brought up. This means that your mother must have a good doctor. Be careful to go to a school where there is what they call a school clinic, where your nutrition and teeth and eyesight and other matters of importance to you will be attended to. Be particularly careful to have all this done at the expense of the nation.*

He added to this advice a message for MOHs that, in view of the enormity of their struggle to redirect medical effort away from treatment towards prevention, a sense of humour was a prerequisite.

This sense of humour is still needed. Many people today ask what public health is, what its boundaries are, what people in public health actually do and what the remit of the minister is. Despite political policies there are still hearts and minds to be won. Part of the problem of raising the profile and identity of the issues core to public health is that other labels are used – for example, the programmes of work subsumed within Health Action Zones, or terms such as 'social exclusion' and 'inequalities'. Welcome that this integration is, it can also create something of an identity crisis for practitioners and public alike. Looking to definitions, one of the most widely used is:

...the science and art of preventing disease, prolonging life and promoting health through the organised efforts of society.[4]

Beaglehole and Bonita recommend this definition since it encompasses the essential elements of modern public health – a population perspective, an emphasis on collective responsibility for health and on prevention, the key role of the state linked to a concern for the underlying socio-economic determinants of health as well as disease, a multi-disciplinary basis which incorporates quantitative as well as qualitative methods and an emphasis on partnership with the populations served.[5]

Whilst practitioners might be comfortable with these concepts, others have suggested that public health should be defined in terms of 'quality of life' because this is more easily understood. The difficulty explaining public health is not unique to the UK. A recent survey in the US found only 3% of the population thought they could define public health, though many more could cite the benefits of clean water and immunisation. The definition used in the US is that public health is:

...what we, as a society, do collectively to assure the conditions in which people can be healthy.

Writing in 1996 in the presidential column for the American Association for Public Health, Barry Levy expressed his view that perhaps the most important challenge to public health is the complacency, and often ignorance, of the public about public health.[6]

...as public health programs and services have succeeded, people have lost sight of the relevance and importance of public health. People take for granted the safety of food, water, air, their workplaces. They take for granted immunizations, seat belt use, family planning options, access to cancer screening programs, healthy attitudes about diet and exercise...

Levy argued that in the US this has resulted in the gradual erosion of the public health infrastructure.

In the light of current policy, it could be argued that such structural erosion is not obvious in the UK. However, behind the rhetoric there have been significant threats – privatisation of water, fears about food safety, BSE – yet there remains public and political support for the Government's commitment to tackling social exclusion and to raising awareness of the social foundations of health.

Whatever the definition and general understanding of public health, it is clear that the task of promoting the public's health lies with many people in many different walks of life. Public health is everybody's business, regardless of whether they are politicians, employers, policy makers, professionals or members of the public. This is not a new idea. *Health for All*, a global strategy developed by the World Health Organisation (WHO) in

1978, recognised that the solutions to ill health did not lie in healthcare alone and proposed a comprehensive collective approach to improving health.[7] This was taken a step further by the Ottawa Charter in 1986 which identified five key areas for action[8]:

• building healthy public policy
• creating supportive environments
• strengthening community action
• developing personal skills
• re-orienting health services.

Furthermore, attention has been recently directed by the Chief Medical Officer (CMO) of England's annual report to environmental perspectives of achieving sustainability by the development of Agenda 21 and the proposal not only for a National Environmental Action Plan but for a local version, a Local Environmental Health Action Plan.[9]

Not only the 'what' but the 'how' are being addressed by public sector policy. Across all sectors, partnership working and community development are being promoted. Redressing inequalities and tackling social exclusion are common themes for the departments of employment, environment, education, transport and health. But common values and policies do not in themselves achieve shared solutions without a great deal of collaboration.

Nor will it be enough to rely on national policy to create change. Public health professionals face a challenging time. They face increased expectations within the healthcare system, where epidemiology is a cornerstone of clinical effectiveness and evidence-based medicine, and will increasingly underpin clinical governance. There are challenges associated with the structural changes within the NHS, and at the same time they must take up the challenges of working in multidisciplinary partnerships on the wider health agenda. This means that different approaches are required, appropriate skills need to be honed and capacity increased. Leadership at national and local level is needed to engage the public and professionals in their health agenda. To do this, public health professionals will need appropriate education, better co-ordination, effective networks and an academic base from which to undertake research and develop appropriate practice not only within the health but also within local government sectors.

These themes, recognised by the former Chief Medical Officer for England, Sir Kenneth Calman, in his report on strengthening the public health function, are reflected throughout the contributions in this book.

Chapter 3 sets the scene. Reflecting on the history of Liverpool, John Ashton traces 150 years of public health from the first MOH, the redoubtable WH Duncan, onwards. For Duncan, the challenges for public health lay in the environment, still a major theme within the *Healthy Cities* approach adopted within Liverpool. Ashton comments on the tension between biomedical and social models, a tension which resonates throughout other contributions, reflecting the increasing demands for public health approaches within the wider agenda as well as the increasing expectations raised by clinical effectiveness and evidence-based care.

Following this historical perspective, authors go on to describe some of the modern challenges – transport, food, housing, inequalities – as case studies for public health action. Duncan faced death rates of 36 per 1000 with one-eighth of the city's population living in underground cellars. Poverty and ill health remain closely linked, as demonstrated by the widening differentials between affluent and less well off populations and communities. Drawing together current threads of thinking on inequalities in health, Benzeval reflects on whether the current government strategies, relying as they do on education and employment, are enough to reach the root cause of poverty and deprivation, particularly with the historical difficulties of co-ordinating policies across government departments. She raises questions not only concerning whether government policies for those living on benefits will bring them out of poverty but also whether the whole issue of addressing inequalities will be of high enough priority when agencies are faced with a long list of areas for action.

Amongst health determinants, food must take high priority. Highlighting that poverty is linked to poor diet and greater ill health, Lang points out that it is not only individual consumption patterns but also the means of production, regulation and environmental impact of distribution which require public health intervention, including action and intervention at a global and European level.

The large vehicles travelling many transnational miles to out-of-town shopping centres, which require shoppers to use their cars, illustrate graphically some of the links between food and transport policy. Transport is a major public health issue and McGrogan discusses the impact of transport policies on health, describing a case study in which changes towards creating a healthy and sustainable local transport policy were made. Another environmental determinant of health is housing, recognised not only by the nineteenth-century but also by the mid-twentieth-century welfare reformers who targeted squalor as one of the five giants to be addressed by the Beveridge reforms. The post-war period was characterised initially by an extensive house building programme, followed by the Thatcher years which brought an emphasis on privatisation and individual ownership of housing. The assets accrued by local councils from the sale of council housing have only just been released in a programme that acknowledges the need to invest in upgrading the quality of housing stock. Better housing will improve health, and Matthews makes a plea for greater clarity about the links between housing and health and the proper integration of housing into public health policy at national, regional, local and individual levels.

Similar need for greater awareness and integration of action exists for health and the criminal justice system. One example of the need for partnership arises from the needs of women who are the victims of domestic violence. A major public health issue, domestic violence requires co-ordination and integration of services but also training and awareness of staff in the healthcare sector. McCartney describes one such approach in Glasgow.

Another major public health problem, not only in the UK but globally, is smoking and the use of tobacco. Since the 1990s have seen an end to the long period of decline in smoking rates, strategies are needed to reduce demand and restrict access, relying not only on individual changes but also on health protection measures, including addressing poverty and creating healthier environments. Reid emphasises that the increasing trend amongst young people is of particular concern in a battle which, it would appear, is being lost.

The public health needs of children and young people could, Macfarlane proposes, be addressed by creating a speciality of child public health. Arguing that poverty is the greatest child health problem, such a speciality could act as a focus for multisectoral partnerships, particularly between health, social care and education sectors. The education sector has a key role to play in promoting health, not only through imparting knowledge but by providing a setting for broader health-related activities and initiatives, such as developing parenting skills and promoting better citizenship. This has been recognised within the new health strategy, *Our Healthier Nation*, in the proposal for healthy settings.[10]

Another healthy setting proposed is the workplace. Identifying occupational health services as primarily preventive and multidisciplinary, Harling suggests that the opportunity could now exist both to reduce the toll of ill health arising from work and work activities and, at the same time, to maximise access to work for all sections of the community, including those with chronic illness and disability. The empirical value of higher levels of employment needs to be matched with greater efforts to provide effective occupational health services – not least within the NHS.

A further challenge to public health is that of an ageing population. Grimley Evans argues that the public health response to the ageing population should be to adjust the environment and lifestyle of the nation to produce the best overall outcome given the genetic propensities of the population. Evidence from the US supports the view that the aim of lengthening life but shortening disability is attainable by a policy of 'postponement as prevention', decreasing disability by reducing the gap between acquiring disability and dying. Within the UK the paucity of data means that more research is needed, particularly to develop a better understanding of the loss of adaptability that occurs with ageing as the result of the interaction between intrinsic (genetic) factors and extrinsic factors in the environment and lifestyle.

The rapidly developing fields of genetics and molecular medicine pose major challenges for public health practitioners and their populations. Zimmern argues that there will be a variety of avenues of development – screening, treatment, phenotypic prevention – which, in the light of increasing public expectation, require that public health practitioners embrace the new genetics with understanding and enthusiasm. It will require education and training as well as serious consideration of the ethical implications both of screening and of the potential to create a new set of inequalities.

Part 2 of the book considers perspectives on the practice of public health from a variety of practitioners. The previous section underlined the essential multidisciplinary nature of public health practice. This is reinforced by the findings of a study by Levenson and colleagues for the King's Fund, which sought to identify good practice, particularly in health authorities, at a time when many public health professionals were involved in purchasing. They found that the benefits of applying knowledge, skills, perspectives and experience from a wide range of different disciplines and professional backgrounds led to greater understanding and involvement of the community and better public health practice. But professional and institutional barriers to change exist, and the challenge of abandoning narrow monodisciplinary ways of working and of improving co-operation are prerequisites for making real progress in improving the health of the public.

The need to adapt practice is amplified by Tony Jewell in his consideration of public health practice in health authorities. Reflecting on the historical development of health authorities, particularly the structural changes of recent years, he explores the current tensions felt by public health practitioners, particularly those of traditional independence, and the expectation by management of corporacy, and the need to take the utilitarian population-based view rather than taking the view of clinical colleagues who focus on meeting the needs of each individual patient. Some of the structural changes and opportunities offered by the new agenda are explored – particularly the Health Improvement Programme – the 'raison d'être of the new authorities' – and the changing relationship with primary care which will increasingly take on population-based responsibilities, including needs assessment.

The need for changes in practice to meet the new agenda is reflected by Anne Davies, who suggests a redefinition of the annual report of the Director of Public Health. Earlier in this Introduction, Shaw's view that the worth of an MOH could be judged by the vital statistics of his population was quoted. Annual reports, initially of the MOHs and more recently of Directors of Public Health, provide both a record of these statistics and an independent assessment of the health of local populations. Davies describes the possible futures for annual health reports in the light of the existing confusion about their role and use, with wide variations in content, style, purpose and dissemination between districts. She proposes that the duty to produce annual reports should be redefined to ensure that comparisons can be made between statistics and also to share experience of what works. She proposes several ways in which reports could become more accessible to the public, becoming standardised while maintaining independence. The impact of this could be a radical change in organisation and accountability for public health, and as such it remains a question for further debate.

This theme is picked up by Colin-Thomé, who develops the strands of health needs assessment, anticipatory care, inter-agency working, community development and clinical governance from a primary care perspective, illustrated by examples of local good practice. The potential for good public health practices lies in primary care, but is as yet unrealised by many. As these five strands are developed, ways of working will change and the potential exists for greater involvement in local communities, particularly through closer relationships between primary care groups (PCGs) and local authorities. Only time will tell whether this aspiration will be realised.

Although the aspirations to work together exist, and the impact of local government policy on health is well recognised, the presence of a national service for health can lead to a gap between this understanding and the need for action by local government. Elson argues that we have to think hard about how to engender true engagement and, by thinking differently, to present a convincing argument that improvements in health are an essential prerequisite for the achievement of some of the primary objectives of local government. The new agenda that requires stronger local government involvement in health strategy also requires a more involved commitment for health in the new local government agenda.

Although the whole of local government policy may be relevant, to some extent, to health, historically there are particularly close links with environmental health. When environmental health and public health were separated by the structural changes in 1974, environmental health officers and public health physicians kept in close contact with their shared responsibilities for health protection, particularly communicable disease control. Jukes comments on the future roles, skills and needs for environmental health and the training implications that follow from adopting a less regulatory and more developmental role.

Many environmental health departments have played an active role in health promotion, employing specialists in this area. Health promoters are an important group of public health practitioners. As described by Black, health promotion is not the domain of one professional group or organisation. Around the country there are many examples of partnerships where health promotion specialists have played a key role in developing shared approaches to policy making and have stimulated community action through community development. However, in common with other practitioners, health promoters are besieged with problems around funding, outcomes, priorities and effectiveness.

Reflecting on the challenges facing public health medicine, Crown stresses that it is not merely more scientific knowledge that is needed but a better understanding of how to bring about change, how to improve methodologies for monitoring and surveillance and how to research persistent public health problems. 'Changing times require new ways of working and it is not good enough to offer more of the same.'

This sentiment is shared by De Witt and Carnell, who review the role of public health nurses. New opportunities are created by the new agenda for nurses, particularly health visitors, to play a leading role in public health. PCGs will, by providing opportunities to work more closely together, enable community nurses to focus on the community and not just individual patients and to develop closer partnerships with social services. This will provide opportunities for effective working across the health and social care spectrum.

Just as public health nurses face the challenge of working in new ways, the role and importance of public health scientists is receiving more attention. Baker describes their important contribution and the challenges faced in achieving training, accreditation and an appropriate career structure. The options for careers can be both within the NHS and in other sectors, and much of the focus of this book is about the broader social agenda. Yet it is important not to belittle the role of clinically effective practice in promoting health gain. This theme is amplified by Hicks, who draws out the importance of the application of epidemiology in promoting effective healthcare, describing the benefits of both public health involvement in clinical care and clinician involvement in public health practice. The application of epidemiology relies on a strong research base. John Gabbay argues that the reliance on the medical model within the research community is too great, but is a result of the structure of the funding mechanisms for research. This needs reappraisal if we are to see the knowledge base for wider public health created, yet there are significant problems in achieving such a shift.

Part 3 of the book looks to the future. In his vision of public health in 2025, Holland describes his ideal public health structure – a structure in which the past lack of democratic governance at regional and local level has been remedied, with a division between public health and clinical responsibilities confirming that clinical services are only one part of the health service equation. Greater sway is given to public information, public health education and public health research. Funding is ring-fenced and there are many more practitioners – playing advisory and participatory roles rather than being engaged in direct management.

Calman's view of the future is less structural and seeks to identify key issues. These include the improved organisation of public health, greater involvement of the public, a better understanding of risk, clarity about good outcomes, effective means of horizon scanning and shared understanding of values. In addition to this he identifies specific areas for development, many of which have been raised as issues by other contributors.

In the final contribution, Hunt looks at the immediate future and how local government and the health service can work effectively together. He describes the opportunities that exist, and the massive modernisation programme that is underway. Initiatives such as Health Action Zones (HAZs) are based on the need to pull policies together from across all sectors – and to find ways of working together. Collaboration is fine in theory but it is difficult to achieve. More exhortations to work together will not be enough. Without integration, commitment and a clear sense of purpose the current opportunities created by political change will disappear and public health will once again take second place to the immediate health service agenda of waiting lists and winter pressures.

References

1 Department of Health (1998) *Modernising Health and Social Services.* No. 13929. DoH, London.

2 Department of Health (1998) *Planning for Better Health and Better Health Care.* Health Improvement Programmes. LAC(98) 23. DoH, London.

3 Shaw GB (1911) *The Doctor's dilemma.* (DH Laurence (ed.) (1957)) Penguin, London, pp. 75–6, 80, 87.

4 Acheson Report (1988) *Public Health in England.* Cmnd 289. HMSO, London.

5 Beaglehole R and Bonita R (1997) *Public Health at the Crossroads.* Cambridge University Press, Cambridge.

6 Levy B (1996) Putting the public back into public health. *The Nation's Health.* **Dec.**

7 World Health Organisation (1985–6) *Targets for Health for All.* WHO, Geneva.

8 World Health Organisation (1986) *Ottawa Charter for Health Promotion.* WHO, Geneva.

9   Department of Health (1998) *Chief Medical Officer's Annual Report on the State of the Public Health.* The Stationery Office, London.

10   Department of Health (1998) *Our Healthier Nation: a contract for health.* The Stationery Office, London.

Acknowledgement

We extend our heartfelt thanks to Jean Carter and Chris Wordsworth for their support work in the preparation of this book.

CHAPTER TWO

Public health policies

David J Hunter

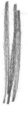

Despite significant improvements in the health of most of the populations of developed countries, including the UK, there continue to be major problems and challenges, principally in the form of a widening health gap. Inequalities in both health status and health service provision between different geographical areas and social groups constitute perhaps the most important public policy challenge confronting governments in these countries. Clearly, public health has a significant contribution to make to the resolution of such inequalities but it cannot do so alone. Tackling inequalities calls for a multi-disciplinary, multi-agency strategy operating at all levels – international, national, regional, local and individual. Although in this book we are concerned specifically with what public health, in all its forms and wherever it resides, can offer to improving the health of our communities at local and national levels within the UK, we should not overlook the fact that, increasingly, the public challenge is a global one, with the European dimension of particular importance for the UK.

This chapter sets the policy context for public health. It is a time of great turbulence not only in the NHS and local government but also in respect of health policy broadly conceived. The Blair project is touching every aspect of public policy and many of its key components, notably its education reforms, Welfare to Work initiative, the 'New Deal', and the work of the Social Exclusion Unit with its indictment of the health gap and of a 'two nation' Britain, are all intended over time to have a profound impact on the public's health.

The policy context is neither straightforward nor always coherent. There is paradox, ambiguity and inconsistency but all policy shares these characteristics. If public health policies appear to have more than their fair share of them it could reflect the very complexity of the public health function itself and the fact that it features in virtually every aspect of our lives. Trade-offs and balances are needed in public health policy over establishing priorities in the use of limited resources as, for example, between prevention or cure, cure as opposed to care, or between health services. Many seemingly intractable problems and challenges facing public health are linked to lifestyle behaviour and political/economic issues, for example, cigarette smoking.

According to Holland, public health possesses the necessary tools to describe the problems and to devise appropriate mechanisms for their solution. But he claims that 'the ability for public health to influence health policy is limited' not only in the UK but elsewhere too.[1] The reasons appear to be twofold: first, for all the rhetoric about the importance of health as distinct from healthcare, successive governments both in Britain and elsewhere have concentrated their attention and resources on curative healthcare services, possibly judging that this is what the public wants and expects.

Second, part of the problem lies in the compartmentalisation of government functions which are organised in vertical silos. As a consequence, although there is substantial investment in education, the health dimension is overlooked or downplayed, as anything with a 'health' label is seen as the business of the Department of Health (DoH). The health focus in public policy is equated with what the DoH does with its resources. Therefore, although education, housing and employment are known to have more profound effects on health status than the use of medical services, there is a failure to link policies in terms of their contribution to health or to recognise the health gains from investments in areas other than the NHS or what the DoH does. It is hardly surprising in these circumstances that the public should equate improved health with better health services.

The compartmentalisation of health policy has, in part at least, been responsible for public health medicine's preoccupation with a largely managerial healthcare agenda focused on contracting, evidence-based medicine and clinical effectiveness. The NHS market-style reforms introduced by the Conservative Government in 1991, in particular the purchaser–provider separation, contributed to the fragmentation that is now a feature of public health. As a consequence the public health effort in promoting health has been dissipated.[2] This could have implications in future for the organisation and location of the public health lead function which presently rests with health authorities. There is much argument over whether this would not be better given over to local government.[3]

There is no denying the contribution that public health can make to the improvement of clinical services, many of which have an important role in promoting secondary prevention, but the downside is that it can, as Scally warns, 'potentially distract attention from the task of addressing the wider environmental and social causes of ill health such as poor housing, poverty and unemployment'.[4] A re-engagement of public health practitioners with the social and environmental determinants of health is therefore both long overdue and welcome.

There are signs that countries, including the UK, are beginning to address the core business of public health, namely, improving the health of populations for which its practitioners, wherever they are located, are responsible. Growing public awareness of, and concern over, public health issues in response, *inter alia*, to a series of crises affecting food safety (i.e. BSE and the *E. coli* tragedy) and the environment (e.g. transport policies and road traffic accidents) is forcing governments to take public health policy seriously and put it higher up the political agenda. As was noted in the Introduction, a particular manifestation of the Labour Government's commitment to public health was the appointment of the first ever Minister for Public Health for England on assuming office in

May 1997. With this appointment, there is no denying that public health policy now has a focus within government at a senior level, although this is not evident elsewhere in the UK. A number of policy initiatives – notably the new health strategy, *Our Healthier Nation* – have been spawned as a direct result of a Minister being in post. It is important to note, too, that although based in the DoH as a member of the health team, the Minister for Public Health has a crucial cross-governmental role in ensuring that the health impact of other departments' policies has been assessed and taken into account in the policy formulation process. Indeed, principally as a result of having this cross-departmental role there is a strong case for having a minister who is not located in a particular department.

The remainder of this chapter reviews recent developments in public health policy in the UK and within the European Union (EU) as a context for the subsequent chapters detailing particular aspects or features of the public health function. The focus is on the broader public health task in improving population health rather than on the narrower, though still important, concerns arising from health services, in particular the quality of healthcare and its pursuance through what in the UK, following the 1997 NHS White Paper, has come to be known as 'clinical governance'.[5] In order to keep the review within manageable proportions, its focus is on issues and themes that are common throughout the UK, rather than a detailed description and analysis of the differences between England, Wales, Scotland and Northern Ireland.

Public health policies in the UK

A large number of strategies and policies to improve health are pursued by the DoH in England and the other health departments elsewhere in the UK. Important differences do exist between the four countries but these are largely about detail rather than about the broad thrust of strategic policy which is essentially indivisible within the UK. Whether greater policy divergence will occur post-devolution in 1999 when a Scottish parliament is established, and assemblies in Wales and Northern Ireland, is a matter for debate, although the accepted view is that initially the differences will not be substantial.[6] In any case, this topic is beyond the scope of the present review. However, it merits close observation as the UK becomes rather less united in future, with implications for regionalisation both within England as well as at a broader European level.

But to return to our theme of the strategies in place to improve health – from 1992 to 1997 these stemmed mainly from the English health strategy, *The Health of the Nation*, and its equivalents elsewhere in the UK.[7] These strategies formed the central plank of health policy in the UK and their importance lay in the fact that they represented the first explicit attempt by government to provide a strategic approach to improving the overall health of the population based on WHO's *Health for All* initiative. In fact, much of the thrust of *Health of the Nation* (and the other strategies) and the focus on health gain can be found in earlier, pioneering work in Wales, where the strategic intent initiative, led by the Welsh Health Planning Forum, proved influential on subsequent developments elsewhere in the UK.

Five key areas of health were identified – coronary heart disease, cancer, mental illness, HIV/AIDS and sexual health, and accidents. They were chosen because:

- they were major causes of premature death or avoidable ill health
- they were ones where effective interventions should be possible, offering significant scope for improvement in health
- it was possible to set objectives and targets in the areas and monitor progress towards them.

The key areas and associated objectives and national targets were tools for achieving the wider strategic aims of the *Health of the Nation* which were to improve the nation's health in terms of life expectancy, reductions in premature death and improvements in quality of life.

An evaluation of the impact of *Health of the Nation* at local level, commissioned by the DoH, concluded that although it had an important symbolic role in putting health, as distinct from healthcare, on the policy agenda, it largely failed over its five-year lifespan to realise its full potential and was handicapped from the outset by numerous flaws.[8] By 1997, its impact on local policy making was negligible. It was not seen to count while other priorities, notably waiting lists, balancing the books, winter emergency pressures, trust mergers – the daily stuff of healthcare delivery which preoccupies most managers most of the time – took precedence.

A particular problem was that *Health of the Nation* was perceived as a DoH initiative that lacked cross-departmental commitment and ownership. At local level, a similar compartmentalisation occurred, with *Health of the Nation* seen principally as a health service document lacking local government ownership. Shared ownership at all levels, both horizontally and vertically, had been stressed as essential for success but was not forthcoming, precisely because of this compartmentalisation and a failure to engage all key stakeholders in fashioning the health strategy. A further problem was that *Health of the Nation* did not change significantly the perspective and behaviour of health authorities. Nor did it cause a major readjustment in investment priorities by health authorities. The strategy also failed to impact in a marked way upon primary care practitioners, either as commissioners or providers. For their part, local authorities perceived *Health of the Nation* to be dominated by 'medical conditions' and heavily 'medically led'. It was a cause for concern among those local authorities that believed they contributed more to a health agenda in its broadest sense than health authorities.

Although the new health strategy, *Our Healthier Nation,* has gone to some length to emphasise the importance of local government, criticisms remain that the document is still disease-focused and continues to give the lead role for health to health authorities. Local government still feels somewhat marginalised. Nor did it appear helpful in presentational terms when the consultation document launching the new strategy carried a foreword signed by two health ministers, without any apparent commitment at this level from other ministers. This was in striking contrast to the equivalent draft documents published in Scotland and Wales, where the entire respective ministerial teams committed themselves to the proposals.

That local government is critical of government health policy, and sceptical of health ministers' overtures concerning the important contribution to be made by local authorities, is borne out in a survey of local authorities' views of *Health of the Nation* conducted for the Health Education Authority and the Local Government Management Board.[9] Much of the criticism of the strategy reported in the survey centred on four main issues:

- the health strategy was too narrowly focused on disease models and failed to promote a positive view of health
- *Health of the Nation* neglected key socio-economic and environmental determinants of health
- the strategy failed to appreciate the potential local authority contribution to a national health strategy
- no new resources were forthcoming to progress the strategy.

There were more general concerns, too, over the preoccupation of *Health of the Nation* with the NHS and DoH, since it seemed to confuse public health with the NHS and, while the latter had a key contribution to make to public health, to give it the lead role seemed curious to many. Few believed that the NHS could detach itself from the pressures of providing health services with all the attendant problems arising.

But, easy though it is to criticise, there is much to welcome in *Health of the Nation*. Nor should it be forgotten that it (and its counterparts elsewhere in the UK) marked the first attempt by any UK government to put in place a coherent health strategy. Nevertheless, by 1997 a fresh start was widely thought to be necessary. It was provided by a new government and a new Minister for Public Health. On 7 July 1998, she announced the Government's new strategy for health, *Our Healthier Nation*. A consultative paper subsequently appeared (again with counterparts published in Wales and Scotland – Northern Ireland had already produced its own strategy in late 1997) and a firm policy statement in the form of a White Paper is expected in 1999. The new strategy seeks to build on *Health of the Nation* rather than start afresh. But it will also set a new direction emphasising social exclusion, inequalities in health, and the importance of housing, employment and the environment in improving health and well being.[10] There will be a greater emphasis on local priorities rather than having too many national ones.

Demonstrating the Government's conviction that 'connected problems require joined-up solutions', there is a strong focus within *Our Healthier Nation* on the cross-governmental dimension to ensure co-ordinated commitment and action across government departments. At local level, the development of Healthy Living Centres and HAZs will serve as innovative mechanisms bringing together a range of partners to improve health and healthcare. Their purpose is to devise new ways of providing support to people in need and to tackle health inequalities in ways which deliberately blur organisational and professional boundaries. These can often become barriers to effective action to effect lasting change in communities. In addition, Health Improvement Programmes (HIMPs), led by health authorities, will bring together all the key stakeholders in a local area, including local authorities, the new PCGs and the public, to agree strategies for improving health as well as healthcare.

Possibly the most significant feature of the new health strategy is its frank admission that the health gap has widened in the UK to unacceptable proportions. Whereas *Health of the Nation* had declined to acknowledge the existence of health inequalities, the new strategy states unequivocally that 'the link between poverty and ill health is clear' with 'the highest incidence of illness ... experienced by the worst off social classes'.[11] Moreover, the responsibility for tackling the causes of ill health rests not with individuals alone but with local communities and government at national level. Hence the Government's proposal for a national contract for better health. Three settings have been identified for action:

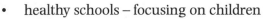

- healthy schools – focusing on children
- healthy workplaces – focusing on adults
- healthy neighbourhoods – focusing on older people.

Four priority areas have been identified, with clear targets to be set for improvements in each by the year 2010:

- heart disease and stroke
- accidents
- cancer
- mental health.

Although generally welcomed for building constructively on *Health of the Nation* and for openly acknowledging the existence of health inequalities, *Our Healthier Nation* has been criticised for its focus on ill health and disease and for failing to adopt a positive approach to health. There is also widespread dismay that a national target in the area of health inequalities has not been proposed.

How far any of these criticisms will be taken into account in the White Paper expected in 1999 remains to be seen. The hope is that at least some of the lessons from implementing *Health of the Nation* will be learned and acted upon. Whatever the outcome, there is at least considerable enthusiasm throughout the public health community for what the new strategy is seeking to do. There is a strong sense that the lack of importance of public health in public policy during the past two decades is finally being challenged.

Linked to the Minister of Public Health's brief and to the new health strategy are other important 'spin-offs' from it. Former CMO, Sir Donald Acheson, has produced a review of the evidence in regard to tackling health inequalities with the aim of establishing what works and what does not. There is also a review of the public health function which the recently retired CMO, Sir Kenneth Calman, initiated. Its purpose is to ensure that a robust public health function is in place to deliver the Government's public health strategy and agenda. An interim report was published in early 1998 and a final report is in preparation.[12]

Other public health policy initiatives include: the setting up of a Food Standards Agency in the aftermath of the public health crises in the 'agribusiness'; a White Paper on tobacco control, published in late 1998; and a consultation document on proposals for new legislation on the control of communicable diseases. In other government department areas for example, a White Paper on integrated transport policy has also been published. Though not emanating from the DoH, the whole issue of transport has important implications for public health. The fragmentation of transport and lack of a coherent policy has been a major cause for concern in contributing to rising car use, an increase in road traffic accidents, and levels of pollution.

Health in an international context

Public health cannot be confined to local or national arenas. A shrinking world in terms of economic development and improved communications brings with it new public health challenges. Public health problems are no respecters of local or national boundaries. Whichever public health issue is selected, whether it be HIV/AIDS, BSE, drug abuse, smoking, toxic waste disposal or global warming, multinational responses are required because these problems are not confined to individual nation states. It is not self-evident that the appropriate institutional arrangements are in place to allow such a transnational dialogue to occur.

In recent years, WHO has been heavily criticised for failing to give a lead on such critical health issues. With a new director general, Dr Gro Harlem Brundtland, in post there are encouraging signs that WHO may be positioning itself to give once again a respected global lead on major health issues. A major reorganisation of WHO's head-quarters in Geneva is underway based on clusters including those dealing with social change and mental health, family and health services, sustainable development and healthy environments, communicable diseases, non-communicable diseases, evidence and information for policy, health technology and drugs. Tackling health inequalities is another key priority for WHO but it will work with other UN institutions, adopting an intersectoral rather than a vertical approach.

In an address to the Harvard University School of Public Health prior to taking up her appointment as WHO's new director general, Dr Brundtland observed that:

> many of our health problems are of a global nature and are closely linked to economic development, the environment and other challenges. They can therefore only be overcome by intensified global cooperation, where strong, efficient and forward-looking international institutions must underpin our common efforts.[13]

If the international aspects of health can only become more important as a result of the pervasive effects of globalisation and the threats it poses to public health, closer to home the European dimension is acquiring greater significance and having a growing impact on EU members. It is to this we now turn in the final part of this chapter.

Public health policies and the EU

For many engaged in health policy and healthcare services, Europe exists in a remote, rather shadowy form. It remains a complete mystery and a source of considerable ignorance. It tends to be viewed, if at all, with mild detached academic interest but is not taken seriously or regarded as central to anyone's business. Such a myopic view is regrettable and probably not an option for much longer. The EU already exerts a significant influence on aspects of health policy through its laws and directives and through the activities of specialised agencies like the European Medicines Evaluation Agency and the European Agency for Health and Safety at Work.[14]

The consequences of developments in European law in areas such as health and safety, trade and competition policy are of growing importance to health policy makers at national level. It would be short-sighted to discount the potential importance of EU public health strategies on health promotion, cancer, AIDS, drug dependency, to name a few priority areas. The emphasis of public health Article 129 (amended to 152 at Amsterdam) on prevention and education means it could play an important role in reducing demand for healthcare services. The specific competence in the field of public health through Article 129 (and now 152) enables the EU to take action to co-ordinate national policies on the prevention of major diseases as well as health information and education.

Probably the most visible example of how Europe is influencing public health practice in the UK has been the European Commission's (EC) worldwide ban on the export of British beef. Another example concerns tobacco. EU health ministers have agreed a ban on tobacco advertising and sponsorship. It will take some years to be fully implemented but, once it is, it will be an example of European policy making preventing thousands of premature deaths.[15]

The consequences of European integration has many consequences for public health, although formally the scope for action by the EU is limited. A recent communication from the EC outlines a possible new EU public health policy based on three strands of action[16]:

- improving information for the development of public health
- reacting rapidly to threats to health
- tackling health determinants through health promotion and disease prevention.

A new public health policy has to await ratification of the Treaty of Amsterdam but a series of events, such as the outbreak of certain infectious diseases, has raised the profile of public health at an EU level which requires extensive public debate. The Commission believes that a new public health policy is now required. While Article 129 emphasises the prevention of disease, the Amsterdam Treaty and Article 152 stress that EU action will be directed towards improving public health, preventing illness and disease, and obviating sources of danger to health. This shift of emphasis requires attending to the determinants of health and not confining attention to disease prevention.

The UK Minister for Public Health has stated her wish to establish a set of priorities for joint action by the Community and the member states on key health determinants.[17] These might include:

• monitoring and surveillance of communicable, rare and emerging diseases
• environment and health
• safeguarding the quality and safety of food and of medicines and medical devices
• ensuring that the regulation of the free movement of health professionals continues to ensure high levels of health protection.

In conclusion, the EU has moved in a short period from a situation in which it had little involvement in public health to one in which it has become a major player in international health. While still at an early stage, it is likely that programmes now being embarked upon will have an increasingly important influence on national health policies.[14] This influence will be exerted not only through obvious health-related activities but also in areas such as health and safety, trade and competition policy. All the more reason, then, to pay close attention to the European dimension and to understand how EU institutions and laws can influence public health policies in the UK.

A related development is the growth of regionalisation within the EU. In the context of devolution to Scotland and Wales and moves in parts of England to develop closer partnerships at regional level between health services and the government offices for the regions and the forthcoming regional development agencies (RDAs), which will have responsibility for sustainable economic development and regeneration, the significance of a regional dimension becomes clear. Although public health is not a core function of the new RDAs, it is included as one of nine additional fields where RDAs will contribute to policies and programmes. Of course, a regional tier need not mean greater devolved responsibility for various functions. As in the NHS, it could result in greater centralisation, which occurred when eight regional offices replaced 14 regional health authorities. But the development of strong links across regional agencies to promote a public health approach is both welcome and overdue. The regional dimension seems likely to acquire greater significance in future as part of the reshaping of governance within the UK. Public health will not be immune from such developments.

References

1   Holland WW (1997) Overview of policies and strategies. In: R Detels, WW Holland, J McEwan and GS Omenn (eds) *Oxford Textbook of Public Health* (3e). Oxford University Press, New York.

2   Holland WW and Stewart S (1998) *Public Health: the vision and the challenge.* The Rock Carling Fellowship 1997. The Nuffield Trust, London.

3   Clarke M, Hunter DJ and Wistow G (1997) For debate: local government and the NHS: the new agenda. *Journal of Public Health Medicine.* **19**(1): 3–5.

4   Scally G (1997) Introduction. In: G Scally (ed.) *Progress in Public Health.* Royal Society of Medicine Press, London.

5   Department of Health (1998) *A First Class Service: quality in the new NHS.* DoH, London.

6   Hazell R and Jervis P (1998) *Devolution and Health.* Nuffield Trust Series No.3. The Nuffield Trust, London.

7   Secretary of State for Health (1992) *The Health of the Nation: a strategy for health in England.* Cm 1986. HMSO, London.

8   Hunter DJ *et al.* (1998) Investing in health? An assessment of the impact of the *Health of the Nation.* In: Department of Health, *The Health of the Nation: a policy assessed.* The Stationery Office, London.

9   Moran G (1996) *Promoting Health and Local Government.* Health Education Authority, London.

10   Calman KC (1998) *The Potential for Health: how to improve the nation's health.* Oxford University Press, Oxford.

11   Secretary of State for Health (1998) *Our Healthier Nation: a contract for health.* A Consultation Paper. Cm 3852. The Stationery Office, London.

12   Department of Health (1998) *Chief Medical Officer's Project to Strengthen the Public Health Function in England.* A Report of Emerging Findings. DoH, London.

13   Brundtland GH (1998) Guest Editorial: Public health: a global challenge. *European Journal of Public Health.* **8**(1): 1–2.

14   McKee M and Mossialos E (1997) Public health and European integration. In: G Scally (ed.) *Progress in Public Health.* Royal Society of Medicine Press, London.

15   McKee M (1998) Editorial: An agenda for public health research in Europe. *European Journal of Public Health.* **8**(1): 3–7.

16   Commission of the European Communities (1998) *The Development of Public Health Policy in the European Community.* Communication from the Commission to the Council, the European Parliament, the Economic and Social Committee and the Committee of the Regions. COM(1998)230 final. Commission of the European Communities, Brussels.

17   Jowell T (1998) Developing EU Public Health Policy. *Eurohealth.* **4**(3): 2–5.

PART 1

Posing the problems: case studies in public health

CHAPTER THREE

Past and present public health in Liverpool

John Ashton

The 150th anniversary of the appointment of William Henry Duncan as Liverpool and England's first MOH was marked in 1997 by a year of celebration, and the opportunity was taken to review the challenges to public health and the responses to them of 'the organised efforts of society' throughout the period from the early 1840s to the present day.[1]* The earliest part of this span of years was characterised by the spectre of cholera stalking the slums of the great towns. With the threat of revolution galvanising the minds of the middle classes it was Chadwick's report on *The Sanitary Condition of the Labouring Population of Great Britain* that provided the stimulus for the development of the Victorian Public Health movement.[2,3] Duncan's part in this has been well described in the writings of Sidney Chave and more recently in those of Gerry Kearns.[4,5]

In his inaugural Duncan lecture delivered at the University of Liverpool Medical School in 1983, Chave described the situation that confronted Duncan in the 1830s and early 1840s, working as a general practitioner in the central dispensaries of what was rapidly becoming the most important port in the British Empire. The population was exploding both from in-migration and natural increase, houses were 'hastily built without regard to suitability of soil or site, for water supply or sanitation', with hundreds of dwellings being packed together in narrow courts and cellars, and dirt, disease and

---

*Public health is the science and art of preventing disease, prolonging life and promoting physical health and efficiency through organised community efforts for the sanitation of the environment, the education of the individual in principles of personal hygiene, the organisation of medical and nursing services for the early diagnosis and preventive treatment of disease, and the development of the social machinery which will ensure to every individual in the community a standard of living adequate for the maintenance of health.

malnourishment flourished. The annual death rate from causes that included dysentery, scarlet fever, measles, tuberculosis and, intermittently and devastatingly, cholera was 36 per 1000, the highest in the country. The task of doing something about the situation was formidable but the crisis in the city elicited a remarkable response from the movers and shakers among the city fathers in the form of the activities of the Health of Towns Association.[6] (In general, the contribution of the city mothers – Kitty Wilkinson, pioneer of public wash-houses; Eleanor Rathbone, Agnes Jones and visiting city mother Florence Nightingale, concerned with community, school and general nursing; and Josephine Butler, the founder of social work and strenuous advocate of fallen women and the dispossessed – came later.) In response to Chadwick's request for evidence to inform his enquiry, Duncan had already conducted a survey of housing conditions in the town and found that one-third of the working-class population was living in the typical narrow and airless courts, and one-eighth in underground cellars, and furthermore that in the many public lodging-houses it was common to find 30 people sleeping in a small cellar room. Duncan's survey and evidence to Chadwick became the basis of a pamphlet 'on the physical causes of the high rate of mortality in Liverpool' which he used to give public lectures and which provided a sound base from which to launch the Liverpool Health of Towns Association in 1845.

The Liverpool Health of Towns Association was formed in April 1845, 4 months after the first association had been established in London. At this first Liverpool meeting, which was convened by the mayor, it was stated that the information provided by Chadwick's Health of Towns Commission Report the previous year had led to the meeting being held. The *Liverpool Mercury* described the attendance at the first meeting as being 'not large, but highly respectable', including leading members of the council and both Protestant and Catholic clergymen, in addition to Dr Duncan and Dr Samuel Holme, or as the *Mercury* put it 'gentlemen of all sects in religion and all parties in politics'. This meeting passed, unanimously, resolutions defining the sanitary objectives to be aimed at and called for legislative action. The duty of the Association should be to 'collect funds, to supply information and to furnish those details which must be the basis of all legislation'. The meeting set up a local committee, which published a monthly journal called *The Liverpool Health of Towns Advocate* for nearly 2 years, 1500 of the first number being distributed free of charge. To cut a long story short, the Liverpool Association, together with its counterparts around the country, played a central part in the struggle for public health legislation, culminating in the Public Health Act of 1848. In the Liverpool case, the Association's work produced the Liverpool 'Sanatory' Act of 1846 which prefigured the national legislation and enabled the town to go ahead with Duncan's appointment. For fuller accounts readers are referred to the writings of Finer, Lewis, and Wohl.[7–9]

Duncan's appointment fulfilled one of the recommendations of Chadwick's 1842 report:

That for the general means necessary to prevent disease it would be good economy to appoint a district medical officer, independent of private practice, with the securities of special qualifications and responsibilities to initiate sanitary measures and reclaim the execution of the law.

In the event his initial appointment at a salary of £300 a year allowed him to continue his private practice and drew a sarcastic comment from *Punch*:

> *By the papers Mr Punch learns that the Town Council of Liverpool intend to appoint an Officer of Health, whose duties will consist in the direction of their sanitary arrangements, and whose services they propose to remunerate by a salary of £300 a year, with the liberty to augment that handsome income, if he can, by private practice.*

> *Mr Punch will engage to find a competent person, who will willingly undertake the responsibilities of this office, on the liberal terms proposed by the Town Council of Liverpool.*

> *Mr Punch, on behalf of the respectable medical gentleman, his nominee, will promise that he, the said respectable medical gentleman, shall devote his full attention to his official duties, and endeavour to make money by private practice only at those few leisure moments when he shall have nothing else to do. For although a practitioner of any eminence expects, generally, to make at least a thousand a year, this gentleman shall regard his situation, bringing him in £300, as of primary importance, and shall look upon his private earning as matters of secondary considerations.*

> *If the Officer of Health recommended by Mr Punch shall have for a patient a rich butcher, with a slaughter house in a populous neighbourhood (not that unlikely since Thomas Fresh, the sanitary inspector for Liverpool reported that in 1851 there were 36 slaughter-houses owned by the Liverpool Abattoir Company and 51 other private slaughterhouses in the borough); an opulent fellmonger or tallow-chandler, with a yard or manufactory in the heart of the town, he shall not hesitate from motives of interest to denounce their respective establishments as nuisances. He shall not fail to point out the insalubrity of any gas works, similarly situated, the family of whose proprietor he may attend; and if any wealthy old lady who may be in the habit of consulting him shall infringe the Drainage Act, he shall not fail to declare the circumstances to the authorities.*[10,11]

After a little over a year the council saw fit to change Duncan's contract to full-time at a salary of £750 per annum on the condition that he give up private practice.

As it transpired, lack of commitment and zeal were not Duncan's problem and he rapidly established a reputation for himself with his frequent letters, not least to the Board of Health and other significant players in London, drawing attention to the dire threats to health in Liverpool. These were subsequently to be greatly exacerbated by the massive influx of refugees from Ireland, escaping the famine (300 000 in the first 6 months of 1847), and it is arguable that his tireless work on behalf of the poor was to contribute to his early death at the age of 57.[4,12] Together with Thomas Fresh and James Newlands, the borough engineer who was responsible for the construction of a total length of 146 miles of sewers and main drains between 1847 and 1858, Duncan contributed in many ways to the effectiveness of what we would now call a multisectoral public health team co-ordinated through the offices of the Town Council. Although Duncan has tended to enjoy a greater prominence than Fresh or Newlands since his death, presumably in no

Table 3.1:   Lessons for the new public health from the work of Duncan, Fresh, and Newlands[4,13]

• An independent voice	• Resourcefulness and pragmatism
• Appropriate research	• The legitimacy of working locally
• Production of reports	• Humanitarianism and a strong moral tone
• Populism	• Cost-effectiveness of prevention
• Advocacy	• The need for organisation

small part as a result of a hagiography to which I have contributed, their relative import-ance and recognition in life was somewhat different. Eastwood has pointed out how this was reflected in their relative salaries, with Newlands being almost on a par with Duncan at £700 a year whereas Fresh received a mere £170; meanwhile the Town Clerk was on £2000, equivalent to £70 000 today.[11]

I have reflected elsewhere on the many lessons to be learned from these early pioneers (Table 3.1).[13] For Kearns much of this can be summarised under the three headings of reporting, certifying and advising: reporting on the state of health of the population; certifying with respect to such matters as overcrowding and the imperatives of providing, among other things, adequate water supply and sanitation; and advising the Town Council, and whoever else seemed appropriate, on the action necessary to improve the public health. It is clear that this 'advising' encompassed the thorny issue of advocacy and lobbying.[14] The second part of this chapter will draw on these themes in exploring how public health in Liverpool today has responded to a very different agenda, albeit subsuming some very familiar themes, such as poverty, inequality and environmental degradation.

The rise and fall and renaissance of public health

There is argument about what constituted the heyday of public health.[13] Certainly, the task changed as the more extreme problems of the great towns began to ameliorate and, in succession, personal preventive services and then personal treatment services were developed on a population-wide basis, culminating in the creation of the welfare state in many European countries and the NHS in Britain. Duncan and his colleagues in Liverpool and elsewhere were very much sanitarians, in that they recognised the central import-ance of environmental factors in the public health problems of the day. The succeeding emphasis on personal prevention threw up a different group of pioneers, of whom the Liverpool 'mothers', or the 'sisters' of public health as they have been called, were a prominent example.[15] The third phase, which began with the discovery of insulin and the sulphonamides and which culminated in the domination of therapeutic thinking for three decades, paradoxically coincided, at least for the first 20 years, with the MOH at the height of his (sic) power, typically with an empire of hundreds of personal health and social workers and environmental health officers under his direction. He also had his feet under the table of the borough council and all its relevant committees, and a direct line from policy making to implementation of programmes of action affecting many of the determinants and predisposing causes of ill health. However, the seeds of the decline were already germinating, not only in the powerful attraction of science-based medicine, but also in the very success of the public health enterprise in controlling the infectious diseases and revealing another set of problems to which the scientists and pharmacologists claimed to have the solutions.[16] The third factor lay in the progressive alienation of colleagues who were becoming fed up of playing second fiddle to medical practitioners.

This last factor had already become apparent many years previously, with concern being expressed in the 1890s about MOHs claiming credit for work done by Inspectors of Nuisances. Eastwood quotes from an editorial in the *Sanitary Inspectors Journal* of 1896 that:

> *whilst we do not counsel insubordination in any respect, we must urge all inspectors to, as far as possible, carry out both the spirit and the letter of the Public Health Acts by preparing and submitting their own reports direct to the Authorities. It is very regrettable to find that in so many cases the Medical Officer of Health obtains the necessary information from the Inspector and dresses it up as his report, when as a matter of fact, the work done by the Inspector he reports upon he knows little or nothing of, but desires to take credit for...*[11]

By 1970 the die was cast when the Seebohm Committee recommended the establishment of separate social services directorates in local authorities. The *coup de grâce* was administered in 1974 with local government reorganisation under which the MOH disappeared both in name and in presence from the local authority, to be replaced by the confusingly titled 'Community Physician' to be situated in the district health authority. To paraphrase Sidney Chave, the MOH was born in Liverpool in 1847, grew up and served his apprenticeship in London, and was killed off in 1974 by a combination of complacency and guild arrogance, on the one hand, and a transient infatuation with the promises of biomedicine for the public health, on the other. During this life span there had been a mere seven holders of the position in Liverpool, beginning with Duncan and ending with the formidable Andrew Semple, a worthy inheritor of the mantle, who, as Duncan himself, had combined service with academic responsibilities.

According to the seminal paper on the matter, the MOH's successor, the Community Physician, was expected to continue the traditional tasks of the MOH 'as teacher, watchdog and troublemaker' ... 'and he will also have new duties in the provision of services as an integral resource of health protection. One of his main tools will be knowledge, a contribution to social policy at every level.'[17] In the event, there was to follow a period of marginalisation and obscurity when, shorn of direct access to local policy and resources in local government and regarded as a failed doctor by clinical colleagues, the Community Physician, rather than being all things to all people, eminent in policy making throughout the health as well as the healthcare system, turned out to be nothing to anybody and thereby finished up claiming territory that s(he) was unable to occupy. Whereas any child growing up in Liverpool in the post-war period would have known the name of Andrew Semple, for it was his name that summoned you to your polio prophylaxis, the obscurity of his immediate successors was indicative of a deep malaise and of a proud enterprise marooned in the mire. It was at this time that Humpty Dumpty truly fell off the wall with a fragmentation of policy making and service provision. This was to exacerbate the challenge of responding to new health issues, such as the provision of community care for the growing numbers of elderly, the mentally ill and disabled on the one hand, and the transformation of thinking about environmental health questions from a sanitary one to an ecological one, grounded in sustainability, on the other.[16,18,19] This situation was generally compounded by the continued domination of the field by medical practitioners at the expense of other relevant disciplines and by the schism that continued to grow between public health academic activity and the real world of policy and practice.[20–23]

The New Public Health, healthy cities, Health Action Zones and all that

The term 'the New Public Health' began to be used in the middle 1980s to describe a myriad of efforts to put Humpty Dumpty back on the wall. Writing in a book of the same name in 1988, I described the New Public Health as '...an approach which brings together environmental change and personal preventive measures with appropriate therapeutic interventions, especially for the elderly and disabled' and went on to state that:

> the New Public Health goes beyond an understanding of human biology and recognises the importance of those social aspects of health problems which are caused by lifestyles, thereby avoiding the trap of blaming the victim by developing Healthy Public Policies – policies in many fields which support the promotion of health'.[16,24]

I concluded by stating that in the New Public Health the environment is social and psychological as well as physical. Much of the thinking behind the New Public Health had been codified in documents from WHO, such as the Alma Ata declaration, the *Health for All by the Year 2000* strategy itself and the *Ottawa Charter for Health Promotion*.[25–27] In turn, these conceptual frameworks, which stressed the importance of public involvement, of public, private and voluntary-sector partnership, of multidisciplinary working and the reorientation of health and healthcare systems, were drawing on day-to-day practical experiences around the world of trying to find relevant solutions to public health problems. Among these were the efforts to establish a health promotion strategy in the Mersey Health Region, centred on Liverpool but containing the counties of Merseyside and Cheshire.

Liverpool, a district of Merseyside – new beginnings

When Duncan was appointed MOH for Liverpool, the town's population was approaching 150 000, compared with the 900 000 it ultimately attained before shrinking back to the 450 000 of today. I make this point because the size of population for which public health is organised in England has fluctuated wildly in the past, with at one time almost 1000 MOHs, often with comparatively small populations, in contrast to the situation in 1998 when there were fewer than 100, with responsibilities typically for populations of 250 000 plus. With the imminent prospect of a move to even fewer large strategic authorities and many more locality health commissions (PCGs) carrying public health responsibilities, we are perhaps about to return to a situation similar to that of 100 years ago. In this apparently continuous process of administrative musical chairs it is as well to remember the adage familiar to physiologists and town planners alike, that 'form follows function', and to be prepared that for a changing set of health challenges, different arrangements will be appropriate.[28] For a brief interlude from the early 1980s until its abolition in 1993 by a centralising national government, the vacuum left by a mal-functioning public health presence at the local level was compensated for by the regional health authority (RHA).

The work of creating a public health strategy and movement within a region of 2.4 million people has been described at some length elsewhere. Suffice it to say that the main elements of agenda setting, consciousness raising and developing models of good practice, to reflect the kind of partnerships with the public and between sectors advocated by WHO, encompassed much of the same territory described by Kearns and myself and drew unashamedly on the work of Duncan, Fresh and Newlands as role models. The demise of the annual report of the MOH in 1974 and its complete disappearance until it was reinstated as a result of the Acheson Enquiry into the public health function in England in 1988, left a huge intelligence gap, which was filled for a time by a major report on health in the region. This report identified 12 priorities for action with specified health targets connected to the process of review (Table 3.2). The report was used to inform key opinion formers and decision makers throughout the health and healthcare system by means of conferences, workshops and other events. The establishment of a Regional Health Promotion Unit sought to compensate for the lack of any dedicated capability for health improvement and lack of direct access to the policy-making committees of the local authorities in the region by providing a focus for the production of strategy documents and for supporting projects and initiatives which illustrated *Health for All* principles in action. Of particular importance was the production of a strategic framework based on the complementarity of policies addressed at the whole population, high-risk groups and health-damaged groups within that population (Figure 3.1). The continuing weakness brought about by the changes of 1974 was the watering down

Table 3.2: Priorities for health in Mersey 1984

- Planned parenthood
- Control of sexually transmitted disease
- Antenatal care, including genetic screening
- Improved child health and immunisation uptake
- The prevention of death and disability from accidents and environmental causes
- Improved dental health
- Some specific aspects of lifestyle related to premature death (including diet, exercise, stress, tobacco, alcohol and drugs)
- The effective control of high blood pressure
- Early detection of cancer
- Reduction of disability in the elderly
- A healthy mind in a healthy body – positive health, especially as it relates to a health strategy for young people
- Dignity and comfort at the time of death

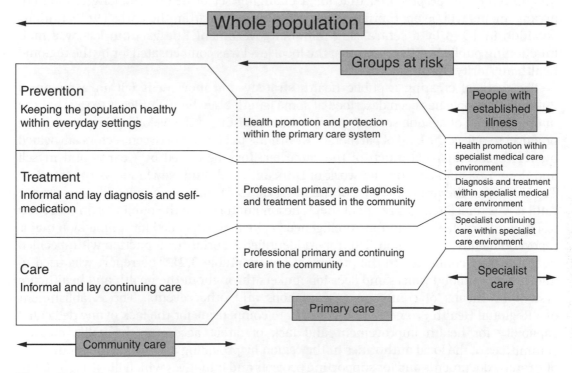

Figure 3.1: The Mersey strategic framework

and fragmentation of powers of certification, something that was highlighted in the Acheson Report with respect to infectious disease control and which seems even more apparent now in the light of the BSE fiasco.

The work in Mersey was recognised as of relevance to WHO's goal of 'taking Health for All off the shelves and into the streets of Europe', and the wheel had come full circle in a sense when Liverpool University and the City of Liverpool found themselves involved in the establishment of the Healthy City Initiative.[19] Not only did this initiative resonate with the experience of the Health of Towns Association in its attempt at bringing together the different sectors of the community for the benefit of the public's health, but it inadvertently revived interest in what has subsequently come to be known as the settings approach to public health, wherein policies to promote and protect the health of a population are grounded in a focus on specific environments. This has proved to be an energising approach for settings as diverse as prisons, schools, hospitals, homes and workplaces. The initiative in Liverpool had some initial teething problems, which were associated with the complexities of the city's politics in the early 1980s as much as the inherent difficulty in establishing effective multi-agency working. In addition, there was a danger that Healthy Cities might lapse into a set of discrete, disconnected projects. It was saved by a reappraisal deriving from the vision of the city's Chief Executive's office and the efforts of the public health directorate, now led by one of a new generation of practitioners schooled in the New Public Health and committed to genuine multidisciplinary partnerships. By 1996 a wide-ranging process of consultation had produced a city health plan, in which if Humpty was not back on the wall, at least all the king's men were signed up to putting him in the most appropriate place.

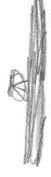

Contrary to popular rumour, history is not a pendulum but a helix. I say this because the time dimension means that you never come back to the same place but to find a new set of problems lodged in a new set of circumstances. The arrangements that were developed by the Victorians were predominantly in response to the threat of infectious disease against a background of poverty, squalor and deprivation, in the context of local economies, albeit with international connections. Today's problems are different, from the demography of collapsed fertility and mass longevity, through chronic, degenerative disease, with HIV/AIDS and drugs thrown in for good measure, together with other social issues connected to the restructuring of the global economy, the changed role and expectations of women, and mass mobility. Today's public health problems can no longer be placed neatly in a box labelled 'the borough council' – some, such as the care of the elderly, need a neighbourhood or locality focus; others, such as transport, crime, drug trafficking or emergency planning, are best dealt with at a level involving several districts, or even at a county, regional or international level. Others no doubt remain best dealt with by the current town or city council. Into this dynamic has now been dropped, in England, the new government's proposals for 'Health Action Zones' and a range of other area-based initiatives, as novel ways of mending Humpty in a new era. The intention of the national public health strategy is to provide an enabling framework in which the public, private and voluntary sectors can find creative solutions to wicked or intransigent problems facing the health and healthcare systems, including those problems caused by

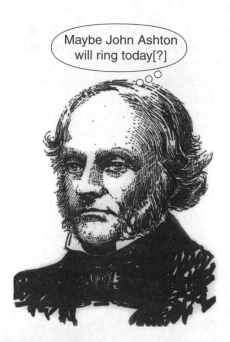

Figure 3.2 (with acknowledgement to Fred O'Brien).

social exclusion and by the failure to implement strategic restructuring of major public services, including specialised medical care. This seems like the Health of Towns Association and Healthy Cities writ large. I wonder if William Henry Duncan and his colleagues are watching? (Figure 3.2).

References

1   Winslow CEA (1920) The untilled fields of public health. *Science.* **51**: 23.

2   Morris CB and Sheard S (1998) *Liverpool 1997 – Celebrating 150 Years of Public Health.* Report of 150 years of public health in Liverpool. University of Liverpool Department of Public Health, Liverpool.

3   Chadwick E (1842*) Report on the Sanitary Condition of The Labouring Population of Great Britain.* Facsimile edition: MW Flinn (ed.) (1964). Edinburgh University Press, Edinburgh.

4   Chave S (1984) Duncan of Liverpool – and some lessons for today. *Community Medicine.* **6**: 61–71.

5   Kearns G (1997) *Dr Duncan sets to work* (address delivered at the Liverpool Medical Institution, January 1997, to mark the 150th anniversary of William Henry Duncan's appointment as Medical Officer of Health to Liverpool).

6   Ashton J and Ubido J (1991) The Healthy City and the ecological idea. *Journal of the Society for the Social History of Medicine.* **4**(1): 173–81.

7 Finer SE (1952) *The Life and Times of Sir Edwin Chadwick.* Methuen, London.

8 Lewis RA (1952) *Edwin Chadwick and the Public Health Movement. 1832–1854.* Longmans, London.

9 Wohl AS (1984) *Endangered Lives. Public Health in Victorian Britain.* Methuen, London.

10 *Punch* (1847) **XII**: 44.

11 Eastwood M (1998) Liverpool: a town ahead of its time. In: *For the Common Good: 150 years of public health.* Chartered Institute of Environmental Health Officers, London.

12 Frazer WM (1947) *Duncan of Liverpool.* Hamish Hamilton, London.

13 Ashton J (1989) Recalling the Medical Officer of Health. *Health Promotion.* **3**(4): 413–19.

14 Crown J and Gunning-Schepers L (eds) (1996) The challenge of public health advocacy. In: M Marinker (ed.) *Sense and Sensibility in Health Care.* BMJ Publishing Group, London.

15 Morris CB and Hutchinson J (1998) Public health practice units. In: *Developing Excellence in Public Health.* Report of a conference. University of Birmingham and NHSE.

16 Ashton J and Seymour H (1988) *The New Public Health.* Open University Press, Milton Keynes.

17 Morris JN (1969) Tomorrow's Community Physician. *Lancet.* **2**(7625): 811–16.

18 Ashton J (1991) Sanitarian becomes ecologist – the new environmental health. Editorial. *British Medical Journal.* **302**: 189–90.

19 Ashton J (ed.) (1992) *Healthy Cities.* Open University Press, Milton Keynes.

20 Ashton J (1992) Institutes of public health and medical schools: grasping defeat from the jaws of victory? Editorial. *Journal of Epidemiology and Community Health.* **47**(3): 165–8.

21 White KL (1992) *Healing the Schism, Epidemiology, Medicine and the Public's Health.* Springer Verlag, New York.

22 White KL and Connelly JE (eds) (1992) *The Medical Schools Mission and The Population's Health.* Springer Verlag, New York.

23 Morris M and Ashton J (1997) *The Pool of Life – A public health walk in Liverpool.* University of Liverpool Department of Public Health, Liverpool.

24 Milio N (1986) *Promoting Health Through Public Policy.* Canadian Public Health Association, Ottawa, Canada.

25 World Health Organisation (1978) *Alma Ata 1977. Primary Health Care.* WHO in conjunction with UNICEF, Geneva.

26 World Health Organisation (1981) *Global Strategy for Health for All by The Year 2000.* WHO, Geneva.

27 World Health Organisation, Health and Welfare Canada, Canadian Public Health Association (1986) *Ottawa Charter for Health Promotion.* WHO, Copenhagen.

28 Ashton J (In press) 1997 Chadwick Lecture – Is a healthy North West Region achievable in the 21st century? *Journal of Epidemiology and Community Health.*

CHAPTER FOUR

Tackling inequalities in health: public policy action

Michaela Benzeval

Introduction

Since the influential Black Report was published in 1980, the international evidence has grown to such an extent that it is now indisputable that social and economic circumstances are the major factors influencing the public's health. People who live in disadvantaged circumstances have more illnesses, greater distress, more disability and shorter lives than those who are more affluent.

Yet, in spite of the wealth of evidence that exists demonstrating the extent and nature of the problem, public policy in Britain has been slow to respond. Under the Conservative Government, policy makers at first rejected evidence about health inequalities, then ignored it, and finally acknowledged the existence of 'variations in health' and tried to identify what the health service could do about them. The new Labour Government has made a much clearer commitment to tackling the root causes of health inequalities. But will this result in real progress in this area? The purpose of this chapter is to trace the development of policies to tackle health inequalities, and in particular to focus on the local response to the problem and how this can be enhanced in the future.

Health inequalities: the problem

Socio-economic differences in health have been recorded in Britain for over a century.[1] However, by far the most significant event in recent history was the publication of

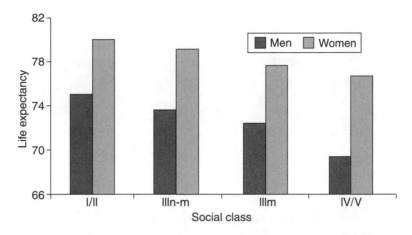

Figure 4.1: Life expectancy at birth by social class, longitudinal study, England and Wales, 1987–91
Source: Hattersley (1997)[6]

the Black Report in 1980, which concluded that 'class differences in mortality are a constant feature of the entire human life-span'.[2]

Throughout the 1980s and 1990s a considerable body of evidence accumulated that showed the poor health experience in terms of premature mortality and excess morbidity of people living in disadvantaged circumstances.[3–5] The latest data on life expectancy at birth by social class[6] are shown in Figure 4.1. For both men and women there is a social-class gradient in health, with men from professional and managerial occupations living, on average, five years longer than men with semi- and unskilled jobs. For women the gap is three years.

Such inequalities can be found for illness, disability and health, and by every measure of social status. For example, Figure 4.2 is taken from the *General Household Survey* and shows the rate of reporting health as 'not good' by respondents' family income. Those respondents in the bottom 20% of the income distribution are four times as likely to say that their health is 'not good' as those in the richest fifth.[7]

In many ways there is nothing especially remarkable about these social variations in health in Britain. They are found in most, if not all, countries.[8–10] However, what is particularly worrying is that a number of studies have begun to show that the health divide has widened in Britain during the 1980s.[11–14]

The causes of health inequalities are complex. The Black Report[2] suggested that they are:

- an artefact of measurement error
- the product of social selection
- caused by individuals' behaviours
- a result of individuals' material circumstances.

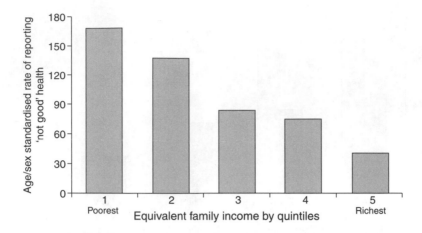

Figure 4.2: Income and health, adults 16–64, *General Household Survey*, Great Britain, 1992/3–1993/4
Source: Benzeval and Judge (1998)[7]

In addition to these explanations, there has been increasing interest in the importance of psychosocial factors for health and investigating the stage of the life course at which inequalities are developed.[1] There has been considerable, and often acrimonious, debate about the relative importance of these explanations. However, the weight of evidence seems to suggest that it is the cumulative effect of people's material and social circumstances that are the most important determinants of health inequalities.[15–17]

The policy response

In spite of the massive accumulation of evidence on health inequalities, until recently government action in Britain to tackle them has been noticeable mainly by its absence. The Black Report, commissioned by the Labour Government in 1977, not only amply demonstrated the existence of health inequalities but also put forward a broad social policy strategy to reduce them. However, when it was delivered to the incoming Conservative Government in 1980, it was published on the August bank holiday weekend with a Foreword by the then Secretary of State for Health, Patrick Jenkins, disclaiming its recommendations.[18]

During the 1980s health policy was preoccupied with managerial concerns about value for money in the NHS rather than the health of the population. Despite signing the WHO *Health for All* strategy in 1985, it was not until the 1990s that policies to improve the nation's health began to be formulated in England. The publication of the *Health of the Nation* Green Paper in 1991[19] and subsequent White Paper in 1992[20] heralded a substantial refocusing of health policy. For the first time a strategy was developed which put improving health rather than healthcare at the centre of the policy debate. The strategy set out a broad framework for improving health which, although overemphasising the role of individual's lifestyles, did acknowledge the wide range of agencies and actors that needed to be involved.

Yet even in these documents the issue of inequalities in health was largely evaded. The 1991 Green Paper[19] only briefly alluded to health inequalities in an appendix, and the 1992 White Paper mainly emphasised the need for monitoring and research to tackle 'variations in health between different groups'.[20] Neither document made any policy recommendations about how to reduce the health divide, although the White Paper did acknowledge that:

> Effective strategies, whether national or local, will need to be sensitive to these variations, and to focus on settings in which they are most evident. It will be necessary to identify the variations that occur in particular health problems in order to concentrate efforts on people at particular risk, and to adopt different strategies for different groups.[20]

Substantial criticism of both the Green and White Papers for failing to pay serious attention to health inequalities led in 1994 to the establishment of a sub-group of the CMO's Health of the Nation Working Group to review variations in health. This group produced a strategy document at the end of 1995 which made recommendations about 'what steps the DoH and the NHS should be taking to tackle variations'.[21] These included, that:

- the DoH must take the lead across all government departments in arguing for *social* policies that promote health, particularly for disadvantaged groups
- purchasers of healthcare must build into their mainstream business plans and activities policies to tackle inequalities in health
- strategic alliances must be developed to improve the health of communities
- specific interventions to promote health among disadvantaged groups must be introduced and evaluated to improve knowledge about what works
- the NHS needs to work much harder to promote equitable access to healthcare, through better resource allocation mechanisms and removing barriers of access to care.

The publication of the report represented a fundamental change in the government's approach to health inequalities.[22] At long last, the existence of 'social variations in health' was explicitly acknowledged by the DoH and a policy response, albeit limited to the NHS, put forward. At the same time the *Priority and Planning Guidance for the NHS*[23] began to identify reducing variations in health as a policy issue. However, before the results of this shift in emphasis could feed through into policy development, there was a dramatic change in political fortunes.

New Labour, new hope?

In May 1997 the Labour Party came to power with a massive majority and an election manifesto with an explicit commitment to tackle inequalities in health.[24] Within months of the election the Government had established an Independent Inquiry into Health Inequalities and launched the development of a new health strategy which has tackling inequalities in health at its heart.[25] In February 1998, the Government published its Green Paper on public health, *Our Healthier Nation*. One of its two principal aims is 'to improve the health of the worst off in society and to narrow the health gap'.[26] It acknowledges the social causes of ill health and inequalities and notes that 'tackling inequalities generally, is the best means of tackling health inequalities in particular'.[26] Two sets of policies, therefore, are vital to this endeavour: general social policies to tackle social exclusion and inequality, and specific health service policies aimed at reducing health inequalities.

Tackling social exclusion

Labour's strategy to tackle social exclusion ranges across a wide spectrum of policies.[27] To co-ordinate these activities, in August 1997 the Government established a Social Exclusion Unit (SEU) in the Cabinet Office.[28] More recently the details of its strategy were set out in the new Green Paper on welfare reform published in March 1998.[29]

The aim of the SEU is to improve understanding of the key characteristics of social exclusion and to promote 'joined up' solutions. Initially, it is focusing its efforts on reducing truancy and rough sleeping, and developing integrated and sustainable models to tackle the problems of the most disadvantaged neighbourhoods.[28] At the same time it has been asked to make recommendations about improving the mechanisms for integration across Whitehall and developing indicators of social exclusion to monitor the Government's effectiveness in this area.[28] *The New Contract for Welfare* aims to 'rebuild the welfare state around the work ethic: work for those who can; security for those who cannot'.[29] Its eight guiding principles place a heavy emphasis on helping and encouraging people into work through the *New Deal* welfare to work schemes, and tackling some of the barriers to work, such as low skills, perverse benefit incentives and access to affordable childcare. Other key aspects of the strategy include: increasing financial support to families with children and reforming pensions to guarantee a decent income for all in retirement.

Although the Government has made a clear commitment to tackling social exclusion and health inequalities, the means it has chosen have been questioned by some and could derail its ultimate success. Two issues are of particular importance.

• First, whether the Government has chosen the appropriate policy levers to address the problem.
• Second, whether the methods for cross-government co-ordination will be effective.

There is not room here to undertake a comprehensive critique of the Government's proposals to reform the welfare state and tackle social exclusion, and it is too early to judge them by results, but a number of warning signals have already been raised.

The Government is building its policies to tackle social exclusion on work and education. No one would argue that the best long-run route to tackling poverty is by ensuring that people are well educated and have decent, well-paid jobs.[4] Policies to establish a minimum wage, improve education and develop welfare to work schemes are all important parts of such an approach. However, there are a number of potential problems. To date, the Government's efforts to promote employment have mainly emphasised supply-side factors, without any explicit effort to increase the overall demand for labour. In times of economic buoyancy this may not be overly important. However, if there is an economic downturn, the Government will need to play a much more active role in creating jobs in order to ensure its welfare to work schemes are effective.

Of bigger concern, however, is the Government's reluctance to improve the living standards of those who remain reliant on benefits. The 1998 budget[30] did make modest improvements, with increases in the child element of income support and in universal child benefit, and the introduction of the new working families tax credit and childcare tax credit. As a redistributive budget, it did much to help families, particularly with young children, and to make the transition from benefits to work much easier. More generally, however, the Government has taken a negative stand against 'cash benefits'. The most stark example of this was the Government's confirmation in autumn of 1997 that it would carry out the Conservatives' decision to cut lone parent benefits. Although the changes in the budget mean that new lone parents will receive the same income as existing claimants by October 1999,[31] the principle of lone parents requiring additional resources because they do not benefit from the same economies of scale as a couple has been eroded.[32] Moreover, other specific groups who were disadvantaged by Conservative benefit changes, for example, 16- and 17-year-olds and asylum seekers, have not seen their situation improved. More importantly, there has never been any official attempt to assess whether the standard of living provided by benefits is adequate, although a number of studies suggest that it is not.[33,34] This means that those who cannot get a job are likely to remain in poverty. In addition, a number of commentators have suggested that the Government's attempts to improve education will be hampered without a more concerted approach to reduce child poverty, and that benefit levels are too low to support people with the costs of finding a job. Ignoring the importance of benefits, therefore, will almost certainly reduce the impact of the Government's attempt to tackle social exclusion.

Even within the confines of the existing focus of the Government's policies to tackle social exclusion and reduce health inequalities, much will depend on its ability to develop much more effective mechanisms for cross-government co-ordination than have existed in the past. The model that Labour has adopted – a special unit within the Cabinet Office to focus on specific topics and try to improve co-ordination – has an earlier precedent in the Joint Approach to Social Policy (JASP)[35] set up in the mid-1970s. JASP was an experiment in rational policy making, providing detailed analysis of social problems to improve collective policy making and priority setting. When it ended it was judged to have had little lasting impact on the co-ordination of central government policies.[36] Those closely involved in its activities put this down to ministerial indifference and departmental obstruction. It proved impossible to develop a sense of collective purpose among Ministers or officials, whose self-interest led them to put the needs of their own departments first, particularly if resource issues were involved.[36] In contrast to JASP, the

SEU does have a strong collective purpose – to reduce social exclusion – and support from the Prime Minister to maintain momentum and 'knock heads together' when necessary. The key question, however, is whether this is sufficient to overcome the blinkeredness of departmentalism or whether more explicit incentives for collective action, for example, an independent budget, will be required.

The role of the health service

More explicitly in relation to health inequalities, the Government has published a number of strategies within the health field, which reiterate its commitment to tackle them and begin to identify how this could be done at the local level.

First, the *Priority and Planning Guidance* issued by the NHS Executive in September 1997 asserted that the 'overall aim of the Government's health policy is to develop a coherent strategy for public health... A key aspect of this will be tackling health inequalities'.[37] The guidance went on to argue that the NHS must promote equity of access to its services and that health authorities must work with partner organisations to tackle the key causes of local health problems.

Second, in December 1997 the White Paper *The New NHS* was published. Again, this made clear that the NHS should 'not just treat people when they are ill but work with others to improve health and reduce health inequalities'.[38] The key catalyst for achieving this would be health authorities. Leaner bodies, freed from the task of direct commissioning, health authorities will have lead responsibility for working with other agencies to improve health and tackle health inequalities. A statutory responsibility for partnership would be placed on them and the key integrating device would be the HIMPs and, in selected areas, Health Action Zones (HAZs).

Finally, in February 1998, as highlighted above, the Government published its Green Paper on public health, *Our Healthier Nation*.[26] At the central government level, it stated that the Minister for Public Health and the Cross-Cabinet Committee for Health will co-ordinate policy across Whitehall and establish health impact assessments on a wide range of government policies to ensure that social policies promote health. At the local level, *Our Healthier Nation* again highlighted the leadership role of health authorities in tackling inequalities in health, with a particular emphasis on the need for HIMPs to focus on improving the health of the most disadvantaged sections of their community. It concluded that:

> *Taken together, the Health Improvement Programmes across the country, combined with the Government's role ... will form a concerted national programme to improve health and tackle health inequalities.*[26]

The success of the Government's strategy to tackle inequalities in health at the local level, therefore, will crucially depend on the ability of health authorities to lead inter-agency action. The next section considers their experience and capacity to do this.

Health authority action

Some, if not all, health authorities have always had small-scale projects to improve the health of disadvantaged communities or increase access to healthcare in deprived areas. In addition, in the mid-1980s many health authorities adopted the *Health for All* targets and/or became Healthy Cities, both of which have reducing inequalities in health as a central component of their aims.[39–41] However, such initiatives have often been at the margins of health authorities' activities, and very few appear to have put equity at the centre of their policy agendas.

During the 1980s there were a number of attempts to assess health authority action in relation to health inequalities. First, Dearden attempted to 'review and evaluate current programmes in the NHS for reducing inequalities in health. ... [but found an] absence of any established programmes dealing with health inequalities'.[42] Second, Castle and Jacobson[43] reviewed the health promotion policies of RHAs and concluded that 'a commitment to the reduction of inequalities in health was not prominent'.[44] Next, the Faculty of Community Medicine in an analysis of public health reports concluded that:

> there are disappointingly few reports that combine epidemiology with social research techniques to pin-point the population groups with the greatest needs ... still fewer reports give information about the implementation of health promotion initiatives in specific social priority areas.[45]

In contrast, Harris and Smith[46] found that over half of the health authorities that responded to their survey about the health problems of unemployment were doing something, including: creating jobs; training healthcare professionals about facilities available for people who were unemployed; and monitoring unemployment and its effects locally.

In the 1990s, Laughlin and Black[47] conducted a survey of community-level projects that had a focus on poverty and health. They identified 94 projects in 50 different areas but concluded that:

> there appear to be few authorities which are seriously addressing the social/political causes of ill health in any systematic or strategic way although many health authorities are linked with the specific work of health alliances such as Healthy Cities project and Health for All initiatives.[47]

A more positive light is thrown on health authority action by the CMO's Working Group on variations in health,[21] which undertook a survey of all Directors of Public Health 'to find out what was currently being done at a local level to address variations in health' and found 'a rich variety of work'. Specific activities cited, included:

- health need assessment
- local targets
- access to effective healthcare
- resource allocation

- purchasing by primary healthcare
- alliances
- public health programmes
- the NHS as an employer.

Unfortunately, the report does not identify whether such activities are widespread among health authorities or whether the specific initiatives are limited to one or two areas. In addition to this survey, the Working Group also commissioned a systematic review of interventions to improve the health of disadvantaged groups.[48] However, one of the main conclusions of the review was that initiatives in this area have been very poorly evaluated in the past. Moreover, most of those interventions identified focus on improving access to healthcare rather than intersectoral action to promote health. Although a few areas[49-51] have established strategic partnerships to tackle inequalities in health, experience and knowledge about the most effective way of doing this is limited, and, unfortunately, guidance in the Green Paper is vague. Nevertheless, there appears to be considerable enthusiasm among both health and local authorities to work in partnerships to tackle inequalities in health.[52] The key question, therefore, is whether they have the capacity to do so, since both health and local authorities are facing significant change agendas in other aspects of their responsibilities.

Local authorities have been the subject of various Green and White Papers and strategy documents – for example, in relation to local democracy and community leadership, sustainable development, best value, education, transport, road safety, housing, environmental health, safeguarding children and better government for older people, to name but a few. While many of the key areas of their responsibilities influence health at the local level, the public health Green Paper is vague as to how local authorities should take this agenda forward or where it fits with their other priorities. In this respect, until a clear co-ordination of policies and priorities can be achieved within Whitehall, there is little hope of clarity at the local level.[36] Much clearer accountability and performance management mechanisms need to be established for local authorities before they can begin to fulfil their potential to tackle inequalities in health.

Redefining the health authorities' role to make working in partnership with local authorities to promote health a much more central part of their responsibilities presents clear opportunities to tackle inequalities in health at the local level. Similarly, the development of HAZs in 11 areas, covering some of the most deprived parts of the country, demonstrates a real commitment to addressing this problem, and the bids show considerable imagination to work across boundaries to tackle some of the root causes of health inequalities.[53] However, there are also considerable barriers that must be overcome.[54] For example, health authorities will also have to develop and manage the devolution of the commissioning process to PCGs. This is likely to be very time consuming, particularly in areas where GP commissioning and fundholding is underdeveloped. In addition, although the Green Paper makes it clear that the public health function will be excluded from the cap on management costs, it is unclear how these monies will be allocated or whether health authorities will receive any additional funding to pump prime initiatives to tackle the wider public health agenda. Moreover, in future PCGs will control much of the health authority's resources, yet traditionally GPs have shown little interest in public health issues. The involvement of community nurses in PCGs may help to balance this situation, but the role of PCGs in relation to *Our Healthier Nation* is still unclear. Such issues must be addressed in order for health authorities to develop their potential to make real progress in reducing the health divide.

Summary

Health inequalities are a serious public policy problem, which the previous government only began to acknowledge in its last few years. While New Labour has made tackling inequalities in health a much more high-profile part of its health strategy, it remains to be seen whether, in practice, this issue will really move up the national and local agenda, which are both crammed with many other priorities. Local enthusiasm to develop strategies in this area and address local issues could make a contribution to reducing inequalities in health. However, as the experience of the Community Development Programme in the 1970s showed, most local problems have their roots in national policies and experiences.[55] As recognised in the recently published review of inequalities in health undertaken by Sir Donald Acheson.[56] Unless these are effectively co-ordinated and focused on the most pressing social and economic problems, health inequalities will remain a scar on British society. National policies to tackle social exclusion must find new ways of co-ordinating policies across Whitehall, and develop policies to ensure that the most vulnerable sections of the population, who cannot work and hence remain reliant on benefits, are not excluded even further.

References

1   Macintyre S (1997) The Black Report and beyond: what are the issues? *Social Science and Medicine.* **44**(6): 723–45.

2   Townsend P and Davidson N (eds) (1982) The Black Report. In: P Townsend, M Whitehead and N Davidson (eds) (1992) new edition, *Inequalities in Health: The Black Report and the health divide*. Penguin Books, London.

 3   Whitehead M (1992) The health divide. In: P Townsend, M Whitehead and N Davidson (eds), *Inequalities in Health: The Black Report and the health divide*. Penguin Books, London.

4   Benzeval M, Judge K and Whitehead M (eds) (1995) *Tackling Inequalities in Health: an agenda for action.* King's Fund, London.

5   Drever F and Whitehead M (eds) (1997) *Health Inequalities: decennial supplement.* Series DS, No. 15. The Stationery Office, London.

6   Hattersley L (1997) Expectation of life by social class. In: F Drever and M Whitehead (eds) *Health Inequalities: decennial supplement.* Series DS, No. 15. The Stationery Office, London.

7   Benzeval M and Judge K (1998) Poverty and health. *Health Variations.* **1**: 12–13.

8   Kunst AE and Mackenbach JP (1994) The size of mortality differences associated with educational level in nine industrialised countries. *American Journal of Public Health.* **84**(6): 932–7.

9   Mackenbach JP, Kunst AE, Cavelaars A *et al.* (1997) Socioeconomic inequalities in morbidity and mortality in western Europe. *Lancet.* **349**: 1655–9.

10   van Doorslaer E, Wagstaff A, Bleichrodt H *et al.* (1997) Income-related inequalities in health: some international comparisons. *Journal of Health Economics.* **16**: 93–112.

11   Phillimore P, Beattie A and Townsend P (1994) Widening inequality of health in Northern England. *British Medical Journal.* **308**: 1125–8.

12   McLoone P and Boddy F (1994) Deprivation and mortality in Scotland. 1981 and 1991. *British Medical Journal.* **309**: 1465–70.

13   Filakti H and Fox J (1995) Differences in mortality by housing tenure and by care access from the OPCS Longitudinal Study. *Population Trends.* **81**: 27–30.

14   Harding S (1995) Social class differences in mortality of men: recent evidence from the OPCS Longitudinal Study. *Population Trends.* **80**: 31–7.

15   Davey Smith G, Blane D and Bartley M (1994) Explanations for socioeconomic differences in mortality. *European Journal of Public Health.* **4**(2): 131–44.

16   Fox J and Benzeval M (1995) Perspectives on social variations in health. In: M Benzeval, K Judge and M Whitehead (eds) *Tackling Inequalities in Health: an agenda for action.* King's Fund, London.

17   Vågerö D and Illsley R (1995) Explaining health inequalities: beyond Black and Barker. *European Sociology Review.* **11**(3): 219–41.

18   Jenkins R (1982) Foreword, in the Black Report (P Townsend and N Davidson, eds). In: P Townsend, M Whitehead and N Davidson (eds) (1992) new edition, *Inequalities in Health: The Black Report and the health divide.* Penguin Books, London.

19   Secretary of State for Health (1991) *The Health of the Nation: a consultative document for health in England.* HMSO, London.

20   Secretary of State for Health (1992) *The Health of the Nation: a strategy for health in England.* Cm 1986. HMSO, London.

21   Department of Health (1995) *Variations in Health: what can the Department of Health and the NHS do?* Variations Sub-Group of the Chief Medical Officers Health of the Nation Working Group, chaired by Jeremy Metters. DoH, London.

22   Benzeval M (1997) Health. In: A Walker and C Walker (eds) *Britain Divided: the growth of social exclusion in the 1980s and 1990s.* CPAG, London.

23   NHS Executive (1996) *Priority and Planning Guidance for the NHS: 1997/98.* NHSE, Leeds.

24   Labour Party (1997) *New Labour: because Britain deserves better.* The Labour Party, London.

25   Jowell T (Minister for Public Health) (1997) *Public Health in England Strategy Speech, Monday 7 July 1997.* Department of Health, London.

26   Secretary of State for Health (1998) *Our Healthier Nation: a contract for health.* A consultation paper. Cm 3852. The Stationery Office, London.

27   HM the Queen (1997) *Opening of Parliament, Session 1997–98.* House of Commons, London.

28   Social Exclusion Unit (1997) *Priority Tasks.* Social Exclusion Unit Home Page, Cabinet Office, London.

29   Secretary of State for Health (1998) *New Ambitions for Our Country: a new contract for welfare.* A consultation paper. Cm 3805. The Stationery Office, London.

30   HM Treasury (1998) *The Pocket Budget 1998.* HM Treasury, London.

31   National Council for One Parent Families (NCOPF) (1998) Budget boost for lone parents. *One Parent Times.* **1**: 3.

32   Sherlock M (1998) Editorial. *One Parent Times.* **1**: 2.

33   Bradshaw J (1993) *Household Budgets and Living Standards.* Joseph Rowntree Foundation, York.

34   Berthoud R and Ford R (1996) *Relative Needs: variations in the living standards of different types of households.* Policy Studies Institute, London.

35   Hunter D (1997) A long life for a quick fix? *Health Service Journal.* **4**(September): 22.

36   Challis L, Fuller S, Henwood M *et al.* (1988) *Joint Approach to Social Policy: rationality and practice.* Cambridge University Press, Cambridge.

37   NHS Executive (1997) *Priority and Planning Guidance for the NHS: 1998/99.* NHSE, Leeds.

38   Secretary of State for Health (1997) *The New NHS: modern, dependable.* Cm 3807. The Stationery Office, London.

39   Ashton J and Seymour H (1988) *The New Public Health: the Liverpool experience.* Open University Press, Milton Keynes.

40   Ashton J (1992) *Healthy Cities.* Open University Press, Milton Keynes.

41   Davies J and Kelly M (eds) (1993) *Healthy Cities: research and practice.* Routledge, London.

42   Dearden R (1985) *Dealing with Inequalities in Health.* HSMC, University of Birmingham, Birmingham.

43   Castle P and Jacobson B (1988) *The Health of our Regions: an analysis of the strategies and policies of regional health authorities for promoting health and preventing disease.* A report for the Health Education Council. NHS Regions Health Promotion Group, Birmingham.

44   Jacobson B, Smith A and Whitehead M (eds) (1991) *The Nation's Health: a strategy for the 1990s.* King Edward's Hospital Fund for London, London.

45   Faculty of Community Medicine of the Royal College of Physicians (1990) *Health for All 2000 News.* **12**: May.

46   Harris CM and Smith R (1987) What are health authorities doing about the health problems caused by unemployment? *British Medical Journal.* **294**: 1076–9.

47   Laughlin S and Black D (1995) *Poverty and Health: tools for change.* Public Health Trust, Birmingham.

48   Arblaster L, Entwistle V, Lambert M *et al.* (1995) *Review of the Research on the Effectiveness of Health Service Interventions to Reduce Variations in Health.* CRD report 3. NHS Centre for Reviews and Dissemination. University of York, York.

49   Benzeval M, Judge K and Whitehead M (1993) The role of the NHS. In: M Benzeval, K Judge and M Whitehead (eds) *Tackling Inequalities in Health: an agenda for action.* King's Fund, London.

50   Nocon A (1993) Made in heaven? *Health Service Journal,* 23 December: 24–6.

51   Costongs C and Springett J (1997) Joint working and the production of a city health plan: the Liverpool experience. *Health Promotion International.* **12**(1): 9–19.

52   Benzeval M, Duggan M and Killoran A (1998) *Our Healthier Nation: a response to the Green Paper.* King's Fund, Association for Public Health and Health Education Authority, London.

53   Department of Health (1998) *Frank Dobson gives the Go-ahead for the First Wave of Health Action Zones.* Press release 98/120, DoH, London.

54   Benzeval M and Coulter A (1998) The health authority's new roles. In: R Klein (ed.) *Implementing the White Paper: pitfalls and opportunities.* King's Fund, London.

55   Taylor M (1992) *Signposts to Community Development.* National Coalition for Neighbourhoods and Community Development Foundation, London.

56   DoH (1998) *Independent Inquiry into Inequalities in Health Report. Chairman Sir Donald Acheson.* The Stationery Office, London.

CHAPTER FIVE

Food as a public health issue

Tim Lang

Introduction

In the mid-1970s, to argue in Britain that food was a public health issue invited a mixed response. Most mainstream medical opinion was either uninterested or sceptical, as were the politicians nominally in control of food and public health policy. True, there was already strong epidemiological and physiological evidence that diet was a major factor in coronary heart disease.[1-3] True, too, bodies in the UK such as the Committee on Medical Aspects of Food Policy had already pronounced concerns,[4] as had other international studies.[5] Nonetheless, although there was strong evidence for changes in direction of food policy and for public health intervention, there was next to no public policy response. By the end of the twentieth century, the gap between evidence for action and state and industrial inaction had taken a high public profile and major changes in institutions in the UK and EU had been set in train, triggered by the BSE crisis.[6] There was widespread public lack of confidence in government, after a series of damaging public health food crises.

Throughout the 1980s and 1990s, the case for public health action was made by a coalition of concerned food and public health specialists, together with a new generation of specialist non-governmental organisations. Persistently, they raised the case that, for all the much-heralded advances in food technology and choice, food was the primary cause of the nation's leading causes of premature death, coronary heart disease and certain cancers. As well as these, there was a rising toll of food poisoning incidence, and other more ill-defined problems ranging from residues from pesticides and antibiotics used in intensive farming to allergies from additives in mass food.[7] By the 1990s, a disparate set of analyses – medical, consumer, environmental, social policy – had been integrated into a new public health perspective on food. This argued that the new public health meant not just human but environmental health, not just equality of access to the

NHS but equity within society, not just risk assessment of food problems but trust in institutions of food governance.

By any account, this food and public health coalition was remarkably successful in taking its case to the public and in winning legal and policy change. Nine years after the Coronary Prevention Group was founded by concerned professionals and held a strategy meeting in 1983 at Canterbury,[8] the government committed itself to reduce heart disease in the 1992 *Health of the Nation* White Paper.[9] Six years after the London Food Commission was founded, focusing on food quality and the new adulteration issues,[10] the Food Safety Act 1990 was passed. Like their forebears, this new public health movement had to learn how to marshal not just facts but public opinion and political force, using media and alliances to do so. Good work though it has done, we should be wary of over-estimating its success. Coronaries continue to take their toll, and food poisoning, to take just one safety issue, has risen inexorably.[11] The challenge today is how to translate concern and evidence of the need for action in food policy into a health-generating food economy; in other words, how to prevent rather than bemoan food-related ill health.

A short social history of food and health

The history of food as a public health issue is an extraordinary tale, of ebbs and flows in public concern, agitation, state response, industrial restructuring. The late twentieth-century period of food and public health scandals are quite in keeping with that tradition and that dynamic.[12] After years of criticism for fuelling heart disease by selling hidden fats, for instance, the food industry has now launched myriad 'low-fat' foods, some of which are high in fat although lower than their generic equivalents. A low-fat spread may be lower fat than butter, but it is still high in fat. Tens of millions of dollars, yen and pounds have been invested to create a new generation of functional foods, so-called designer foods with specific health attributes. A visit to the supermarket or pharmacy or health food shop will illustrate their arrival. Even as these products arrive, concerns from researchers and health specialists are being voiced – that they are technical 'fixes' which do not resolve underlying problems or, in the case of a new generation of 'non-fat fats' (which pass through the intestines undigested), that they actually fuel fat intake by encouraging people to think they are cutting back everywhere on fat intake. Such arguments constantly rage in food and health policy. It was ever thus.

From the eighteenth century to the end of the nineteenth, food and its impact on health peppered the public policy agenda. Whether through bread riots or political upheavals about the cost of food in relation to wages or about food quality, these episodes were all associated with the transition from a rural to industrial economy.[13] The first Public Health Act in the UK was in 1848. Although not a food act, there had already been a quarter century of public turmoil about the quality and health impact of food. Routine adulteration and high food prices sparked a vibrant anti-adulteration movement and the co-operative movement.[12,14,15] Both argued that the unfettered market could not be relied upon to produce safe or affordable food and successfully campaigned for new laws to protect public safety and new practices to give the public food it could trust and afford. The 1875 Food Act is still the legal foundation on which current laws are based.

When the public health perspective is broadened to include social policy aspects of food, the health toll lengthens. Poverty, in particular, has always been the ultimate discriminator of health.[16,17] Diet is a key factor in this relationship. The better a population's diet, the longer it tends to live, and the higher an individual's income, the better his or her diet is and the longer he or she tends to live. This applies even in an affluent country such as the UK.[18] The British battle over industrialisation's legacy of food poverty, ranging from facilities in towns to cooking skills and facilities in houses, raged until the twentieth-century welfare reforms began to right the gross inequities.[19] Arguably, it was the 1906 Education (Provision of Meals) Act, introducing the right for local authorities to pay for school meals, which ushered in the welfare state itself, although it was not until the Second World War that full provision was made, and then only because women were wanted in the waged labour force.[20]

The Second World War marked a watershed in British food and health policy. A Ministry of Food was set up to implement health-derived planning, more overtly through the rationing scheme.[21] This crisis-generated interventionism convinced many that, unpalatable though such controls may be in economic orthodoxy, they did generate better health. Post-war food and agriculture underwent a radical change of policy. After a century of reliance on colonial cheap food, the 1947 Agriculture Act symbolised a shift to support British farming. Production was to be encouraged. The close relationship forged in the war between food capital and government was to be continued. This policy change enabled a scientific revolution to be more systematically applied, both on and off the farm.[22] Intensification was the theme, getting more from capital, labour and animals. War controls were relaxed. The Ministry of Food was disbanded and its rump merged into the productionist Ministry of Agriculture and Fisheries to create MAFF, with food coming symbolically last.

Thus in the 1950s, just as the 1930s-inspired food and health movement grew old, a modern food revolution began, bringing to market new foods, new ways of growing, transporting, packing and cooking food. Production gradually took command, and it was decades before the epidemiological studies provided the dietary connection with degenerative diseases and before a 'big picture' made the connection with other diseases and reasserted the public interest.[23] The ill-health list now associated with food is wide-ranging: heart disease, cancers, food poisoning, allergies from additives, risks from residues from intensive production (antibiotics, pesticides, nitrates), contaminants and, of course, BSE. After decades in which those in control of food production and retailing had basked in consumer glory at successfully increasing production and reducing the amount of money people spend on food from 30% in 1950 to 10% in 1990, by the late 1990s few could deny the powerful evidence that productionism may have filled shelves but it also brought a new wave of food-related ill health. In particular, attention should be directed to the issues of cost and inequality. Cheap food has a high health cost.

The costs of public health are left out of the image of 'efficient' production

Behind the astonishing efficiencies of modern food production, the costs of protecting public and environmental health are externalised. The 1996 edition of the DoH's *Burdens of Disease* calculated that heart disease drugs cost the NHS £500 million a year, bowel cancers £1.1 billion, and diseases of the circulatory system cost 12.1% of the total health and social services budget.[24]

Based on 1993–94 figures, the British Heart Foundation Research Group at Oxford University[25] calculated the costs of coronary heart disease as:

- 66 million lost working days, equivalent to 11% of all days lost due to sickness
- £858 million in invalidity benefits
- £3 billion for lost production in British industry
- a minimum of £1420 million in direct treatment costs to the NHS; of this the bill for drugs alone was £650 million; there are 23 000 coronary bypass operations annually
- total costs of approximately £10 billion per year; this includes NHS costs.[26]

There are also high externalised costs from food poisoning. Food poisoning figures, whether reported or proven, are rising inexorably.[11] The costs have been estimated as £1 billion per year.[27] The care costs to the NHS for 100 000 people treated in 1991–94 was £83 million.[28] There are two main possible causes for this rise. Food may be more contaminated – due to cross-contamination or to more pathogens in the 'reservoir' or even to the complexity of food system. The other cause could be changed consumer behaviour due to new technologies, shopping patterns or lack of knowledge. The latter interpretation, which has often been promoted by food industry interests understandably wishing to divest themselves of responsibility, has a sting in its tail. If consumer responsibility is generally accepted, what happens when it can be proven that the consumer was *not* responsible? In the USA, where a litigation-oriented consumerist culture is furthest advanced, the annual cost of food-borne illness from pathogens has been estimated as between US$7.7 billion–$8.4 billion.[29] Each case of salmonellosis, for instance, is estimated to cost US$500–$1350, with a case of botulism working out as US$322 000. Legal fees account for a heavy proportion of these costs.

Obesity is a risk factor in heart disease, and its reduction was one of the targets set in the 1992 *Health of the Nation* White Paper.[9] Exercise is a key to reduction of obesity, yet figures continue to rise. Gyms abound and the public are invited to buy stationary running and rowing machines to work off excess diets. The food industry also supports the need for more exercise, perhaps in part as this focus shifts attention from the fats and heart disease story. Meanwhile exercise is being structured out of people's lives by the car. It is hard to build exercise into one's daily life, for instance, when shopping for food. Shopping assumes a car rather than walking. Food retailers promote the car (and sell petrol). Above all, the siting policy of the big chains has been premised upon having ever larger stores serving more customers. Hypermarkets are more profitable per sales area than smaller stores.[30] Retailers have actively pursued this approach.[31] One of the big four supermarkets in the UK is on record as saying, 'new sites are located where safe and convenient access is obtained by car' and that 'today, we would not open a store which did not have a large surface level car park'.[30]

Besides shopping, the environmental impact of the food system is extensive. On pesticides, for instance, the simplest calculation is the cost of clean-up. In 1997 Ofwat, the water industries regulator, calculated that the capital costs of installing activated carbon to reduce residues to permitted levels is £1 billion.[32] The combined capital and running costs of reducing pesticide residues is currently being spread at an annual £100 million. Water consumers pay for this but the problem stems from farming. One private sector is externalising its 'efficiencies' onto a public one.

Another illustration of environmental health carrying hidden health costs is the 'food miles' problem, the distance food travels before consumers eat it. Over the period 1979– 93, although the tonnage of food, drink and tobacco transported has remained remarkably constant, the distance it has travelled within the UK (let alone before it gets there) has risen by a third.[35] Not only is the food travelling further, but consumers are travelling further to get it. The distance they travel to shop in general rose by 60% between 1975–76 and 1989–91, but the travel taken by car more than doubled.[30] Far from hypermarkets being convenient, they in fact generate more, not fewer, trips for food shopping. Instead of shopping being factored into other daily routines, it now is a dedicated operation on its own. The mileage of trips to town-centre food shops is less than half that taken to edge-of-town stores.[34]

Another environmental externality is the so-called 'Ghost Acres' phenomenon in which an 'efficient' developed food system uses additional distant land in developing countries.[33] Food imports into the UK in 1995 represented the equivalent of 4.1 million hectares of productive land.[35] Much of the produce is for animal feed for intensive husbandry. Pig and poultry meat prices may have fallen considerably over the past four decades in Europe, bringing them routinely into the mass diet, but the full cost of land utilisation on other populations is rarely included. Brazil, for instance, is a major exporter of soya and citrus fruits, yet has the world's second highest rate of child malnutrition. There is concern, too, that the seas are being excessively harvested. Cod is almost fished out.[36] According to Food and Agriculture Organisation figures, 32% of the current fish catch of the world ends up as fishmeal for meat production.[35]

Since its earliest days, the public health movement has been motivated by a humanitarian desire to reduce waste and help populations achieve their full potential. The new public health analysis of food faces a considerable challenge in this respect. The modern food economy is, in fact, not without systematic waste. An illustration is what happens to fruit and vegetables. The population of the UK has a relatively low intake of fruit and vegetables. To tackle cardiovascular disease, the Government estimates that the population of England needs to increase its intake by half[37] and that of Scotland needs its intake to double.[38] Yet in 1993–94 the EU spent 390 million ecu (*c.* £230 million) to buy and destroy 2.5 billion kg of fruit and vegetables.[39] It would have been better for health if schoolchildren were given the 980 million kg of apples or 312 million kg of oranges destroyed. Although the UK is blessed with a benign climate, ideal for growing many fruits and vegetables, its food sector is in fact in a deficit with the world. The food trade gap is immense and growing. The total food and drink trade deficit has risen from £5.5 billion in 1989 to £7.7 billion in 1996; by 1996 the deficit for fruit and vegetables was nearly half of that figure.[40]

According to National Food Survey data, the percentage of household expenditure on food between 1950 and 1990 has dropped from a third to a tenth, but the averages disguise class differences.[18] Today, the poorest tenth of households spend one-quarter to one-third of their incomes on food, while the richest spend nearer 10%. The children of families in the lowest socio-economic groups eat less than half the fresh fruit and vegetables that those of the richest eat. After years in which both rich and poor classes consumed more fruit, the gap recently grew again. Concerned about the trade rather than social-class deficit, from the early 1980s Mrs Thatcher's government espoused a nineteenth-century food trade policy: export more to cover the cost of the enormous import bill. Unfortunately the policy failed to stem the deficit. In the health-critical sector of fruit and vegetables, the trade gap grew from £2.5 billion in 1989 to £3.84 billion by 1996. Yet agriculturally and climatically, the UK is well suited to grow such products. It may not be able to grow mangoes or pineapples but is wonderful for soft and top fruit and for many vegetables. If such products are being imported, with even inadequate demand and with attendant employment and health losses, agricultural policy cannot surely be judged a health success. It is sometimes hard to disentangle to what extent this is the fault of the Common Agricultural Policy (CAP), national policies or the logic of intensive development.

Food and public health are European and global issues

The main positive contribution of the CAP to health has been to ensure security of supply in Europe from the ashes of the Second World War. While this is a definite gain, the re-emergence of food poverty in Europe suggests that there are some serious deficiencies in how the CAP works today.[41] No calculations of CAP costs in relation to health in general, or to low-income consumers in particular, have been made, other than general calculations about costs to 'average' consumers or taxpayers.[42–44] The burden of CAP on low-income consumers is proportionately considerably greater than on the more affluent, because the poor spend a higher percentage of their expenditure of food,[18] yet CAP institutionalises inequality of support. Eighty percent of EU support that actually goes to farmers goes to the largest 20%.[45] Agricultural support costs the average EU family with two children up to £20 per week in taxes.[46] With estimates such as the one showing that the weekly food bill is £7.75 higher than it need be, one could appreciate that pressure to reform the CAP is intense but the situation is immensely complex.

Variation in eating patterns between EU member states suggests that there is no simple, unidirectional effect of the CAP on either diet or health. Despite EU member states sharing the same CAP regime, there is considerable variation in diet-related ill health. While reviews of premature mortality in Europe conclude that diet is a factor in the leading causes of death,[47–49] they do simultaneously note that within the EU there is 'a remarkable variability ... in the causes of premature deaths'.[50] There is also considerable variation in what proportion of income is allocated to food, with Portugal spending 33% and Greece 31% but the UK 12% and the former West Germany 12% in 1990.[51]

Although the CAP is usually depicted as one policy, it is in fact a web of diverse public policy measures. No comprehensive review of its effects on health in general or inequalities in health in particular has been undertaken.[52] This should be a priority within the Commission, since Article 129 of the Maastricht Treaty accorded the Commission more power to consider health impacts of its policy. The Amsterdam Treaty promised a strengthening of this commitment.[53] The health audits now being produced by the Directorate for Public Health[54] are welcome, but there has been reluctance to review the CAP despite it being by far the greatest budget within the EU.[55] According to the 1997 Court of Auditors' report, in 1996, CAP's total cost was 39.080 billion ecu, 54% of a total EU budget of 72.793 billion ecu.[56] Although the trend is for CAP's share of EU expenditure to fall, its 1998 EU budget was still a commitment for 40.437 billion ecu, 44% of a total of 91.012 billion ecu.[57]

The total cost of CAP is immense, but it should be remembered that its focus is on raw food production. CAP's origins lie in ensuring security of supply after Europe's dire experience of shortage in the Second World War.[58,59] The primary commodity tends to be a small element of the final cost that the consumer pays for food in the shops. Most value is added off the farm, by processing, packaging, transport and retailing. For instance, farm-gate cereal prices account for only 16% of the consumer cost of a loaf of bread.[60] Nevertheless, it should also be remembered that the CAP is a public policy – a choice of how to spend money. In the new public health terms, the funds could, and perhaps should, be better spent on direct support for environmental protection or for the poor, to enable them to eat more healthily. In 1991, half CAP's budget was spent on storage of surpluses and on export restitution to subsidise the gap between the CAP's high price regime and lower world prices, i.e. to fund exporters to dispose of surpluses.[45]

The health impact of various CAP commodity regimes is itself complex and varied. Of the 39 billion ecu that CAP cost in 1996 according to the Court of Auditors, 16.9 billion ecu was used to subsidise arable crops; 8.3 billion ecu subsidised meat, eggs and poultry; 1.8 billion ecu, sugar; 1.5 billion ecu, fruit and vegetables; and 1 billion ecu, tobacco.[56] Those studies that have reviewed CAP's health impact have focused upon single commodity regimes such as dairy fats, tobacco, alcohol, and fruit and vegetables.[39,61,62]

Whereas tobacco funding is deleterious in its health effects, in the case of dairy fats, the figures can be interpreted to suggest that by maintaining a high price regime for dairy fats, the CAP reduces the potential for a high uptake, i.e. is relatively beneficial for health. One study[61] stressed that butter consumption is relatively price elastic (i.e. sensitive) and that CAP policies, by raising these prices, depressed demand, which is a good thing given overall health targets.[9] It suggested that there is limited substitution between butter and margarine. Low-income consumers, however, are more price sensitive in their behaviour, and the study found that EU schemes for disposing of butter at reduced prices displaced other sales and led to an increase in overall consumption of yellow fats. This sector policy, therefore, seemed to be pulling in both directions. By funding marketing to increase uptake, the CAP undermined its own price signals and undermined clear health promotion messages.

In the case of fruit and vegetables, half the regime's expenditure in some years has been spent on destroying edible fruit. In 1993–94, for example, the EU spent 390 million ecu to buy and destroy 2.5 billion kg of fruit and vegetables.[39] No estimate has been made of the health gain that could accrue from the transfer of these products to schoolchildren or to low-income consumers. This could be a fruitful line of research. School fruit, from CAP sources, could do for children's health what school meals and milk offered in the 1940s – a better mix of production and health.[63]

Conclusion

Recent experience of conflicts over food and public health have been salutary reminders of some old public health lessons. Public health is never given, it has to be gained. In industrial societies where the vast majority of the population is urban, the consuming classes are dependent upon a food industry which, if unchecked, will understandably push food policy in its own favoured directions. For centuries, experience shows that power between grower, processor, seller and purchaser/consumer can easily swing in the producers' favour, unless the state, having set health and trading standards, then monitors and enforces them. To rely upon self-regulation or deregulation to achieve high standards of public protection is not a strategy that has stood the test of time. For a food policy to work relatively well to the general good, attention has to be directed on three core issues:

- institutions of food governance – to ensure that they work in the public interest, are flexible and are appropriate
- food policies – to ensure that health is a priority over industrial or sectoral interests
- food culture – to support the enjoyment of food and the popular understanding of what is needed to gain the maximum benefit from food, through education, advice and information.

Over the past two centuries, food concerns have had an impressive capacity to unseat orthodoxies and to unsettle governments. Food is a great leveller. No one likes to think that his or her food is adulterated or causes ill health. All people, of whatever class, politics, age, gender and ethnic culture, like to think they choose their food. Food is a deeply personal affair. While people are remarkably resistant to change their diet in some circumstances, they are also remarkably fast to do so on other occasions. In 1950, who would have thought that pizza would be the favourite food of children in the UK in the 1990s? Or that sun-dried tomatoes would sell in British stores? Taste, in other words, is malleable. Hence the challenge to food and health policy: if change can be driven in one direction, why not another? Why not choose health rather than ill health?

References

1   Keys A (ed.) (1970) Coronary heart disease in seven countries. *Circulation.* **41**(S1): 1–211.

2   Burkitt D (1973) Some diseases characteristic of modern Western civilisation. *British Medical Journal.* **1**: 274–8.

3   Trowell HC and Burkitt DP (eds) (1981) *Western Diseases: their emergence and prevention.* Edward Arnold, London.

4   Department of Health and Social Security (1974) *Diet and Coronary Heart Disease: Report of the Advisory Panel of the Committee on Medical Aspects of Food Policy.* DoH, London.

5   Cannon G (1992) *Food and Health: the experts agree.* Consumers' Association, London.

6   Lang T (1998) BSE and CJD: recent developments. In: S Ratzan (ed.) *The Mad Cow Crisis: health and the public good.* UCL Press, London, pp 65–85.

7   Lang T (1997) Going public: food campaigns during the 1980s and early 1990s. In: DF Smith (ed.) *Nutrition in Britain: science, scientists and politics in the twentieth century.* Routledge, London, pp 238–60.

8   Coronary Prevention Group (1983) *How to Prevent Heart Disease.* Proceedings of a conference of the Coronary Prevention Group, 28–30 September, Canterbury, Kent. Coronary Prevention Group, London.

9   HM Government (1992) *Health of the Nation.* HMSO, London.

10 London Food Commission (1987) *Food Adulteration.* Unwin Hyman, London.

11 Parliamentary Office of Science and Technology (1997) *Safer Eating: microbiological food poisoning and its prevention.* Houses of Parliament, London.

12 Paulus I (1974) *The Search for Pure Food.* Martin Robertson, Oxford.

13 Thompson EP (1993) The moral economy of the English crowd in the eighteenth century. In: EP Thompson (ed.) *Customs in Common.* Penguin, Harmondsworth.

14 Birchall J (1994) *Co-op: the people's business.* Manchester University Press, Manchester.

15 Redfern P (1938) *The New History of the CWS.* JM Dent, London.

16 George S (1976) *How the Other Half Dies.* Penguin, Harmondsworth.

17 Wilkinson RG (1996) *Unhealthy Societies.* Routledge, London.

18 Leather S (1996) *The Making of Modern Malnutrition.* Caroline Walker Trust, London.

19 Lang T (1997) Dividing up the cake: food as social exclusion. In: A Walker and C Walker (eds) *Britain Divided: the growth of social exclusion in the 1980s and 1990s.* Child Poverty Action Group, London, pp 213–28.

20 Webster C (1997) Government policy on school meals and welfare foods, 1939–70. In: DF Smith (ed.) *Nutrition in Britain: science, scientists and politics in the twentieth century.* Routledge, London.

21 Beveridge W (1928) *British Food Control*. Oxford University Press, Oxford.

22 Lang T (In press) The complexities of globalisation: the UK food system as a case study of tensions within the UK food system and the challenge to food policy. *Agriculture and Human Values*.

23 Cannon G (1987) *The Politics of Food*. Century, London.

24 NHS Executive (1996) *Burdens of Disease*. Department of Health, London.

25 British Heart Foundation (1996) *Coronary Heart Disease Statistics*. British Heart Foundation, London.

26 British Heart Foundation (1998) *CHD Statistics – Economic Costs*. British Heart Foundation Research Group, Oxford.

27 Roberts J (1995) The socio-economic costs of foodborne infection. Paper to Oxford Brookes University conference Foodborne disease: consequences and prevention, St Catherine's College Oxford, April. Oxford Brookes University, Oxford.

28 Communicable Diseases Surveillance Centre (1995) The cost of in-patient care for acute infectious intestinal disease in England, 1991–1994. *Communicable Report*. **6**, Review no 5.

29 El-Gazzar FE and Marth EH (1992) Foodborne disease: investigative procedures and economic assessment. *Journal of Environmental Health*. **55**(2): 24–7.

30 Raven H and Lang T (1995) *Off our Trolleys?* Institute for Public Policy Research, London.

31 Wrigley H (1998) European retail giants and the post-LBO reconfiguration of US food retailing. *International Review of Retail, Distribution and Consumer Research*. **8**(2 April): 127–46.

32 Ofwat (1997) *1996–7 Report on the Financial Performance and Capital Investment of the Water Companies in England and Wales*. Ofwat, London.

33 Paxton A (1994) *The Food Miles Report*. Sustainable Agriculture, Food and Environment Alliance, London.

34 Whitelegg J (1994) *Driven to Shop*. Eco-logica and Sustainable Agriculture, Food and Environmental Alliance, London.

35 McLaren D, Bullock S and Yousuf N (1998) *Tomorrow's World: Britain's share in a sustainable future*. Earthscan, London.

36 Kurlansky M (1998) *Cod*. Jonathan Cape, London.

37 Department of Health (1994) *Nutritional Aspects of Cardiovascular Disease*. Report of the Cardiovascular Review Group of the Committee of Medical Aspects of Food Policy. HMSO, London.

38 The Scottish Office (1994) *Eating for Health. A Diet Action Plan for Scotland*. Scottish Office, Edinburgh.

39 Whitehead M and Nordgren P (eds) (1996) *The Health Impact of CAP*. National Institute of Health, Stockholm.

40 Food from Britain (1997) Personal communication, based on calculations from HM Customs figures, in Office of National Statistics (1997) *Overseas Trade Statistics*. Department of Trade and Industry, London.

41 Lang T (1998) Time to reform CAP on health grounds? *Eurohealth*. **4**(2, Spring): 1–3.

42   Johnson M (1995) *Comparative Social Measures of Subsidies to Agricultural Production.* US Department of Agriculture, Economic Research Service, Staff paper AGE-9509, April, Washington DC.

43   CEG (1997) *The Common Agricultural Policy, Diet, Nutrition and Health.* Proceedings of a seminar held at the Commission of the European Communities, London, 26 February 1997. Consumers in Europe Group, London.

44   OECD (1997) *Agricultural Policies in OECD Countries: measurement of support and background information 1997.* Organisation for Economic Co-operation and Development, Paris.

45   House of Lords (1991) *Development and Future of the Common Agricultural Policy.* HL Paper 791. HMSO, London.

46   CEG (1996) Paper CEG 96/20. Consumers in Europe Group, London.

47   James WPT, Ferro-Luzzi A, Isaksson B and Szostak WB (1988) *Healthy Nutrition: preventing nutrition-related diseases in Europe.* World Health Organisation Regional Publications, European Series, No. 24. Copenhagen.

48   James WPT, Ralph A and Bellizi M (1997) Nutrition policies in Western Europe: national policies in Belgium, the Netherlands, France, Ireland and the United Kingdom. *Nutrition Reviews.* **55**(11): S4–S20.

49   STOA (ed.) (1997) *Nutrition in Europe.* European Parliament Scientific and Technological Options Assessment, Directorate General for Research, PE Number 166.481. European Parliament, Brussels.

50   Ferro-Luzzi A and James WPT (1997) Diet and health. In: STOA (ed.) *Nutrition in Europe.* European Parliament Scientific and Technological Options Assessment, Directorate General for Research, PE Number 166.481. European Parliament, Brussels.

51   CEC (1992) *Agricultural Situation in the Community 1991.* Office for Official Publications of the European Communities, Luxembourg.

52   Lang T (1998) *Food and Nutrition in the EU: implications for public health.* Report to Société Francaise de Santé Publique, the European Public Health Association and the Directorate of Public Health of the Commission of the European Communities. Centre for Food Policy, Thames Valley University, London.

53   Belcher P (1997) Amsterdam 1997: a new dawn for public health. *Eurohealth.* **3** (2, Spring): 1–3.

54   CEC (1995) *On the Integration of Health Requirements in Community Policies.* First report. COM(95) 196 final. Commission of the European Communities, Luxembourg.

55   EPHA (1997) *Public Health and the EU: an overview.* European Public Health Alliance, Brussels.

56   Commission of the European Communities (1997) *Official Journal,* C-348, volume 2, p. XXI.

57   EU (1998) *European Union Budget 1998.* Publications Office, Luxembourg.

58   Neville-Rolfe E (1984) *The Politics of Agriculture in the European Community.* Policy Studies Institute/European Centre for Political Studies, London.

59   Tracy M (1982) *Agriculture in Western Europe: challenge and response 1880–1980*. Granada, London.

60   NFU (1998) Personal communication, calculated from figures from Home Grown Cereals Authority and Office of National Statistics, November 1997 prices, National Farmers Union Economics Department, London.

61   Henson S and Traill B (1994) *The Common Agricultural Policy and Consumption of Yellow Fats*. Report on a project for the British Heart Foundation. Department of Agricultural Economics and Management, Reading.

62   Henson S and Swinbank A (1997) CAP and health. In: CEG *The Common Agricultural Policy, Diet, Nutrition and Health*. Proceedings of a seminar, 26 February 1997, European Commission, London. Consumers in Europe Group, London.

63   Boyd Orr, J (1943) *Food and the People*. Pilot Press, London.

CHAPTER SIX

Transport

Gary McGrogan

Introduction

The relationship between transport and health is becoming one of the most talked about issues within the UK and is something that both national and local government are trying to tackle. Everyone can relate to it and everyone has their say about it.

The positive aspect of transport is that it opens up access to a range of resources and services, including employment, leisure, healthcare, and participation in social and community life. Walking and cycling provide direct health benefits in terms of increased physical activity and the subsequent reduced risk from heart and circulatory problems. However, the negative health impacts of motor transport are many and wide ranging, from death and injury on the roads, to the effects of poor air quality; from increasingly sedentary lifestyles to social fragmentation and loss of neighbourliness; from the destruction of green spaces and tranquillity, to the global environmental threat of climate change.

Making the links

Accidents

Two-fifths of accidental deaths result from road-traffic accidents.

Stress, fear and danger

Fear of traffic, accidents and unsafe pedestrian routes causes stress. It also results in reduced mobility and access to services, facilities, social and community life, particularly for those already experiencing disadvantage.

Air quality

Traffic-related pollution is now the prime cause of poor air quality in towns and cities. In the past, the major air pollutants were sulphur dioxide and smoke emitted from industry and domestic fuel. These have decreased markedly, while nitrogen dioxide, ozone and small particles, known as PM10, all largely traffic-related, have increased dramatically. Traffic-related air pollution exacerbates a range of respiratory problems and is also linked with heart disease. Some of the pollutants involved have also been shown to be carcinogenic. The Department of the Environment, Transport and the Regions have recently issued consultative proposals on a national air quality management strategy, including new air quality standards. However, concerns remain that the proposed standards may not adequately safeguard health. In many cases air quality standards may have been met, yet there will still be observable health effects caused by severe but short episodes of poor air quality.

Environmental damage

Air pollution is only one of the many ways in which motor transport causes environmental damage, which affects health. Today most people live their lives with a background of noise, two-thirds of which is caused by traffic. The transport sector produces nearly a quarter of the UK's emissions of the major greenhouse gas, carbon dioxide. Global warming brings with it many potential health impacts. Unpredictable weather patterns disrupt food production and water supplies. Extreme weather events such as floods and storms lead to disasters with physical and mental health impacts. Changing temperatures will also affect the distribution of many communicable diseases.

Social interaction

Access to appropriate transport is an important factor in the development and maintenance of social and community life, which is known to be a determinant of health. However, many road-building schemes since the 1960s have resulted in the destruction of town and city neighbourhoods. Communities have quite literally been severed, with people cut off from local schools, shops and other facilities. Car use and public transport may enable some people to meet their needs further afield rather than locally, but others such as young people, older people, people with disabilities and those at home caring for small children, feel the loss of neighbourliness and social support most keenly.

Physical activity

Walking and cycling as a means of getting from 'a to b' has declined over the past 20 years. Physically active people are less prone to anxiety and other mental ill health, and have half the risk of coronary heart disease and up to one-third the risk of stroke, compared to inactive people. In children, physical activity is important for normal development and with increasing numbers travelling even very short distances to school by car, there is real cause for concern.

Inequalities

Access to a whole range of important resources and services for health, including employment, leisure, family and friends, education and healthcare, increasingly depend on the availability of appropriate means of transport. However, many people who are often already vulnerable, are further discriminated against by years of planning and transport policies which have failed to promote choice and have tended to assume car use as the norm. Many groups in society suffer from social exclusion due to a lack of appropriate and accessible means of transport. Such groups rely heavily on public transport, where fares have increased and services have often declined, or are inadequate. The same groups are also more vulnerable to the ill-effects of motorised transport. Lower-income groups are more at risk from road-traffic accidents as they are more likely to be pedestrians. They are also more likely to live close to heavy traffic and are therefore more exposed to poor air quality.

Transport policies

The importance of transport policies at a national and local level that take account of health issues cannot be overemphasised. Towns and cities are fast moving towards the situation where they are becoming so severely congested, polluted and environmentally damaged that they require a drastic change in transport policy to prevent health and well being being severely affected.

The Local Government Association advocates the replacement of existing transport policies and programmes with Local Transport Plans, which are five-year action plans. However, it must be stressed that the proposals will not be successful unless they are couched within a strategic framework for planning and transport policies which is consistent with regional guidance, structure plans, unitary development plans and district plans. Central government needs to contrive to promote integrated transport policies which will encourage people to switch from private car to public transport use and to provide fiscal incentives for industry to use rail and waterways freight.

The challenge

The challenge is to promote more sustainable, health-enhancing forms of transport and thereby reduce the damage caused by the present car-based transport systems to our health and environment. This means increasing the attractiveness, accessibility and use of healthier ways of getting about, reducing the need to travel and cutting dependence on private cars. Above all, it is vital that these challenges are met in ways that reduce rather than perpetuate social inequalities in health.

The key challenges are:

- to ensure that transport policies do not exacerbate social inequalities in health
- to reclaim the streets for social interaction, walking and cycling
- to increase the use of public transport
- to reduce dependence on cars
- to reduce the need to travel
- to create partnerships and collaborative working for change.

The Sheffield and Rotherham transport challenge

This challenge encouraged debate within Sheffield and Rotherham (adjacent large metropolitan areas with a combined population of over 800 000) concerning the impacts of transport and health, and allowed the sharing of ideas about the development of a healthy and sustainable transport policy for the area.

Health in its broadest context is a state we value, and it is something to which all of us have a right. It can affect our ability to realise aspirations, satisfy our needs and to feel at ease in our environment. Good health helps us to realise our sense of mental, emotional, physical and spiritual well being. A wide range of factors – biological, social, economic, environmental and psychological – influence health.

Local Transport and Health Group

A transport and health group was formed in Sheffield and Rotherham, with representation from the statutory sector, environmental health, health promotion, transport planners, transport providers, and from university, business and voluntary sectors. The *Health for All* partnerships and the partnerships for social and economic regeneration from both areas were also represented.

Since 1995 the Transport and Health Group has been an energetic and productive alliance. A public consultation document and accompanying leaflet were produced in

September 1996, and over the next nine months members of the group were involved in a wide-ranging, facilitated, public consultation process.

The group has been able to take advantage of the opportunity presented by the broad consensus which now exists for change in our patterns of transport provision and use. Interests as diverse as those represented by the Council for the Protection of Rural England, Royal Automobile Club, Confederation of British Industry and government departments covering transport, environment and health all agree that current trends in traffic growth are unsustainable.

Production of the public consultation document

As members of the group began to work on different sections of the consultation document, very disparate views emerged. Health was a key concept where different interpretations were held. Some members of the group felt uncomfortable with the broad view of health that others were taking. Instead of a focus on traffic, air quality and (mainly physical) ill health, they were looking at something much broader, encompassing mobility, access, sustainability, well being and social inequalities.

A first draft was produced using some material from group members. Despite reservations, the vision section was especially well received, and the group wanted more emphasis in the document on the positive role that wider access and mobility could play in improving and sustaining health for all. Consensus was finally achieved and, with hindsight, this process was clearly crucial to the group, establishing collective ownership of the document and support for its broad interpretation of both health and transport.

Much of the literature on intersectoral working stresses the importance of the gradual process of building relationships and trust, and common understandings. The group also felt a collective sense of achievement, having produced in a relatively short time some tangible outcomes in the form of the consultation document and accompanying leaflet.

The public consultation process

In addition to a wide distribution of 150 000 leaflets and 1500 copies of the full document, a number of targeted groups were approached with the offer of a facilitated consultation session. Groups traditionally marginalised in decision making and who are most vulnerable to discrimination and health inequalities were targeted. Sessions were also offered to the business sector, transport providers, service providers and environmental groups.

Public consultation outcomes

Forty written responses were received, together with a number of indirect replies through the local press. Between 70 and 80 people also took part in the consultation via a variety of meetings, where there was strong consensus around the key themes and recommendations of the document. Many respondents pointed out other issues and actions that they felt also needed to be addressed. Several felt that there was a need for more emphasis or exploration of the impact of transport of goods or freight, with global food transportation being particularly highlighted. Key challenges identified included the need for transport policies to: reduce social inequalities in health; reclaim the streets for social interaction, walking and cycling; increase the use of public transport; reduce the dependence on cars; reduce the need to travel; and create partnerships and collaborative working for change.

What happens next?

Many ideas for action to be taken by the voluntary and community sectors, business employers and service providers, transport providers, planners and regulators were identified in the consultation. There were also suggestions for action at national level. All these suggestions were relayed to the appropriate agencies and organisations.

Two of the key themes of the document, addressing health inequalities and promoting participation and planning, have been progressed through a significant development resulting from the consultation. The funding of a community Health and Transport Project based within Sheffield Community Transport will aim to work with specific communities in the city to identify their needs relating to transport and health.

The project has identified two areas where significant improvements can be made, particularly within marginalised communities:

- create a mechanism to ensure that statutory organisations become aware of their needs
- develop policies and initiatives to involve marginalised communities in the decision-making process.

It is vital that the views gathered by the consultation process influence the actions of a wide range of organisations that have a bearing on transport policy and activities, both locally and nationally. The key players in local transport provision also received the outcome document in order that they could consider the views expressed and the suggestions made for the future.

The Government Office for Yorkshire and Humberside has expressed its support for the aims of the document and offered its assistance in taking forward local work in the future. This has encouraged the Sheffield and Rotherham Transport and Health group to develop links with the other two South Yorkshire District Councils to develop country-wide policies.

Postscript

Since this chapter was written, the Government's integrated transport strategy has been written. Local action described above fits with its recommendations, particularly making explicit the links between transport and health.

Further reading

Health Education Authority (1998) *Transport and Health: a briefing for health professionals and local authorities.* HEA, London.

Local Government Association (1998) *LGA Response to DETR Consultation Paper 'Opportunities for Change'.* LGA, London.

Sheffield and Rotherham Transport and Health Group (1996) *Improving Health in Sheffield and Rotherham: the transport challenge.* SRTHG, Sheffield.

CHAPTER SEVEN

Why should public health include housing?

Geoff Matthews

Introduction

The purpose of this chapter is to assert the continuing importance of housing in public health policy. The answer to the question posed in its title will not be a technical one (although reference is made to other more technical work). The difficulties of assessing the evidence of the housing/health link, of defining and quantifying its influence, and of translating it into practical terms are acknowledged, but they are not taken as a reason for inaction. We know, even if we do not understand fully, that poor housing causes poor health, that better housing leads to better health and that housing inequality promotes health inequality. For many housing and health agencies 'on the ground', which are providing services often to the same groups of people, working together on these issues is a simple fact of life.

This chapter will summarise research evidence of the links between housing and health, broadening the discussion to consider links with housing services; it will suggest the obstacles that may have inhibited the influence of these links on service provision; it will briefly give good practice examples of good work which has already been done; and it will consider what action is necessary to ensure the proper integration of housing into public health policy at national, regional, local and individual levels.

Links between housing and health

There is extensive evidence of the relationship between housing and health.[1-5] The areas of influence most commonly discussed are homelessness and poor conditions inside and outside the home (see Appendix A). This chapter will describe these areas of work, but will also consider the relevance of housing-related services and housing service co-ordination to public health. A further approach influenced by health and safety considerations is summarised in Appendix B.

The influence of housing on health is strongest in two areas: homelessness and housing conditions, and research has of course focused on these.

Homelessness

The major impact of homelessness on health[7,8] is summarised in Table 7.1. These issues are particularly marked in street homelessness. Life expectancy is 42 years amongst those sleeping rough, as against the national average of 74 for men and 79 for women.

Table 7.1: The health impact of homelessness

Mental health problems
  risk of suicide
  drug and alcohol abuse
  loneliness, boredom, loss of self-esteem, relationship breakdown
  behavioural problems in children
  delayed child development
Physical health problems
  TB
  asthma
  heart disease
  infection, especially gastroenteritis among children
Other
  limited access to health education and primary care
  increased level of home accidents in temporary accommodation
  increased levels of domestic violence, risk of assault
  emotional and relationship problems

Conditions inside the home

The official measure of conditions inside the home is the standard of fitness for human habitation. This covers: serious disrepair, structural stability, dampness prejudicial to health, lighting, heating, ventilation, water supply, drainage, WC facilities, bath/shower/handbasin, hot and cold water, and facilities for cooking and preparation of food. To these influences on health should be added the four most important health and safety hazards – poor energy efficiency, radon, poor internal arrangement and poor fire safety. Overcrowding exacerbates the influence of most of these factors.

Table 7.2:   The health impact of conditions inside the home

Physical health
   respiratory illness, coughing, asthma, TB
   hypothermia
   ischaemic heart disease
   diarrhoea, gastroenteritis, dysentery
   a range of general poor health, such as headaches, allergic responses and infections
   nervous-system damage, slowed mental development in children (connected with lead water pipes)
Mental health
   stress
   depression
Other
   increased risk of accidents due to structural hazards, poor internal layout and poor home safety. The risk
      from fire in the private rented sector is well documented. The risks are greater for older people
   increased risk of illness and death associated with passive smoking, carbon monoxide, asbestos and
      radon gas

Statistics taken from the major national government surveys of housing conditions in 1991 suggest that there were 1 638 000 houses unfit for human habitation in the UK – 1 in 14. Though unfit owner-occupied houses are more numerous, houses in the private rented sector are more likely to be in poor condition. There is also a link between the age and income of occupants and poor housing conditions.[9]

The fitness standard has been the subject of much criticism and it is currently under review by government. Significant change is likely – probably to a fitness rating approach that assigns points to different elements of unfitness.

The main health impacts of poor conditions inside the home are summarised in Table 7.2.

Conditions outside the home

The health impact of the environment outside the home has received less attention than the internal environment. However, the immediate surroundings of a home can exert a powerful influence on health and quality of life more generally. They will also require very different policy responses to the problems identified above. Little statistical evidence is available, but the most recent English House Condition survey[10] found that nearly 1.3 million households were living in 'poor living conditions' (areas where there are concentrations of poor housing and/or environmental problems) and they were more likely to be dissatisfied with their home.

Design and layout

Victorian public health action focused on a number of planning and design issues that affect health. Key issues still relevant include playspace, defensible space, location of facilities such as shops and recreation, accessibility, space standards and the density of permitted development. These factors may lead to increased stress and depression, violent behaviour and longer-term mental health problems. Design and layout may impact particularly upon those unable to leave the immediate vicinity of the home – older people and children.

Air quality, pollution and neighbouring uses

Planning policy aims to separate housing from other uses, but is not always successful. Health may be prejudiced by specific pollutants from local industrial processes or from the presence of contaminants in the soil. Prominence has been given recently to issues of noise pollution which may impact significantly on quality of life.

Security

The relevance of crime, the fear of crime and antisocial behaviour has achieved prominence recently. The planning, design, allocation and management of housing can all have an influence here. It is important to note that these are issues not only for the management of local authority and housing association homes – areas of private housing experience problems at least as serious.

High-rise accommodation

Design and security issues can be concentrated on unpopular high-rise estates. Particular problems associated with this building type are: quality of service provision (e.g. communal area cleaning and facilities maintenance), lack of playspace, insulation and noise insulation, structural issues and fire safety, and accessibility.

Housing-related services

The research summarised above focuses rightly on the relationship between a traditional definition of housing need (homelessness and house conditions) and health. It considers a home in terms of its adequacy as a unit of accommodation and the policy prescriptions that follow typically stress the need for more affordable housing and the need for more public subsidy of repairs in local authority housing and private housing.

Arguments for including housing in public health should also go wider. There are a number of services closely related to the provision of housing which exert a key influence over health.

Disabled Facilities Grant and adaptations

Where people need adaptations to give access to and to improve movement around their home, they may be entitled to a local authority Disabled Facilities Grant. This grant covers all works to make the home suitable for the accommodation, welfare or employment of a disabled person – not just to bring it up to the fitness standard. Adaptations are also funded by local authority social services departments and from Registered Social Landlords (housing associations). This type of work is particularly relevant to elderly disabled people.

Minor repairs

Small repairs can have a disproportionate impact on the adequacy of a home, and on the independence and well being of the person living there. The new Home Repair Assistance Grant is available at a local authority's discretion. Many local authorities are now also looking at other ways of helping people carry out and finance their own repairs. As well as disrepair, insulation or security may be addressed. Small repairs may be particularly important for home safety.

Housing management

Access to local authority and housing association homes may be particularly important for those suffering from serious ill health and for this reason most local authorities give a specific weighting to applicants with health problems. However, practice varies considerably and is widely thought to be unsatisfactory. Particular issues are how far mental health needs are taken into account and what knowledge a local authority has of adaptations in its property. The management of tenants' antisocial behaviour makes an important contribution to community safety policies generally and can be key to mental health.

Housing costs

There is a well-established link between poverty and health. Housing costs are a significant part of household expenditure and contribute to poverty and employment traps. Much debate has surrounded rent levels in social housing and rent allowances in private rented accommodation.

   Poverty is also found amongst marginal home owners, who are vulnerable to changes in income, employment status and interest rates. Heating costs and issues of fuel poverty/ energy efficiency are also a direct influence on health and household income.

Housing service co-ordination

Without good links between housing services and other services – especially social services and health – gaps, overlaps and inconsistencies are likely to result. Recent reports[11,12] have found that current services are generally far from 'seamless' and that this is true both at the strategic and operational levels.

Examples of key areas where liaison is essential to the health of service users are:

Housing needs assessment

Health service and social services staff are frequently involved in making medical assessments of applicants for local authority and housing association homes. Conversely, it is also important that housing needs are taken into account in needs assessment for community care, and in preparation for hospital discharge, or for leaving local authority children's homes.

Support services

A range of support services are provided by different agencies in conjunction with housing. For example, the responsibility of wardens in sheltered accommodation has increased considerably: liaison with health and social services is now integral to their work. Various agencies are involved with the successful resettlement of groups such as young people leaving care, ex-offenders and those with drug- or alcohol-related problems. Independent living schemes meet a range of different needs, either in the home, in the building, close to it, or offering a 'floating' service. The adequacy of the home is clearly dependent on the successful provision of such support.

Registered Social Landlords (housing associations) have traditionally fulfilled a role that is complementary to the mainstream housing of local authorities. Despite their current role as the sole providers of new social housing, many retain this character and have particular expertise in providing accommodation for people with support needs. Frequently, housing associations will work with voluntary organisations who will provide management and support services in housing association property.

Liaison with primary care services

Liaison between housing and primary care services has been touched on above in relation to assessment issues. There are also important issues with a public health dimension relating to the inadequate access of homeless people to GPs and to the closure of large psychiatric hospitals.

The proposals in the recent NHS White Paper for PCGs[13] are an opportunity to enhance and support existing relationships at locality level. It will be important to ensure that the groups address the wider health gain/health inequality agenda and that they relate to the whole local authority rather than solely to social services.

Conclusion

To summarise, there are five key areas in which housing can make a contribution to public health:

- homelessness
- conditions inside the home
- conditions outside the home
- housing-related services
- housing service co-ordination.

It is also possible to present the above analysis in terms of health priorities. Public health policy should take housing into account because it can make an impact on:

- heart disease
- mental health
- respiratory problems
- home accidents
- digestive system disorder
- child development
- cancer.

It is worth noting that this list includes all of the national targets proposed by the current Green Paper on public health.[14]

Why doesn't public health include housing?

Given the weight of the arguments above, the inclusion of housing in public health might appear to be as inevitable as it was to the Victorians. The fact that the links are not always made is important. There are a number of contributory factors, but key issues include the following.

- The housing/health link is notoriously difficult to establish conclusively as bad housing is often found alongside a number of other causes of ill health; its incidence is difficult to isolate; the causal relationship between poor housing and other disadvantage is complex; and there may be ethical problems in researching people in poor housing without linking this with action to improve house conditions.
- It is particularly difficult to *quantify* the housing/health relationship, and therefore the benefits of housing activity for other services are difficult to measure and, in

particular, the cost is difficult to estimate. This causes difficulty in setting spending priorities between different areas of social policy.

- Difficulty measuring the health impact of housing activity means that it is also difficult to set realistic targets and difficult to monitor progress against them. Problems with the fitness standard mentioned above may not have helped. There are also some doubts over the official measures of homelessness, and particularly with regard to homelessness which does not attract statutory priority under the homelessness legislation.

- Housing and health services have different legislative powers and duties, different financial accountability, and different cultures and professional traditions: they may define problems and solutions in distinctively separate terms. Joint working may in some cases literally be unthinkable.

- The policy environment is itself often hostile to joint working. Despite the increased emphasis on holistic, intersectoral thinking, promoted in particular in relation to urban regeneration, many obstacles remain: accountability mechanisms, which emphasise internal performance measures and cost; increasing diversity of service providers ('fragmentation'); financial uncertainty caused by reduction/changes in funding; and the promotion of competition between providers.

It is important for policy makers looking to integrate housing into public health to take account of these difficulties and to find ways of avoiding them.

Good-practice examples

A review of inter-agency work between health and housing[11] concluded that 'although inter-agency working between health and housing is recognised as important, it is, in practice, very limited'. A further study of inter-agency working to address housing, health and social care needs of people in ordinary housing[12] was only slightly more positive: it found few three-way links, only *ad hoc* links at service delivery level and significant gaps in service provision. However, the national picture should not obscure a wealth of innovative activity taking place locally. An extensive range of good practice examples is found in *Housing and Health*.[5] More information can be found in the Chartered Institute of Housing's Good Practice Guide No. 13.[15]

For present purposes it might be most useful to give examples focusing on the operational level – the service delivery resulting from the strategic thinking considered above. What follows is far from systematically collected, but gives some idea of the main direction initiatives have taken. It is clear that more is happening at local level than is generally acknowledged, and it is to be hoped that the HAZ initiative and the new HIMPs will both encourage more such examples and provide the basis for sharing them more effectively.

Aligning housing-led activity with health priorities

Health impact has been used in various ways to prioritise housing activity. One authority is considering building health criteria into its capital programme assembly. Others have used health criteria to target capital work, e.g. on the basis of a MORI survey on health, Croydon increased its discretionary grants budget for elderly owner-occupiers in poor housing; Bexley targeted the council's housing association development programme to meet the need for group home development and wheelchair-accessible housing. In an interesting piece of lateral thinking, Bexley has used property from its empty property scheme as temporary accommodation for high-rise residents experiencing emotional difficulties.

Aligning health-led work with housing priorities

A number of authorities locate health facilities in areas of poor housing or with services for homeless people. A joint community health development project involving health, housing and social services has been undertaken on a Housing Action Trust estate in Waltham Forest to establish a community health advice shop, a counselling service, intensive domiciliary support service and a training project. Birmingham runs Well Women and children's clinics at homelessness centres. It is relatively common to move health staff to provide jointly a service to homeless people (Birmingham, Newcastle). Health staff can also be trained in housing issues, e.g. health workers with home-safety expertise (North Tyneside).

Joint funding/commissioning

Joint funding of staff who work across organisational boundaries is now not uncommon, often making use of joint finance. Birmingham uses joint finance for a programme of small grants for frail elderly people nominated by GPs. It has also vired Transitional Grant monies to fund additional Disabled Facilities Grants. Health authority funding has been used elsewhere for the conversion of private rented property for people living with HIV and AIDS (Kensington and Chelsea), for the support elements of supported housing schemes and for funding GP advice for medical assessment purposes. Frequently, the housing contribution to joint schemes takes the form of land or accommodation for services funded by other agencies. An innovative partnership has developed in Newcastle where the community alarm system is run jointly with the local NHS trust, so that elderly people can access community nursing services directly.

Sharing staff resources

Several local authorities have now brought together multidisciplinary teams with members from health, housing and social services. As well as the services to homeless people mentioned above, these have been used to deal with Disabled Facilities Grant applications (Kirklees, Calderdale) and complex community care needs (Bexley). Secondment has also been used in a similar way to share expertise, e.g. a public health nurse, a community psychiatric nurse and an occupational therapist are seconded in Newcastle to help with medical priority assessment under its allocation scheme. Various ways of increasing staff's mutual understanding have been used: housing staff have shadowed health staff in Hammersmith and Fulham. In Hillingdon, the housing service has provided training to hospital trust staff in the role and procedures of the service, and housing staff have been trained by the Trust regarding people with a mental illness who 'fall through the net'.

What should be done and by whom?

Housing needs to be integrated into the public health agenda and the lessons of the good practice given above disseminated and built on.

The CMO's report of emerging findings from the project to strengthen the public health function in England[16] identified four levels at which action is needed: the individual, local, regional and national. These are considered in turn.

National level

Public health policy

Although the majority of activity may be at local or individual level, its effectiveness will be dependent on action and leadership at regional and national level. National leadership is crucially important where activity is needed which crosses the boundaries between agencies and across government departments. The Government must get its policy framework right. It has begun to do this with the Green Paper on public health.[14] However, if the focus is to be on causes of ill health, then *causes* should feature in the targets and contracts to promote public health. This might be done by expanding the targets proposed to cover 'process' issues – the action necessary to achieve the stated target. Targets would include homelessness and house condition.

In addition, *the home* could be added as a 'healthy setting' and its relevance to the health of elderly people emphasised.

Health Improvement Programmes

HIMPs and the new local authority duty to promote economic, social and environmental well being will be key mechanisms in making the link between health and housing. They will need to be guided by a very clear government policy framework. From housing's point of view, it will be important to communicate clearly and strongly the Government's expectation that housing is integral to the new public health agenda. Experience gained in relation to community care and housing shows that without an explicit, concerted, determined and cross-departmental effort to foster joint working, it will be slow to take effect. Although health authorities will have the leadership role in relation to HIMPs, it will be important to challenge as early as possible the assumption that these pro-grammes are primarily health-led.

Local housing strategies

Housing Improvement Plan guidance issued by the Department of the Environment, Transport and the Regions is taken into account by local authorities when setting their local housing strategies. The guidance also provides the criteria against which local authority performance is assessed by government offices for the regions when allocating the discretionary part of local authority Housing Improvement Plan borrowing approval. It is therefore essential that due weight is given to the need to take into account public health issues as an integral part of the strategy to consult with health authorities on the strategy and to co-operate with them on its delivery.

Legislative/regulatory obstacles

Legislation/regulation should facilitate local joint working on housing and health, and existing obstacles should be removed. Key issues might include the following.

- The regime for Compulsory Competitive Tendering established definitions of housing management performance which deter joint working and operational liaison. It will be important that these difficulties are not replicated by the proposals for Best Value. An insistence upon a narrow definition of performance may leave little flexibility for innovative joint working which may be deemed to promote 'inefficiency'.
- Mechanisms for bringing in private finance to repair private housing are inflexible and prevent the development of leasing schemes in the private rented sector and equity release schemes for owner-occupiers.
- Regulation of private rented sector properties is necessary to improve standards and management, and also a necessary precondition for encouraging investment and the professionalisation of the sector.

Good-practice dissemination

Good practice on the integration of housing and public health needs to be developed in order to clarify the key issues and to disseminate innovative ways of working across disciplinary boundaries.

Research

Research into the public health benefits of housing activity should continue to be undertaken.

Regional level

Government offices for the regions

These have a key role in promoting health issues as an integral part of successful local housing strategies (as mentioned above).

Regional housing/health issues

A regional approach may be developed to address specific housing and support needs:

- where regional facilities are closed (e.g. 'spikes')
- where people with specific needs converge on urban centres (e.g. asylum seekers).

Local level

Integration between housing and public health at local and individual levels is essential as it is here that the majority of services are delivered. Some key issues:

- the analysis of a district's public health needs can often include reference to poor housing and homelessness: this should be reflected in practical action to meet these needs
- strategic and operational levels should both reflect housing/health integration. Strategic planning often fails to affect service delivery and individual initiatives at operational level are often not taken up at more senior levels
- it is not enough simply to insert relevant housing activity piecemeal into health planning (or vice versa): real integration implies joint planning, joint funding and joint working between staff.

A checklist for housing/health joint working might be adapted from the AMA publication (Table 7.3).[5]

Table 7.3:   Key areas for local housing/health joint working

Strategic planning
- local housing strategy, housing association business plans
- specification of housing management
- Best Value proposals
- housing needs research
- Local Agenda 21, Health of the Nation/Health for All/Healthy Alliances/Healthy City Strategies
- Director of Public Health annual report/health commissioning plans
- joint consultative committee/joint funding
- regeneration/community development/economic development strategies
- business plans of health provider units
- GP funding and locality planning
- health promotion

Operational co-ordination
Health issues should be considered in policy/service delivery covering:
- homelessness
- adaptations
- allocations
- private sector renewal
- Capital Programme assembly

Housing issues should be integrated into policy/service delivery covering:
- elderly people
- mental health
- hospital discharge/resettlement
- joint assessment
- home visits
- user/carer involvement

Housing and health might work together on
- planning timetables
- joint training

Individual level

Expertise on consulting over public health issues will need to be developed quickly. It will be important to use the existing consultation mechanisms. Housing has developed a range of these in relation to the local housing strategy and housing management with tenants, housing providers and funders, landlords, etc.

References

1   Department of the Environment (1997) *Housing Digest*. The Stationery Office, London.
2   Smith S (1991) *Housing and Health: a review and research agenda*. ESRC Discussion Paper 27, University of Glasgow Centre for Housing Research, Glasgow.

3   Lowry S (1991) Housing and health. *British Medical Journal*.

4   Ambrose P (1996) *The Real Cost of Poor Homes*. Royal Institute of Chartered Surveyors, London.

5   Association of Metropolitan Authorities (1997) *Housing and Health: getting it together*. AMA, London.

6   Department of the Environment, Transport and the Regions (DETR) (1998) *Housing Fitness Standard: consultation paper*. The Stationery Office, London.

7   Connelly J and Crown J (1994) *Homelessness and Ill Health*. Royal College of Physicians, London.

8   Nuffield Provincial Hospital Trust (1994) *Housing, Homelessness and Health*. Standing Conference on Public Health. Nuffield Provincial Hospital Trust, London.

9   Leather P and Morrison T (1997) *The State of UK Housing*. The Policy Press, Bristol.

10   Department of the Environment, Transport and the Regions (1998) *English House Condition Survey*. The Stationery Office, London.

11   Goss S and Kent K (1995) *Health and Housing: working together?* The Policy Press & Joseph Rowntree Foundation, Bristol.

12   Arblaster L, Conway J, Foreman A and Hawkins M (1996) *Asking the Impossible*. The Policy Press, Bristol.

13   Department of Health (1997) *The New NHS: modern, dependable*. The Stationery Office, London.

14   Department of Health (1998) *Our Healthier Nation: a contract for health*. The Stationery Office, London.

15   Chartered Institute of Housing (1998) *Housing and Health*. Good Practice Guide No. 13. Chartered Institute of Housing, Coventry.

16   Department of Health (1998) *Emerging Findings from a Project to Strengthen the Public Health Function in England*. The Stationery Office, London.

Appendix A: The health implications of poor housing (source Association of Metropolitan Authorities (1997)[5] with additional comments from P Molyneux and J Palmer)

Housing issue	Health implications	Evidence and costs (where available)	General blocks to effective action
Homelessness	1 Mental health problems	Increased risk of severe mental health problems, suicide, drug and alcohol abuse	Disorganised/disrupted lifestyle of many homeless people makes reliable follow-up difficult
	2 Increased level of physical problems	Increased risk of TB, asthma, heart disease, diarrhoea and sickness	Where housing decisions depend upon assessment by health and social care agencies, poor inter-agency co-ordination and time taken to make assessment mean that homeless person has often broken contact before a decision is made
	3 Evidence of poor child development	25% of children in bed and breakfast hotels classified as having below birth weight against 7% norm	
	4 Limited access to health education and primary care	53% of children in temporary accommodation immunised against diphtheria against 90% norm: levels of emergency (acute) admissions 2.4 times more frequently than average families; only 63% registered with a GP against 97% norm	Lack of appropriate supported housing options for individuals and families in many areas mean that a referral into unsupported general needs housing is common
	5 Increased level of home accidents in temporary accommodation		Lack of resettlement and ongoing tenancy support to help sustain person in temporary accommodation, and in their home once housed
	6 Increased levels of domestic violence and emotional and relationship problems		If homeless person has previously had a social housing tenancy, lost through rent arrears or nuisance, may be treated as 'intentionally homeless' by housing authority and offered unsupported hotel or private sector tenancy
			Housing agencies may find difficulty in helping homeless person to obtain specialised medical care, e.g. for mental health, drug or alcohol abuse, etc.

Appendix A: *continued*

Housing issue	Health implications	Evidence and costs (where available)	General blocks to effective action
Poor conditions inside the home	1 Dampness and condensation	Increased respiratory illness, coughing, asthma, diarrhoea and gastroenteritis, headaches and tiredness – DoH estimated cost of treating illness resulting from condensation: £800 million per annum	Backlog of major repairs in council housing, and growing problem in housing association homes, due to government spending restrictions means progress in dealing with these problems is slow
	2 Poor heating and insulation	Illness and death from hypothermia, ischaemic heart disease and respiratory illness. 8000 extra deaths for each degree Celsius the temperature falls below average in winter months	Poverty and unaffordable central heating (inc. VAT on fuel) systems leads to use of paraffin heating and no heating at all
	3 Poor ventilation	Increased risk of transmission of infectious disease such as TB, as well as illness caused by damp and condensation	
	4 Disrepair, unfitness, and lack of amenities	Disrepair can make houses cold, dangerous and difficult to heat. Lack of basic amenities leads to increased rates of gastrointestinal illness such as dysentery. Both increase levels of stress, long-term depression and anxiety	Growth in marginal home ownership makes maintenance and improvement unaffordable to some owners Cuts in grants to private home owners
	5 Lead water pipes	Cause damage to the central nervous system, affect the mental development of children and cause a general reduction in the speed of reaction and reflex, possibly increasing risk of accident in the home	Water companies and householders slow to replace lead pipes
	6 Inadequate noise insulation	Causes short-term physiological responses such as increased blood pressure and pulse rate, and long-term chronic stress, increasing anxiety, headaches, depression, etc. Increases the risk of accidents in the home: estimated to cost the NHS £300 million per annum	
	7 Structural hazards, internal layout, home safety		
	8 Air quality – passive smoking, carbon monoxide, asbestos, radon gas	The increased risks of illness and death from these sources are well documented	Public health education on smoking, heating and ventilation widely ignored

Appendix A: *continued*

Housing issue	Health implications	Evidence and costs (where available)	General blocks to effective action
	9 Houses in multiple occupation	Risk of death by fire increases by about 10 times; increased risk of a range of health problems due to layout and standards increase anxiety, stress, depression, increased blood pressure, respiratory illness and transmission of infectious disease	Inadequate regulation and control of HMOs
	10 Overcrowding	Increases the risk of respiratory infection, infectious diseases such as TB and digestive-tract infections such as dysentery; lack of space increases risk from accidents and levels of stress	Inspection programmes less rigorous than they were
Poor conditions outside the home	1 Design and layout	Poor design and layout of housing may lead to increased stress and depression amongst residents, prompting violent behaviour and contributing to longer-term mental health problems; poor design and layout may also inhibit child development	Estate action is beginning to deal with the design and layout problems of the 1960s and 1970s but the scale of the problem is immense
	2 Air quality, pollution and neighbouring uses	Concentrations of outdoor air pollution and noise from neighbouring uses affect the quality of life and may cause anxiety, stress and depression. Specific pollutants that are harmful to health may be passed into local ecosystems via industrial process or accidents. Contaminated land can endanger health through the escape of contaminants into the soil	Pressure to develop local economies and create/preserve jobs may hamper planning/environmental health efforts to improve environment
	3 Security	A secure environment gives comfort and confidence to residents, while poor security can lead to stress, anxiety, depression and potentially violent behaviour. There is also the possibility of physical harm to residents from intruders in the home or from street violence outside	
	4 High-rise housing	The design and layout, and the associated quality of service provision, can have an impact on a variety of conditions including stress, anxiety, depression, violent behaviour, increased blood pressure, isolation, inhibition of child development, presence of infectious diseases and respiratory problems	See design and layout above

Appendix A: *continued*

Housing issue	Health implications	Evidence and costs (where available)	General blocks to effective action
Links between housing costs, poverty and poor housing	1 Poverty and employment traps	Recent government policy of decreasing capital subsidy and increasing rents deepens poverty and employment traps. Residents become dependent upon benefits and find difficulty in increasing personal income	Recent government policy on capital subsidy in housing increased rents, but income support and housing benefit were not increased in line. Social housing rents taking a higher proportion of disposable income than previously. Poverty and employment traps deepening
	2 Housing benefit changes	Changes in the housing benefit regulations are already causing increased levels of homelessness and causing people to leave good-quality housing and move to cheaper bedsits often in HMOs; proposed changes will increase these trends	Cost of housing benefit doubled between 1989/90 and 1994/95 and still increasing
	3 Marginal home ownership	Almost 50% of those owning their home outright and 15% of those buying with a mortgage had an income of less than £150 per week in 1991 (OPCS). Renovation grants to help with basic repairs have been cut back	See comments in sections above
	4 Heating costs	Heating costs influence available income. One study showed tenants facing a choice between 'heating and eating'	
	5 Areas of concentrated deprivation	High concentrations of low-income households result in social exclusion, and in high demands on housing, health, social welfare and police services	See comments in sections above
	6 Links between poverty, housing, and ill health	A limited income determines access to housing, which in turn influences health. Poor health restricts earning capacity and hence access to housing	'Social exclusion' means that people are not only in poverty but outside accepted norms, creating their own moral and social norms – crime, drug and alcohol abuse, domestic and street violence, dual incomes from benefits and an 'undeclared' cash economy, multiple demands on education, housing, social care, health and police services, etc.

Appendix B: Fitness rating – health and safety hazards and related matters (source DETR (1998)[6])

Health/safety hazards	Relevant matters to be assessed	Health/safety hazards	Relevant matters to be assessed
Risk of falls	Design and layout Disrepair Structural stability Lighting	Falling objects and explosion	Structural stability Disrepair Design (HW appliances, etc.)
Fire safety risks	Fire separation Fire precautions Means of escape Landfill gas	Injury from doors and windows	Design and layout Disrepair (Architectural glass) Lighting
Exposure to cold and excessive heat	Heating system and controls Insulation and heat loss Disrepair (energy rating, if needed)	Sanitation and drainage	Water closets, etc. Design and layout Disrepair Drainage (foul/waste water)
Exposure to radon	High radon area Remedial measures (measurement, if needed)	Personal hygiene	Bath/shower and washbasin Hot and cold water supply Design and layout Disrepair
Burn and scald hazards	Design and layout (e.g. kit) Heating system and controls Disrepair (services, etc.) Outlets	Food safety	Kitchen facilities, sink, etc. Hot and cold water supply Design and layout Disrepair
Electric shock	Heating system Ventilation	Other sources of infection	Infestation Design and layout Disrepair Refuse containment
Mould growth and damp	Heating and insulation Design and disrepair Drainage (surface water) Ventilation	Exposure to noise	Sound insulation Design and layout Disrepair
Indoor air pollutants, CO, etc.	Design and layout Disrepair (appliances) Water supply Disrepair	Crime and fear of crime	Basic security Design and layout Lighting Disrepair
Exposure to lead	(Old paint and wiring) Disrepair (services, etc.) Outlets	Space and privacy	Design and layout (Ceiling heights) Disrepair
Asbestos and other pollutants	Heating system	Lighting (depression, etc.)	Design and layout Disrepair (Natural and artificial light)

CHAPTER EIGHT

Domestic violence

Siobhan McCartney

Introduction

The 49th World Health Assembly in 1996 agreed that violence is a public health priority. Resolution 49.25 endorses recommendations made at prior international conferences to tackle the problem of violence against women and girls, and to address its health consequences.[1]

There has been growing recognition on an international and national level of the impact of domestic violence on the health of women and its importance as a public health priority. This has been marked most recently internationally at the 1993 World Conference on Human Rights,[2] the 1994 International Conference on Population and Development[3] and the 1995 Fourth World Conference on Women.[4] At a national level, the recent Green Paper consultation document, *Working Together for a Healthier Scotland* (1998),[5] draws attention to domestic violence as a major public health problem. Domestic violence, however, is not highlighted in the Green Papers for England, Wales or Northern Ireland. The recent British Medical Association Report (1998) highlights the need to develop strategies to reduce the health implications of domestic violence.[6] The *Scottish Needs Assessment Programme Report* (1997)[7] outlines the role of public health in terms of taking the lead to build 'healthy' public policy, reorienting health services and strengthening community action. Action at each of these three levels may help to reduce the prevalence of domestic violence and diminish the long-term impact of violence on women and their children.

This chapter will:

- outline its working definition of domestic violence
- explain the nature of domestic violence
- explore why domestic violence is a public health issue
- outline the implications for health services
- describe one example of attempts at the city-wide level in Glasgow to reorient health services.

What is domestic violence?

It is of crucial importance to clarify what is meant by the term 'domestic violence', in order to determine both the extent of the problem and the subsequent action required to tackle the issue. The definition adopted in this chapter, informed by the *Scottish Needs Assessment Programme Report* (1997),[7] is: 'domestic violence is psychological, emotional and economic, as well as physical and sexual abuse of women by male partners, or ex-partners'.

Domestic violence refers to a particular power dynamic within the context of a particular relationship. Therefore, domestic violence cannot by seen as synonymous with other forms of intrafamilial abuse including abuse of the elderly, child abuse and abuse by women against men.

The Declaration on the Elimination of Violence Against Women passed by the United Nations General Assembly (Vienna Declaration 1993)[8] states that:

> violence against women is a manifestation of historically unequal power relations between men and women ... and that violence against women is one of the crucial social mechanisms by which women are forced into a subordinate position to men.

The nature of domestic violence

Domestic violence can take a number of forms and includes physical, emotional, economic and sexual abuse.

- Physical: punching, slapping, choking, hitting with objects or weapons, threatening with a knife or gun, stabbing, shooting, throwing out of cars, drowning.
- Emotional: verbal abuse, constant criticism, distorting women's sense of perspective, playing mind games, undermining self-confidence, humiliation in front of others, monitoring women's movements.
- Economic: withholding of money, denial of opportunity to work, denial of economic independence.
- Sexual: rape, sexual assault, penetration with instruments, unwanted sexual intimacy.

Domestic violence is a very different form of violence from 'stranger' violence. It is rarely a single attack and is much more likely to be repeated over a number of years. It is also often controlled in that it almost always occurs in private and physical violence is usually directed at those parts of the body which are generally concealed. The violence usually starts early in a relationship and almost always escalates in frequency and severity over time.[9,10] Dobash and Dobash reported that half of a sample of 108 women staying in refuge accommodation had been assaulted within the first year of living with their husband, and in most cases the violence had emerged within the first three years of marriage.[9]

Domestic violence can be fatal. In England and Wales, 40–45% of female homicide victims have been killed by present or former partners. This compares with 6% of male homicide victims.[11] A recent report from HM Inspectorate of Constabularies for Scotland (1997) indicates that 50% of women victims of homicide in Scotland are killed by their partners.[12]

Why is domestic violence a public health issue?

Domestic violence is a matter of public health. Violence debilitates women and girls physically, psychologically and socially, sometimes with lifelong results.[13]

The extent of domestic violence and its subsequent effect on the health and well being of women makes it a significant public health issue. Domestic violence has a number of implications for health services, as part of a range of relevant support services in the statutory and voluntary sectors.

The extent of domestic violence

The Home Office report on domestic violence (1989)[14] states that 'domestic violence constitutes a pervasive problem' in Britain, the study of which has not received systematic attention in the academic world. The report estimated that 1.25 million women in England and Wales may have experienced domestic violence within a 12-month time period.

The health effects of domestic violence

There are a number of health problems associated with the violence which make it an important issue for public health. Women who have experienced domestic violence are more likely to have poor health, chronic pain problems, depressions, addictions, difficulties in pregnancy and to have attempted suicide than women who have not experienced such violence.[15]

Physical health problems

The most common form of physical injury is bruising, followed by cuts.[9] Domestic violence is also associated with high rates of internal injuries and unconsciousness.[16] Burge found that women survivors of domestic violence were more likely than accident victims to have multiple injuries.[16] Ruddle and O'Connor showed that women often suffered injuries that left them with permanent scars and disfigurement. Often these injuries are untreated.[17]

The American Medical Association (AMA) has suggested that there may be a number of delayed physical effects associated with domestic violence, including arthritis, hypertension and heart disease.[18] Pregnancy is also a time of vulnerability for women and estimates suggest that 15–17% of women are assaulted during pregnancy.[19]

Emotional and mental-health problems

There are also a number of emotional and mental-health problems associated with domestic violence. Walker documents high levels of anxiety, fears, panic attacks, depression and an increased sensitivity to further impending abuse.[20] Jaffe *et al.* showed that abused women experienced higher levels of anxiety and depression than a comparable sample of women who had not experienced domestic violence. Women were matched for family income, length of marriage and number of children.[21] In a study in 1993 by Mooney, 40% of abused women stated that they had trouble sleeping and 46% felt depressed and had lost confidence.[22]

The risk of suicide attempt is much higher amongst women who have experienced domestic violence than those who have not. In a study in 1990 by Amaro *et al.*, 17% of women who had experienced domestic violence had attempted suicide, compared to 5% in the control group.[23]

The effect on children witnessing domestic violence

Domestic violence has serious effects on children. Reports indicate that as many as 90% of children are witness to domestic violence against their mothers, often without the realisation of parents.[24] A range of emotional difficulties have been identified amongst children whose mothers are experiencing domestic violence. These include increased levels of anxiety, psychosomatic illness, depression, sadness, withdrawal, disruption to their education and lower rating in social competence.[25]

There is also evidence to link perpetrators of domestic violence with physical and sexual abuse of children in the same family.[26] This can be either as part of the violence directed at their mothers, on separate occasions, or a combination of both scenarios.

Implications for the health service

Help-seeking behaviour of women

Large numbers of women experiencing domestic violence make contact with the health service. A study by Dobash, Dobash and Cavanagh found that amongst the group of women interviewed, 80% had sought medical attention for injury, chronic illness and pain at least once while they were in the violent relationship. In contrast, only 2% of women in the same group had contacted the police.[10] In the USA, the FBI states that domestic violence is the most unreported crime and estimates that it is probably more unreported than rape.[27]

The response of services – women's experiences

Research suggests that although abused women are making contact with the health service, healthcare professionals are not identifying a large proportion of women experiencing domestic violence who contact them.[9,28,29] Research indicates that women may not voluntarily disclose the violence for a number of reasons: difficulty in raising the subject, fear of partners finding out or that their actions would be judged.[9,29]

Research has suggested that there are five key elements that women utilising health services due to domestic violence find helpful, as follows[30]:

- awareness that domestic violence may be a possibility
- recognising the signs and symptoms of domestic violence
- initiating discussion about domestic violence by asking direct questions in a sympathetic and non-judgemental way
- willingness to listen and make time within a busy schedule
- giving advice and information about support services.

Attempts to improve service delivery

There is an increasing level of awareness of the impact of domestic violence on health and the need to create a more systematic and effective response within health services. However, this has not yet led to the creation of a systematic approach to the issue across the NHS.

The situation in the USA is very different from that in the UK. In 1991, the AMA launched a major campaign to educate the public and healthcare professionals about domestic violence. The Joint Commission on Hospital Accreditation also issued new standards requiring that all hospitals develop protocols and provide training for their staff on how to respond to different forms of abuse.

The Home Office report on domestic violence (1989)[14] recommends a number of steps for development within the NHS. These include:

- developing a standard protocol for identifying women who are experiencing domestic violence
- developing training programmes for staff

- encouraging staff to liaise with and refer to other agencies
- developing data recording systems to estimate the extent of the problem.

However, despite these recommendations, the NHS response to domestic violence has been relatively slow to develop.

Action to address domestic violence at the city level: the Glasgow experience

In recognition that domestic violence is a large public health issue with a number of implications for health services, there have been a number of initiatives produced at the city level in Glasgow with a particular health focus.

The Glasgow policy framework

In June 1992, the Women's Health Working Group of the Glasgow Healthy City Project launched the Glasgow Women's Health Policy,[31] with the overall aim of improving the health and well being of the women in Glasgow. The policy was adopted by Greater Glasgow Health Board, Strathclyde Regional Council, Glasgow District Council and the other partner organisations of the Healthy City Project. The policy identified five priorities for action, which included the issue of women's safety in their home and in the community. As part of its commitment to the implementation of the Women's Health Policy and in recognition that domestic violence is a large public health issue, Greater Glasgow Health Board set up a commissioning team to investigate the problem.

The Health Gain Commissioning Team on domestic violence

The remit of the team is to review the response of a number of different health service settings to women experiencing domestic violence. In addition, the group has to produce a series of recommendations to inform the planning process. The work of the team has focused on attempting to implement the recommendation from the Home Office report on domestic violence (1989).[14] Therefore, attempts have been made to introduce and evaluate the impact of introducing guidelines on domestic violence supported by staff training into a number of key health service settings.

Health service audits

Pilot audits have been completed within Accident and Emergency (A&E) and family planning settings, are ongoing in an obstetrics setting and are being developed within primary care settings. The audit process involves:

- determining current detection rates, current practice and attitudes of staff
- training staff on protocol introduction
- introducing protocol over a fixed time period
- assessing the impact of intervention.

Protocols on domestic violence

Considerable time was taken in drawing up the protocols on domestic violence in conjunction with service providers and women's organisations. Home Office recommendations[14] and AMA guidelines[18] informed the protocols. The protocols were designed to:

- describe how to identify domestic violence through routine screening and recognition of clinical presentations
- provide examples of how to ask questions in ways that can elicit meaningful responses and help women explore their options and take action
- provide information about options and resources for women experiencing domestic violence
- describe how to ensure clear documentation of the abuse for the purpose of monitoring and prevention of further abuse.

Training programmes on domestic violence

Both pilots in A&E and family planning presented a number of logistical and organisational problems which resulted in alternative scenarios being developed for training purposes. For example, difficulties in releasing staff in the selected A&E department led to the development of an open learning pack.[32] The pack relied on staff motivation, managerial support and staff release from duties for completion. The training programmes were designed to introduce the protocol on domestic violence and, drawing on staff's experience and expertise, to:

- improve their awareness and understanding of domestic violence
- improve their awareness and understanding of agencies that provide support for women experiencing domestic violence
- consider their attitudes to domestic violence
- acquire the tools to implement the protocol effectively and systematically as applied to their work setting.

In both settings, knowledge and attitudes of staff were found to have shifted but there was no significant difference in detection rates after the introduction of the protocols.

Conclusions from the pilot audits

The Health Gain Commissioning Team reached the following conclusions about the prerequisites for improving service delivery to women who have experienced domestic violence:

- there is a wide variety of attitudes to, and levels of knowledge about, domestic violence, which can affect service delivery
- protocol introduction may overcome these variables, but the support of senior management for training, which explores attitudes to domestic violence, and current practice of operational staff is required
- once agreement has been reached to introduce change, careful consideration and attention must be given as to how this is communicated to staff at every level of the organisation
- service providers need to consult closely with outside domestic violence specialists in order to introduce appropriate training and provide appropriate referral information to women.

The health service has a distinct and important role to play in identifying women experiencing domestic violence, providing information, referring to support agencies and documenting the abuse. This role must be set in the context of a national policy framework. However, the health service cannot tackle the issue of domestic violence alone, and it must begin to work with other agencies and women's organisations to develop a strategic approach to domestic violence at the national level which can save lives, lessen injury and diminish the long-term impact of violence on women and their children.

References

1 World Health Organisation (1997) *Violence Against Women: a priority health issue.* Women's Health and Development, Family and Reproductive Health. WHO, Geneva.

2 United Nations World Conference on Human Rights (1993).

3 International Conference on Population and Development (1994).

4 Fourth World Conference on Women (1995) Beijing, China.

5 Secretary of State for Scotland (1998) *Working Together for a Healthier Scotland. A Consultation Document* (1998). The Stationery Office, Edinburgh.

6 British Medical Association (1998) *Domestic Violence: a healthcare issue.* The Chameleon Press, London.

7 Scottish Forum for Public Health Medicine (1997) *Scottish Needs Assessment Programme Report.* Scottish Forum for Public Health Medicine, Glasgow.

8 United Nations (1993) *Declaration on the Elimination of Violence Against Women.* United Nations General Assembly, Vienna.

9   Dobash RE and Dobash RP (1979) *Violence Against Wives*. The Free Press, New York.

10   Dobash RE, Dobash RP and Cavanagh K (1984) The contact between battered women and social and medical agencies. In: J Pahl (ed.) *Private Violence and Public Policy*. Routledge and Kegan Paul, London.

11   Mirrlees-Black C (1995) *Estimating the Extent of Domestic Violence: Findings from the 1992 British Crime Survey*. Home Office Research and Planning Unit, London.

12   Report of HM Inspectorate of Constabulary (1997) *Hitting Home: a report on the police response to domestic violence*. HM Inspectorate of Constabulary, Edinburgh.

13   Bunch C (1997) *The Intolerable Status Quo: violence against women and girls*. Progress of Nations. UNICEF.

14   Smith LJF (1989) *Domestic Violence: an overview of the literature*. Home Office Research Study No. 107. HMSO, London.

15   Plichta S (1992) The effect of woman abuse on health care utilisation and health status: a literature review. *Women's Health International*. **2**: 154–63.

16   Burge SK (1989) Violence against women as a health care issue. *Family Medicine*. **21**: 368–73.

17   Ruddle and O'Connor (1992) Quoted in: M McWilliams and J McKiernan (1993) *Bringing it Out in the Open: domestic violence in Northern Ireland*. HMSO, Belfast.

18   Council on Scientific Affairs, American Medical Association (1992) Violence against women. Relevance for medical practitioners. *Journal of the American Medical Association*. **267**: 3184–9.

19   Bewley CA and Gibbs A (1991) Violence in pregnancy. *Midwifery*. **7**: 107–12.

20   Walker LE (1979) *The Battered Woman*. Harper and Row, New York.

21   Jaffe P, Wolfe D, Wilson S *et al.* (1986) Emotional and physical health problems of battered women. *Canadian Journal of Psychiatry*. **31**: 625.

22   Mooney J (1993) *The Hidden Figure of Domestic Violence in North London*. Islington Council, London.

23   Amaro H, Fried L, Cabral H *et al.* (1990) Violence during pregnancy and substances abuse. *American Journal of Public Health*. **80**: 575.

24   Mullender A and Morley R (1994) *Children Living with Domestic Violence*. Whiting and Birch, London.

25   Jaffe PG, Wolfe DA and Wilson SK (1990) *Children of Battered Women*. Sage, Newbury Park, California.

26   Kelly K (1994) The interconnections of domestic violence and child abuse: challenges for research, policy and practice. In: A Mullender and R Morley (eds) *Children Living with Domestic Violence*. Whiting and Birch, London.

27   Durbin K (1974) Wife beating. Ladies journal. Quoted in: LJF Smith (1989) *Domestic Violence: an overview of the literature*. Home Office Research Study No. 107. HMSO, London.

28   Borkowski M, Murch M and Walker V (1983) *Marital Violence: the community response*. Tavistock Publications, London.

29 Pahl J (ed.) (1985) *Private Violence and Public Policy*. Routledge and Kegan Paul, London.

30 McWilliams M and McKiernan J (1993) *Bringing it Out in the Open: domestic violence in Northern Ireland*. HMSO, Belfast.

31 Glasgow Women's Health Working Group (1992) *Women's Health Policy*. Glasgow Women's Health Working Group, Glasgow.

32 McCartney S, Munro K and Dickie J (1995) *Protocol on Domestic Violence: an open learning pack*. Accident and Emergency Department, West Glasgow Hospitals NHS Trust, Glasgow.

CHAPTER NINE

Tobacco control: a losing battle?

Donald Reid

Why smoking is a public health problem

Despite the substantial decline in its use over the past 30 years, the smoking of tobacco, chiefly in the form of cigarettes, remains the largest single preventable cause of ill health in the UK, as well as a major cause of health inequality. Currently, nearly 3 in 10 adults smoke, of whom half will die from their habit, one-third before the age of 65 years,[1] from cardiovascular and chronic respiratory diseases and cancers of the lung and other sites.[2] There are about 120 000 smoking-attributable deaths annually, or 20% of all deaths[2]; smoking during pregnancy is a cause of low birth weight and miscarriages.[3] Quitting smoking at any age reduces the risks, although earlier quitters benefit most.[3]

Most of the harm is caused by the carbon monoxide and carcinogenic tars present in tobacco smoke; nicotine increases the risk of coronary heart disease but is otherwise much less dangerous.[2,4] However, it is highly addictive, which explains why quitting can be so difficult.[2,4]

Environmental tobacco smoke causes several hundred lung cancer deaths annually, increases the risk of chronic respiratory illness and ischaemic heart disease in adults,[2] and is especially damaging to children under 5 years of age.[5]

The prevalence of adult male smoking has fallen by half since 1948[3]; adult female smoking rose until 1966 but has since declined to the same level as that of men (Figure 9.1).[3] However, adult prevalence increased for the first time in 1966, chiefly among young men.[6] Teenage smoking, which had remained static since 1982, began to rise, especially among girls, in 1994.[3] In the UK, 1 in 4 teenagers become regular smokers by the age of 16, most of whom take up the habit between the ages of 12 and 15.[7]

Smoking was originally a relatively classless habit, but a marked social-class gradient has developed since 1948,[8] due to a decline in prevalence among non-manual workers[3]; a similar gradient appeared among English teenagers in the 1990s.[3]

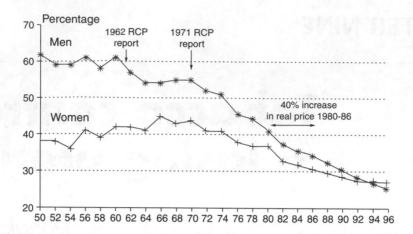

Figure 9.1:   Prevalence of cigarette smoking in adults 16 and over in the UK, 1950–96
Source: 1948–70 Tobacco Advisory Council, 1972–96 OPCS General Household Survey

Prevalence is closely related to deprivation[9]; Graham (personal communication) found that prevalence among deprived women increased with cumulative disadvantage. Smoking among ethnic groups is lower than the average for the UK population as a whole, although there are wide variations.[3]

Two contrasting, but complementary, strategies are available to prevent smoking-related disease (Table 9.1):

- addiction control, focusing on reducing the prevalence of smoking
- harm reduction, focusing on developing safer tobacco products.

Reducing prevalence: preventing teenagers from starting

Strategies to prevent teenage smoking include actions to reduce the demand for cigarettes through education, and to restrict supply through price increases and preventing sales to under-16s.[7,10]

Reducing demand through education

Although knowledge of the health risks has no effect on teenage smoking, sophisticated school programmes based on social learning theory can, under favourable conditions,

Table 9.1: Summary of available interventions

Intervention	Effects on smoking behaviour	Cost effectiveness from an NHS perspective	Comments
Reducing prevalence: preventing teenagers from starting			
School health-education programmes	Under favourable conditions, can delay recruitment to smoking	Minimal costs to NHS	Results under real-life conditions have been disappointing
Cessation programmes for teenagers	Poor long-term outcomes; unpopular with smokers	Poor	Brief GP advice is a better alternative
Non-smokers' clubs	None	Poor	Not recommended, except for publicity generation
Bans on smoking in schools	Effects on teenagers doubtful, but beneficial to teachers' health	Minimal costs	Recommended for teachers' benefit
Banning advertising	Some effect on recruitment	No cost to NHS (apart from advocacy)	Highly recommended
Mass campaigns	Results have been mixed	£86 per life year saved in Vermont[14] – if effects are permanent, which is uncertain	Worth further experimentation
Enforcing legislation banning sales to under 16s	No evidence for an effect on behaviour	High cost to other sectors[7]	Politically popular but benefits are small
Price increases through taxation	Likely beneficial effects	No cost to the NHS	See below
Reducing prevalence: helping adults to quit			
Brief advice from health professionals, especially GPs	Up to 5% quit rate	£12–£95 per year of life saved (pyls)[21]	Large-scale implementation is difficult to achieve
Smokers Advice Clinics	10–24% quit rate	Less cost effective than simpler interventions	Not suitable as a mass method because difficult to recruit smokers
Nicotine replacement therapy	Doubles effectiveness of other interventions; also effective in isolation	£20–£200 pyls for GP time alone (not available on NHS prescription)[21]	Should become available on NHS prescription, at least for those on income support
Advice to pregnant smokers	5–12% quit rate	Much cheaper than the costs of dealing with low weight births	Only 55% report receiving advice

Table 9.1: *continued*

Intervention	Effects on smoking behaviour	Cost effectiveness from an NHS perspective	Comments
Health warnings on packets	Small effect on consumption likely	No costs to NHS	Well worth strengthening
Unpaid media publicity, e.g. No Smoking Day (NSD)	Up to 5% fall in consumption, 0.3% quit rate for NSD	NSD: £22–£111 pyls[21]	Essential for its effects on public opinion, as well as on smokers' behaviour
Mass campaigns	0.44% quit rate in Scotland	£350–£650 pyls[31]	Apart from tax, the only method available for achieving rapid nationwide declines in prevalence – but best combined with other actions
Ban on all forms of advertising	Effects on adult consumption and teenage prevalence are likely	No costs to NHS except for media advocacy	Highly desirable
Price increases through taxation	Price elasticity of 0.5% for consumption; effects on prevalence also	No costs to NHS	Highly effective but scope limited by smuggling and concern over effects on deprived smokers
Socio-economic policies to reduce deprivation	Smoking rates among long-term unemployed and those on benefit are much higher than average	Should reduce NHS costs	Essential to prevent growing inequity
Restrictions on smoking in the workplace	Up to 15% fall in consumption, and some effect on prevalence also	Small costs to NHS	Highly desirable, but focus must be on small businesses to avoid inequity
Harm-reduction strategies			
Reducing tar and nicotine levels	May reduce quit rates if smokers believe that low-tar cigarettes are 'safe'	No costs to NHS	Probably has resulted in some gains to health, but much reduced by compensatory smoking
Developing NRT products as permanent substitutes for smoking tobacco	As yet untried on a large scale; health risks would be much reduced	No costs to NHS at present	Controversial but may be necessary if all else fails

delay recruitment to smoking for several years, but not indefinitely.[7] They are most effective at age 12–13, but not with established smokers.[7] However, it has not been possible to replicate these results on a large scale under real-life conditions, as the most effective programmes are also the most difficult to implement.[7] Consequently, although programmes for younger children can influence parental smoking,[7] the contribution of school health education appears to be relatively limited.

The same applies to school-based cessation programmes for teenagers, whose impact is limited both by difficulties of recruitment and poor long-term outcomes.[7] Brief advice from a GP is likely to be more cost effective.[11]

Clubs for non-smoking teenagers ('Smokebusters') can be highly popular, and therefore costly to service.[7] However, they have no effect on teenage prevalence,[12] although they can provide valuable media publicity.[7]

The influence of adult role models could be reduced by banning smoking on school premises, although this does not necessarily reduce prevalence and has proved difficult to implement in secondary schools.[7] A ban on all forms of tobacco advertising and sponsorship is desirable for the same reason, especially as a 1992 cohort study concluded that 'tobacco advertising promotes smoking among young people ... [though] the effect appears to be small in comparison with other influences'.[13]

Mass campaigns aimed at youth have had mixed results; significant declines in prevalence were achieved in trials in Vermont[14] and Norway,[15] but not in regional programmes in Minnesota and England.[7] Comprehensive mass media and community programmes aimed at all age groups were associated with declines in teenage smoking in Australia[7] and Finland,[16] but similar programmes in California[7,10] and Massachusetts[17] have had little effect on youth. However, in the absence of other options, the encouraging results from controlled trials[14,15] justify further experiments with this intervention.

Restricting access

Although extensive efforts have been made in the UK to enforce the legislation banning sales to children under 16, overall ease of purchase by minors has changed little since 1986.[7] A controlled study in Massachusetts found no link between increased compliance with legislation and prevalence of teenage smoking.[18]

The effects of increased price on young smokers are difficult to measure, but it probably reduces consumption (i.e. the total number of cigarettes smoked), though not necessarily prevalence, in the UK.[7,10]

Preventing teenage smoking – conclusions

Although politically popular, interventions intended to prevent teenage smoking have had little effect in the UK (or elsewhere) in recent years.[7] The more effective measures have proved difficult to implement on a large scale and generally have a delaying effect only – although delay is beneficial as late recruits are also early quitters.[19] However, for the NHS at least, a better return on investment can be achieved by concentrating resources on adults.

Reducing adult prevalence

Actions to reduce adult prevalence include provision of encouragement to give up, together with bans on smoking in public and the use of fiscal policy to increase price.

Reducing the demand for cigarettes – helping adults to quit

At any given time, 6 million, or 40% of the UK's 15 million smokers are contemplating quitting, while 12 million have already given up.[8] The most common reasons cited for trying to quit are: health (87% of current or ex-smokers), expense (51%), family pressure (43%) and restrictions at work (16%).[8]

Advice from health professionals

Health professionals have a potentially major role to play in helping adult smokers to give up, since even brief advice from a GP during a routine consultation can lead up to 5% of smokers to quit.[8,20] Although more sophisticated GP interventions achieve a higher quit rate, they are less cost effective[21] and are unlikely to be used on a large scale by hard-pressed practice teams.[22]

If every smoker was advised to quit at every consultation, up to 500 000 might give up each year.[20] However, less than half of all British smokers report receiving advice from their GP or other health professionals,[23] and only 7% report that doctor's advice helped them to stop.[20] As with school health education, there are many reasons why the full potential of this intervention is unlikely to be realised in practice.[24]

Smokers' cessation clinics, providing specialist courses for groups of smokers, have one-year quit rates in the range 10–25%, but are often unpopular with smokers[3] and are not as cost effective as other interventions.[8]

Nicotine replacement therapy (NRT), i.e. the use of patches and gums, etc. to deliver nicotine alone, can double the effectiveness of GP advice.[4] However, it is not available on NHS prescription and is less cost effective than brief advice, both to the GP and the smoker.[21] In the USA, NRT purchased over the counter is estimated to have increased by 10% the number of smokers who quit annually[25] – so this may be a valuable intervention for those who can afford it. Nevertheless, NRT should be available on NHS prescription – at least for those entitled to income support since universal access might cost the NHS up to £120 million annually.

Interventions during pregnancy

Given the risks to the fetus, it is disappointing that only 55% of pregnant women in the UK report receiving advice to stop, and only 5–12% succeed,[20] the majority of whom relapse after the birth.[20] A low-budget mass campaign in the UK had no discernible effect on prevalence among pregnant smokers.[20] Fortunately, many women seem able to quit successfully either before conceiving or very early in pregnancy, prior to receiving professional advice.[26] However, a major decline in smoking during pregnancy can probably only be achieved through broader interventions aimed at the community as a whole.

Mass communications

The simplest form of mass communication is to print health warnings on cigarette packets, as occurs in the UK under a voluntary agreement with the tobacco industry. Their effect on prevalence is unknown, but the 1995 introduction of stronger warnings in Australia probably reduced consumption to some extent.[27]

The creation of unpaid publicity may also encourage smokers to quit – for example, the annual No Smoking Day in the UK. Since the cost of delivering the message is mainly borne by the media, NHS participation in this event may be as cost effective as brief GP advice, even with a quit rate as low as 0.3%.[21]

Other examples of effective antismoking publicity include the pioneering reports of the Royal College of Physicians of London in 1962 and 1971 on the health effects of smoking. Media coverage of these was the principal cause of the 30% decline in male prevalence of smoking in the UK between 1962 and 1980 – despite a concurrent fall in the real price of cigarettes.[8] The publication of major reports of this kind can have an elasticity of response of up to –0.05, i.e. they can reduce per capita consumption of cigarettes by up to 5%, at least in the short term.[8,20] Investment in the creation of publicity should therefore by given serious consideration by health authorities[28] – especially as it is essential for the creation of public opinion favourable to effective political action to control tobacco use.[7,8,20]

Mass campaigns involving paid advertising have also been associated with rapid, major declines in prevalence in the USA,[8] Australia,[8] California[29] and Massachusetts.[30] In England, a Health Education Authority controlled trial found significant increases in cessation rates in regions with the most intensive television campaigns (D McVey, personal communication).

In Scotland, the Health Education Board's 1992 mass campaign helped 0.44% (or about 5000) of all smokers to quit, at an estimated cost per year of life saved between £350 and £650.[31] Though not as cost effective as brief GP advice or No Smoking Day, this compares well with more sophisticated interventions; furthermore television mass campaigns are the cheapest, most equitable[8,20] and practicable way to persuade several thousand people to give up smoking within a few months from launch.

Advice can also be given to smokers via telephone 'quit lines', but these are often little used except in conjunction with a mass campaign.[8,20] A free quit line promoted as part of the Health Education Board for Scotland campaign was called by 80 000 smokers, or 6% of all adult smokers, in 1992–93.[31]

Since antismoking campaigns are more likely to succeed in the absence of tobacco advertising and sponsorship, a complete ban is likely to lead to a fall in consumption as well as removing a significant influence on adolescents.[7,8,20]

Restricting smokers' access to cigarettes

Effects of increased price

For every 1% increase in real price, per capita consumption of cigarettes typically falls by about 0.5%, provided real disposable income remains constant.[8,20] A sharp decline in 'affordability' in 1980–82 was associated with one of the fastest falls in prevalence and consumption ever seen in the UK[8,20] (Figure 9.1) especially among manual workers.[3,32]

However, the scope for increasing taxes may ultimately be limited by smuggling, much of it with the tobacco industry's connivance,[33] and by concern over its effects on deprived groups.[34] Although price increases do cause some of the poorest smokers to quit, they worsen the plight of those who cannot – who must then spend an even larger proportion of their limited income on cigarettes. Opinion is therefore increasingly divided as to whether further real increases are justified.[34]

Restrictions on smoking in public

Over 90% of the largest companies in the UK restrict smoking to protect staff from environmental tobacco smoke.[8] This reduces environmental tobacco smoke, together with consumption (by up to 15%) and probably also prevalence.[35]

Restrictions should therefore be actively promoted in all workplaces, especially smaller businesses which are both more likely to employ smokers and to allow unrestricted smoking. Restrictions on smoking in shops and places of entertainment will have less effect on prevalence generally, but are necessary for the protection of employees from environmental tobacco smoke, as well as helping to establish non-smoking as the norm.[8,20]

Harm-reduction strategies

A harm-reduction strategy has been pursued by the UK government since the 1960s, in the form of a voluntary agreement with the industry to reduce tar and nicotine levels in cigarettes. This has probably led to some overall gains to health,[20] though these are much reduced by compensatory smoking behaviour,[36,37] and are trivial compared to the benefits of giving up altogether.[20]

However, the advent of NRT offers the prospect of developing products intended for use as long-term substitutes for cigarettes, rather than as aids to cessation.[4] If so, all products that deliver nicotine, including cigarettes, must be brought under a uniform system of regulation.[4] At present, the safest products (NRT) are licensed as medicines, while the most dangerous (cigarettes) are controlled on a voluntary basis only.[4]

Discussion and conclusions

It is evident from the recent increases in prevalence in the UK, especially among the young, that smoking is a battle which is no longer being won. It is not entirely clear why the 1990s have seen an end to the long period of declining prevalence in many industrialised countries, but one obvious cause is the increase in smoking in films – no doubt with tobacco industry support.[38]

All this has occurred at a time when fiscal policy, one of the UK's principal weapons against smoking in the past, is under threat both from increasing smuggling and concerns over its effects on the most deprived. The former could be resolved by harmonisation of taxes across Europe, but the latter requires a major effort to alleviate deprivation, especially unemployment.[39]

However, the UK government made a promising start in 1998 with the announcement of an annual £33 million programme. For England, this is intended to reduce the prevalence of smoking among adults from 28% to 24%, and among teenagers from 13% to 9%, by the year 2010.[40] It includes increased funding for mass campaigns and NHS smoking cessation services, and free provision of a week's supply of NRT for smokers in deprived areas. These will be supported by tax increases, further restrictions on advertising, and various voluntary actions to discourage smoking in public.

The principal criticism of this otherwise imaginative and comprehensive strategy lies in its funding, which is only one-third of the highly successful California State campaign. Furthermore, it will do little to reduce health inequalities unless accompanied by a major effort to tackle poverty and deprivation. Those who rely on nicotine to anaesthetise them against the stresses of lone parenthood or long-term unemployment, are unlikely to turn to free NRT as an effective substitute. While the cost of effective anti-deprivation measures would amount to several £ billion annually, the health benefits would be far wider than the prevention of smoking related disease.[39]

Should the new UK programme fail, the only option will be to develop nicotine delivery systems for long-term maintenance, rather than as an aid to cessation. If neither rising prevalence nor the harm done by tobacco can be reversed, a decline in UK peace-time life expectancy, for the first time in living memory, is inevitable in the long run.

Thanks are due to Dr Jennifer Mindell for her helpful comments on an earlier draft. However, the opinions expressed are those of the author alone, who writes in a personal capacity.

References

1   Wald NJ and Hackshaw AK (1996) Cigarette smoking: an epidemiological overview. *British Medical Bulletin.* **52**: 3–11.

2   UK Departments of Health (1998) *Report of the Scientific Committee on Tobacco and Health.* The Stationery Office, London.

3   Health Education Authority (1996) *Health Update: smoking.* Health Education Authority, London.

4   Raw M (1997) *Regulating Nicotine Delivery Systems.* Health Education Authority, London.

5   Royal College of Physicians of London (1992) *Smoking and the Young.* RCP, London.

6   Department of Health (1998) *Health Survey for England, 1966.* DoH, London.

7   Reid DJ, McNeill AD and Glynn TJ (1995) Reducing the prevalence of smoking in youth in Western countries: an international review. *Tobacco Control.* **4**: 266–77.

8   Reid DJ, Killoran AJ, McNeill AD and Chambers JS (1992) Choosing the most effective health promotion options for reducing a nation's smoking prevalence. *Tobacco Control.* **1**: 185–97.

9   Marsh A and McKay S (1994) *Poor Smokers.* Policy Studies Institute, London.

10 McNeill A (1997) Preventing the onset of tobacco use. In: CT Bolliger and KO Fagerstrom (eds) *The Tobacco Epidemic.* Kargel, Basel.

11 Walhgren DR, Hovell MF, Slymen DJ *et al.* (1997) Predictors of tobacco use initiation in adolescents: a two-year prospective study and theoretical discussion. *Tobacco Control.* **6**: 95–103.

12 van Teijlingen E, Friend JAR and Twine F (1996) Evaluation of Grampian Smokebusters: a smoking prevention initiative aimed at young teenagers. *Journal of Public Health Medicine.* **18**: 13–18.

13 Goddard E (1990) *Why Children Start Smoking.* OPCS for the Department of Health. HMSO, London.

14 Secker-Walker RR, Worden JR, Holland RR *et al.* (1997) A mass media programme to prevent smoking among adolescents: cost and cost effectiveness. *Tobacco Control.* **6**: 207–12.

15 Hafstad A, Stray-Pedersen B and Langmark F (1997) Use of provocative emotional appeals in a mass media campaign designed to prevent smoking among adolescents. *European Journal of Public Health.* **7**: 122–7.

16 Vartiainen E, Paavola M, McAlister A *et al.* (1998) Fifteen-year follow-up of smoking prevention effects in the North Karelia Youth Project. *American Journal of Public Health.* **88**: 81–5.

17 Hamilton W and Harrold L (1997) *Independent Evaluation of the Massachusetts Tobacco Control Program, Third Annual Report.* Abt Associates for the Massachusetts Department of Public Health.

18 Rigotti NA, di Franza JR, Chang Y-C *et al.* (1997) The effects of enforcing tobacco-sales laws on adolescents' access to tobacco and smoking behavior. *New England Journal of Medicine.* **337**: 1044–51.

19   Breslau N and Peterson E (1996) Smoking cessation in young adults: age at initiation of cigarette smoking and other suspected influences. *American Journal of Public Health.* **86**: 214–20.

20   Reid DJ (1996) Tobacco control: overview. *British Medical Bulletin.* **52**: 108–20.

21   Buck D and Godfrey C (1994) *Helping Smokers Give Up – Guidance for Purchasers on Cost Effectiveness.* York University Centre for Health Promotion, for the Health Education Authority, London.

22   Lennox AS and Taylor R (1995) Smoking cessation activity within primary health care in Scotland: present constraints and their implications. *Health Education Journal.* **54**: 48–60.

23   Office for National Statistics (1997) *Smoking Related Behaviour and Attitudes.* From the 1996 Omnibus Survey for the Department of Health (ONS 97 182). ONS, London.

24   Coleman T and Wilson A (1996) Anti-smoking advice in general practice consultations: general practitioners' attitudes, reported practice and perceived problems. *British Journal of General Practice.* **46**: 87–91.

25   Shiffman S, Gritchell J, Pinney JM *et al.* (1997) Public health benefit of over the counter nicotine medications. *Tobacco Control.* **6**: 306–10.

26   Mindell J (1995) Timing of pregnancy related changes in smoking habit in Derby. In: K Slama (ed.) *Tobacco and Health.* Plenum Press, New York.

27   Borland R and Hill D (1997) Initial impact of the new Australian tobacco health warnings on knowledge and beliefs. *Tobacco Control.* **6**: 317–25.

28   Mindell J (1997) An assessment of the feasibility of health authorities generating unpaid mass media publicity in the long term. *Health Education Journal.* **56**: 125–33.

29   Hu T-W, Sung H-Y and Keeler TE (1995) Reducing cigarette consumption in California: tobacco taxes vs an anti-smoking media campaign. *American Journal of Public Health.* **85**: 1218–22.

30   Harris JE, Connolly GN, Brooks D *et al.* (1996) Cigarette smoking before and after an excise tax increase and an antismoking campaign – Massachusetts, 1990–96. *Mortality and Morbidity Weekly Reports.* **45**: 966–70.

31   Ratcliffe J, Cairns J and Platt S (1997) Cost effectiveness of a mass media-led anti-smoking campaign in Scotland. *Tobacco Control.* **6**: 104–10.

32   Townsend J, Roderick P and Cooper J (1994) Cigarette smoking by socio-economic group, sex and age: effects of price, income, and health publicity. *British Medical Journal.* **309**: 923–7.

33   Joossens L and Raw M (1995) Smuggling and cross border shopping of tobacco in Europe. *British Medical Journal.* **310**: 1393–7.

34   Townsend J (1995) The burden of smoking. In: M Benzeval, K Judge and M Whitehead (eds) *Tackling Inequalities in Health.* The King's Fund, London.

35   Evans WN, Farrelly MC and Montgomery E (1996) *Do Workplace Smoking Bans Reduce Smoking?* National Bureau of Economic Research, Working Paper 5567. NBER, Washington DC.

36   Forst C, Fullerton FM, Stephen AM *et al.* (1995) The tar reduction study: randomised trial of the effect of cigarette tar yield reduction on compensatory smoking. *Thorax.* **50**: 1038–43.

37   Jarvis M and Bates C (1998) *Low Tar Cigarettes and Smoker Compensation*. Action on Smoking and Health, London.

38   Stockwell TF and Glantz SA (1997) Tobacco use is increasing in popular films. *Tobacco Control*. **6**: 282–4.

39   Benzeval M, Judge K and Whitehead M (eds) (1995) *Tackling Inequalities in Health*. The King's Fund, London.

40   DoH and Scottish, Welsh and NI Offices (1998) *Smoking Kills: a White Paper on tobacco*. The Stationery Office, London.

CHAPTER TEN

Children and young people

Aidan Macfarlane

Definition of child public health

A definition of public health as it applies to children's issues would be:

The organised efforts of society to develop healthy public health policies to promote the health of children and young people, to prevent disease in children and young people and to foster equity for children and young people within a framework of sustainable development.

What's different about the public health needs of children and young people?

Children and young people up to the age of 18 represent approximately 1 in 5 of the entire population. As a group they have significantly different health needs from that of adults, because:

- they represent the most vulnerable members of society, due to their relative physiological, emotional and psychological immaturity
- they lack political power, resulting from their lack of voting rights
- their primary healthcare providers are their parents, with the result that children are dependent on their parents' socio-economic circumstances without having any power in changing those circumstances
- the prevalence, expression and management of disease and other health problems in children are significantly different from those in adults.

How in practice are these issues addressed?

The vulnerability of children

This has been accepted and addressed by the UN Convention on the Rights of the Child, to which the UK along with most other countries, has signed up.[1] These rights include:

- a family which has suitable socio-economic resources so as to provide a warm, loving, secure environment, with adequate food, housing, clean water, etc.
- recognition that 'the child, by reason of his physical and mental immaturity, needs special safeguards and care' and which provides accurate and appropriate information and medical facilities for parents and children
- freedom from congenital abnormalities or preventable infections
- parental ability to plan their families
- freedom from prejudice 'of any kind, such as race, colour, sex, language, religion, political or other opinion, national or social, origin, property, birth or other status'
- freedom from violence, conflict and pollution.

Children and young people's lack of political power

This will remain an issue, but it is worth noting that in the UK, what evidence there is suggests that, in general, young people aged 12–19 do not feel that lowering the voting age further is desirable.[2] This does not negate the need to take into account the views of young people on the delivery of health services, and the UN Convention on the Rights of the Child, covering, as it does, three main aspects of children's lives – participation, provision and protection – reflects this. In relation to participation, Article 12 of the convention provides for children to have the right to express an opinion and to have that opinion taken into account in any matter or procedure affecting the child.

Legislation and circulars and guidance in the UK have required that local authorities and health authorities should ensure that systems are in place to allow young people, as users of services, to be consulted, and to have their views taken into account in a non-tokenistic way.

The rationale for consulting children and young people is summarised by the Local Government Information Unit, in their resource guide, *Hear! Hear! Promoting Children and Young People's Democratic Participation in Local Government*:

> *There are three arguments for involving young people in council deliberations; political, legal and social. Services can be improved and democracy strengthened; the UN Convention on Rights of the Child demands it; and young people as members of society share a fundamental right to participate.*[3]

Parents as primary healthcare providers

That parents are the primary healthcare givers is shown by:

- the fact that 80% of all illness in children (fevers, rashes, diarrhoea and vomiting, coughs, etc.) is dealt with by parents without going anywhere near the medical system
- the huge increase in basic child health knowledge which parents now have and have access to.

Support for this parental role includes:

- the development of a national, parent-held 'personal child health record', which acts as the major record of a child's health and development
- support for the role of parental observation in child health surveillance
- development of increasing appropriate literature on child health matters for parents, in magazines, on television and on websites.

Children and young people suffer from different health problems than adults

This is easily demonstrated by examining the causes of death of children and young people:

- for children under 1 year they are sudden unexpected deaths, congenital abnormalities and diseases of the nervous system
- for children aged 1–4 years they are congenital abnormalities, accidents, cancer and diseases of the nervous system
- for children aged 5–17 years they are accidents, cancers and diseases of the nervous system.

Child public health is intimately involved in preventative aspects of all these causes of mortality, from the monitoring of congenital abnormalities through to the distribution of new vaccines to prevent meningitis. Furthermore, the recognition of these differences has led, over the years, to increasing paediatric specialisation and now to increasing specialisation within the field of 'child' public health (see below).

The major 'child' public health issues

Political power

Political power and political opinions remain the most powerful tools that could operate towards better child health, but they also remain the greatest stumbling blocks, due to the continuing absence of radical political thinking aimed at bringing about greater equality of distribution of wealth within the UK. The health of children remains dependent mainly on the socio-economic status of their parents, which remains mainly dependent on the political system.

Poverty

Both relative and absolute poverty remain the greatest child public health problem, as it has done from time immemorial, though our ability to bring about change, given the political will, has greatly increased.

Prevention

Much work has been done in the field of child health in primary prevention. The three successes of particular note being immunisations, prevention of accidents and the prevention of sudden unexpected infant deaths. On the one hand, although much work has been done and an enormous amount of time and effort have been spent in health promotion to young people, there has been a notable lack of success in the fields of preventing smoking, preventing drug taking and preventing unwanted pregnancies.

Parenting

The overall role and value of 'parenting' relative to child health (and to other aspects of their existence) is beginning to be the focus of increasing political and media attention. Attitudes are moving away from seeing 'parenting' as simply an 'instinctual' or 'learnt on the job' spare-time occupation, towards the recognition of parenting as a highly skilled, mainstream occupation which, for almost all people, will be the single most important professional job they will be required to carry out during their lifetime. Further, it is a skill for which there is increasing evidence that training can play a useful and effective role. However, without tackling the problems of poverty and social inequality, the abilities of people's parenting skills will remain a lower area of interventional priority.

Who has been, is and might in the future be responsible for the public health of children?

Involvement in, and delivery of, the multivarious aspects of child-related public health (outlined below in further detail) is, or should be, the remit of a broad range of professionals. Other than parents and children themselves, they are: global organisations, including WHO and UNICEF; other international and national non-governmental organisations; the EC; politicians and legislators; professionals in education and social services; health service professionals in medicine and nursing at primary-, secondary- and tertiary-care child health and paediatric levels; health promotionists; public health professionals and those involved in environmental health; architects, town planners, etc. This is much the same kind of group that is involved, one way or another, in public health in general, as each of the above professionals may be involved in aspects of child public health to a greater or lesser degree, but very few of them will be involved in the subject as their main speciality.

The challenge for child public health, as in so many other similar areas, is therefore to have relatively few specialists being responsible for disseminating appropriate knowledge and training, in appropriate ways, to the appropriate people – most of whose main jobs and thinking will be in other areas of speciality.

Who are, or might be, these 'relatively few specialists' at the present time?

Public health as it relates to children remains, with a few exceptions, mainly within the provenance of overall public health, both in the UK and in Europe. These 'exceptions' are nonetheless becoming more common, with academic specialists in *child* public health already in place in the Nordic countries, Spain, Portugal and France. In the UK, with the recent introduction of the academic title and post of 'Professor in Child Health', there has been growing expertise in the field amongst academically trained paediatricians and a considerable increase in the number of epidemiologists specialising in aspects of child health and care.

At a service level, professionals specialising in child public health alone are still rare, especially in the UK, although one or two do exist. More common are paediatricians working outside of hospitals, within communities, and here the relative terms in Europe include:

- 'social paediatricians', a term used in most European countries except the UK for a group of health professionals initially trained in paediatrics, working mainly outside of hospitals, who have received some further training in population child health and illness
- 'community' paediatricians, a term used in the UK for paediatricians working mainly outside of hospitals, with populations of children with chronic disorders in the community, but who may also have a variable degree of training and interest in aspects of child public health.

Within the health services, along with these doctors are other professionals, including nurses, health promotionists and health services managers, who are beginning to realise that an increasing amount of their work involves concepts developed in the field of child public health.

The future of child public health within primary care groups

Some of child public health will, in the future, have to become the remit of PCGs. Of particular relevance to these will be:

- understanding and supporting parents in their role as the primary health carers of children
- supporting primary prevention initiatives relative to childhood illnesses, e.g. immunisations, 'back to sleep' campaigns, etc.
- understanding and acting on the social context of child health in co-operation with local council services
- accessing contemporary information relative to effective interventions in the field of child health
- understanding the prevalence of childhood disability and the community management needed to care for these children
- basic understanding of the 'rights of the child' and child protection issues.

Basic training

Basic training in child public health for members of PCGs might therefore cover: immunisation; social, economic and demographic factors affecting child health, including mortality and morbidity; factors relating to the physical, mental and emotional growth and development of children; communication skills for health professionals when dealing with parents and children; general child protection and health promotion; factors relating to lifestyles of young people (diet, exercise, drug abuse, etc.); the role of the family in influencing child health and development; trends in childhood mortality and morbidity (including physical and mental disability); promotion of breast feeding; screening and surveillance methodologies in childhood; effects of violence within families; principles of multidisciplinary working to meet children's health needs; prevention of illness in adults by prevention in childhood and adolescence (diet, exercise, smoking, etc.).

How will public health develop in the future relative to children as an issue?

The most major needs for further improvement in overall child health in the twenty-first century continue to lie mainly in the political field, and include:

- parental, and therefore child, access to decent socio-economic circumstances
- parental and child access to a good general education

- parental access to specific education on parenting, including knowledge relating to the latest research on the effects of parenting on mental health outcomes in children
- access to information about their own individual child's health and development
- well-informed and interested media and politicians, compassionate to the interests of children and their parents
- an easily accessible medical care system for all children and young people, irrespective of their economic situation, culture, gender or race.

However, those specialising in *child* public health have a clear role in helping to achieve these ends by:

- the collection and distribution of relevant child health mortality and morbidity statistics
- adding value to these statistics with appropriate explanations of their relevance to specific groups of users (politicians, legislators, local authorities, etc.)
- adding value to such statistics by advising on the effectiveness of interventions (medical and otherwise)
- using such data for political advocacy on behalf of children and young people
- appropriately identifying and filling gaps in available information concerning child health
- supporting research into the effectiveness of interventions used in the field of paediatrics and child health
- ensuring parental and child participation in the decision-making processes involved in the planning and delivery of health services for children and young people
- ensuring equity of access to health services for children and young people
- ensuring the provision and distribution of accurate and appropriate information about child care and health via a variety of methods (media, primary care, schools, etc.)
- involvement in training appropriate professionals whose work includes aspects of child public health.

Conclusion

In our global society, in which knowledge and facts are accumulating at an increasing rate, created by and creating increased specialisation, it is inevitable that *child* public health is becoming a specialist subject in its own right. Whatever the terminologies used for the various professions involved, to varying degrees, in the multivarious aspects of child public health, it will remain a specialist profession with relatively few producing appropriate information for the many.

At a service level the success of these few specialists should, and will, be judged on:

- the quality of information that they are able to accumulate relative to the health of children and young people
- their ability to 'add value to' and to disseminate this information in an appropriate format to the appropriate organisations, such as the new PCGs

- the influence they are shown to have on improving the health of children and young people in the future.

For the foreseeable future, equity of distribution of the gross national wealth will remain the single issue that will most influence the health of children. Without a move towards greater equity, those working in child public health can continue to have a secondary role by mitigating the effects of social inequalities.

References

1   United Nations (1990) The Convention on the Rights of the Child. Adopted by the UN General assembly on 20 November 1989, entered into force on 2 September 1990.

2   Roberts H and Sachdev D (eds) (1996) *Young People's Social Attitude. Having Their Say: the views of 12–19 year olds*. Barnados Publications, London.

3   Local Government Information United (1996) *Hear! Hear! Promoting Children and Young People's Democratic Participation in Local Government* (resource guide). LGIU, London.

CHAPTER ELEVEN

Occupational health

Kit Harling

Introduction

Contemporary occupational health has been described as the reversible relationship between work and health.[1] The discipline is as much concerned with the impact of health on an individual's capacity for work as it is on the impact of work on the health of an individual or population.

This was not always the case. Although the first significant legislation affecting the lives of workers (Health and Morals of Apprentices' Act 1802) includes the term 'health', for much of the nineteenth and early twentieth centuries what is now recognised as occupational medicine focused simply upon those diseases that were caused by environmental factors at work. Health in its broader context was seen as the preserve of the social reformers.

The medical context of the time, and the appalling toll of industrial injuries and diseases, made this preoccupation with occupational conditions inevitable. It is only as society has developed and the prevalence of occupational diseases has reduced that we are able to take a more rational view of the health of the workforce. Occupational health is interested in the health of working people. In reality, however, the interest of occupational physicians extends beyond a simple consideration of the workforce.

The Health and Safety at Work Act 1974 placed duties on employers to safeguard as far as possible the health of people at work. An additional duty, less frequently reported, was also placed upon employers to safeguard the health of 'other persons not being employees' but likely to be affected by the work activities. It is from this beginning that occupational physicians developed their interests 'beyond the factory fence' and became involved in the impact of work activities amongst the wider community.[2]

Up to this point, occupational health interest in the health of the wider population was focused entirely upon the effects of work on health. In its most extreme form, the release of toxic substance from the Union Carbide factory in Bhopal, India, represents the damage that industrial processes may do in the general population. Less extreme examples, such as the release of dioxin from a plant in Derbyshire in the 1960s, have occurred in the UK.

Another facet of this problem is the anxiety engendered within a population from their perceptions of the adverse impact of emissions from industrial plants. Waste-disposal sites have, over many years, generated scare stories about the impact of their emissions both on animals and humans. The impact of these emissions on reproduction is a recurring anxiety, guaranteed to stimulate media interest.

The relationship between poverty and health has been well described and is once again a live political issue. This poses a number of challenges for occupational physicians. Lack of access to work, particularly for those with chronic illness or disability, ensures continuing poverty. Promoting fairness in recruitment and continuing employment is now one of the key roles of an occupational physician. The use of a medical procedure, be it a simple pre-employment health questionnaire or the most advanced genetic testing, in selection for employment or promotion has a huge potential to discriminate unfairly within a population. Preventing this discrimination and actively assisting employers to modify work and workplaces to increase opportunities for access to employment are key roles of occupational medicine as we approach the new millennium.

In addition to the effects of poverty, work *per se* is an important part of maintaining health. In addition to monetary rewards, employment offers status, a feeling of self-worth, stability, structured activity and companionship. A healthy workplace is a positive contributor to the mental health of the workforce and has even been shown to reduce the prevalence of physical illness, such as lower back pain.

Work, then, is a central feature in the life of the population. Whether it is directly by its effect, either positive of negative, on the life of the worker, or indirectly on the lives of those dependent upon the worker, the health implication of work is all-pervasive. No arrangements for improving the health of the public can afford to ignore the occupational health aspects.

Who does what

Occupational health as a speciality has developed slowly in the UK. Perhaps the single most important factor preventing growth was the exclusion of occupational health services from the NHS in 1948. Of course, there was considerable worry about the cost of the new NHS, which was at that time primarily a service for the treatment of illness. It was a convenient argument to point out that, as the employer had always been responsible for funding occupational health services, there was little point in incorporating such provisions into a national health service as they could be developed equally well on a local basis. This had the effect of removing occupational medicine from the mainstream of developing British medicine and preventing the development of any clear or effective links between the evolving NHS and the workplace.

This effect was compounded by the overwhelming change in employment patterns that has occurred over the past 40 years or so. After the Second World War, work largely revolved around being an employee. More often than not, this involved working for a large company and nationalisation in the post-war era grew the massive smoke-stack industries. Coal, steel, gas, railways and other nationalised industries employed a huge proportion of the working population. That working population was still largely male and the existence of two earners within a conventional family was unusual.

Large firms, and in particular the nationalised industries, employed substantial medical services. Indeed, the very success of these services, which provided care to a significant proportion of the population, was very much in keeping with the social development of the time and obscured the impact of the lack of communication with the rapidly developing NHS.

More recently, employment patterns have shifted dramatically. There has been an explosive growth in self-employment and work in small and medium-sized companies. Added to this, the use of part-time, temporary or contract staff has fundamentally altered the traditional relationship between employers and employees. The medical services of the nationalised industries have disappeared and, in many large employers, outsourcing has been a euphemism for dismantling many (though not all) private-industry occupational health services. There has been a growth in individual private practitioners providing occupational health services under contract. We have also seen the emergence of companies specialising in the provision of occupational health services to a wide variety of industries, again under contract.

The other growth area for occupational health has been in the NHS and local author-ities. The development of occupational health services in the NHS, which started with a health circular in 1982,[3] has led to the creation of specialist services throughout the country. This growth has been patchy and a recent estimate suggests that even in 1998, less than one-third of NHS staff have access to a specialist occupational health service.

NHS occupational health departments were created to care for NHS employees. Many (though by no means all) departments provide occupational health services to non-NHS employers. Such work increases the variety of employment and offers enhanced training opportunities for those holding senior or specialist registrar appointments. The process was accelerated by the notion of income generation put forward at the end of the 1980s.

Such external work is on a contract basis, negotiated individually with specific employers. The temptation has been to provide those services that employers want, irrespective of proven benefit, rather than basing services on an integrated assessment of health need. Introduction of occupational health services should be preceded by an assessment of the customer's needs. There has been a lack of focus on 'who is the customer' and too often this has been seen as being a requirement to meet exclusively the needs of the organisation rather than the needs of the workforce or even the local community.

Our Healthier Nation

For perhaps the first time in half a century, the Green Paper *Our Healthier Nation*[4] offers a blueprint, or at least an opportunity, for improving the health of people at work. The

Green Paper offers the prospect of the healthier workplace becoming a key feature of health planning. Making the health authority responsible for the health of the population naturally draws the workplace into the planning process. At a stroke, this would significantly reduce the professional isolation that has so hampered the development of occupational healthcare, and indeed health itself, at work.

The two major contributions to the health of the population would be to reduce the toll of ill health arising from work and work activities, coupled with arrangements to maximise access to work for all sections of the community, including those with chronic illness and disability.

Dealing first with reducing work activities as a cause of ill health, the major challenge relates to those working for small and medium-sized companies or those who are self-employed. There is no requirement for such employees to have access to occupational health advice although such rules are common in Europe.

There are at present a multiplicity of providers. Many services are provided by GPs working on a very part-time basis. Recently, the Faculty of Occupational Medicine has introduced a Diploma in Occupational Medicine, the syllabus of which lays out the basic principles of the speciality. It allows any doctor to demonstrate both to employers and employees a certain level of achievement. Individual occupational physicians, either alone or working in partnership, will provide services to employers; and, more recently, large companies, often on a national basis, will provide similar services. As noted above, many occupational health departments in the NHS will provide such services, as do some occupational health departments in large companies.

If the benefits of an occupational health service are to be expanded to cover the majority of the working population, some form of incentive for employers will be required. Failure to safeguard the health of people at work is a criminal offence and may give rise to civil litigation. However, the likelihood of such enforcement actions remains low and most company managers are more concerned with the immediate rather than distant threats.

It is possible that in time a European-wide directive may transfer the continental system of compulsory occupational health services to the UK. This would not be helpful if at the same time this simply resulted in a requirement to carry out 'routine medicals' on otherwise fit and healthy people. Occupational health services are primarily preventive and involve a multidisciplinary team, including nurses, occupational hygienists, ergonomists, psychologists and safety professionals. It would be an irony if the mechanisms to extend occupational healthcare also damaged this protective effect.

It may be that some sort of financial incentive would be a better carrot for the improvement of occupational health services. The government is an obvious contender for such a mechanism through the corporate tax system. Although not widely seen in the UK at present, employers' liability insurers may also have a role to play. Premiums for this compulsory insurance have risen way ahead of inflation in recent years, reflecting the increasing costs of personal injury and other litigation. A reduction in premiums for those companies who are able to demonstrate an effective occupational health and safety system would be a significant push in the right direction.

The second contribution that a healthier workplace can make to the health of the public lies in the benefits of properly organised working systems and increasing the access to work for the disadvantaged in society. The occupational health team, and in particular occupational psychologists, can make a substantial contribution. It could be seen as a logical extension of an occupational health department, developing from the prevention of ill health caused by work. It is perhaps the other end of the same spectrum.

Widening access to work is rather more difficult. There is, with the occasional exception, little enthusiasm within the NHS to see return to work and rehabilitation towards this end as being an important 'outcome measure' for the success of medical intervention. Once again, the separation of occupational health services and healthcare at the workplace from mainstream medicine has been the main cause of this failure.

We were all taught at medical school to ask our patients: 'What is your occupation?'. On the very rare occasions that this is actually done in practice, one or two words are written down. Rarely, if ever, does it appear that the doctor has understood the full implications of the job title, and they instead rely upon misleading stereotypes.

There is a need to develop within healthcare a mechanism for providing sound occupational medicine advice for patients recovering from serious illness or who have a chronic disability. This will not be required in every case, but the poor access to work and the rapidity with which employment can be lost in these circumstances has a major impact on the health of the population at large.

Occupational health services within the NHS are ideally placed to take up this challenge. It is to be hoped that pilot studies will emerge soon to demonstrate the effectiveness of this type of approach. However, the major difficulty is that the NHS does not have sufficient occupational health services to meet its own needs as an employer, let alone to take on additional responsibilities. There is, however, an argument for refocusing the activities of NHS occupational health services so that professional variety is achieved by innovative schemes in rehabilitation, rather than the provision of basic occupational health services simply to improve the finance of the employing Trust.

In terms of the promotion of health, the workforce has in the past simply been viewed as a captive audience for traditional, general health promotion activities, perhaps with the employer picking up the bill! The benefits of such activities in the workplace have not been rigorously assessed, particularly in terms of their impact on employment. I have heard it argued, in a presentation to health service managers, that by altering the diet at work, a reduction in the prevalence of ischaemic heart disease and sickness absence will be achieved. Such arguments devalue the real benefits that such activities may produce.

There has also been a lack of clarity about the meaning of the term 'health promotion'. An integral part of the running of any business is the need to provide information, instruction and training to staff. Where this has involved matters of health and safety, there is sometimes a claim that this is 'health promotion'. There are fundamental differences in the skills and competencies required when discussing workplace-specific health issues when compared with general health promotion. Where work-related health information is being produced, a clear understanding of work and work processes is required as well as knowledge of the health issues.

There are benefits to the health of a workforce from general health promotion events. These may be a simple manifestation of the Hawthorn effect.[5] This effect, named after a factory where it was first described, involves an improvement in performance and staff morale that is achieved by the management taking an interest in the workforce. In this example, productivity increased when the lighting was improved. Initial claims that this was a direct effect were refuted when a further increase in productivity was achieved by reducing the lighting levels.

When linked to national campaigns, the workplace does offer another medium through which to sell the 'healthy' message. There can be little doubt that a smoke-free workplace is rapidly becoming the norm and there is a growing realisation that alcohol and work do not mix safely. Carefully dovetailed into national campaigns, health promotion at work can enhance the public health message and improve the lives of the workforce.

Conclusion

We must not forget that perhaps a quarter of the workforce does already have access to occupational health services at their place of work. An immediate benefit to the health of the population could be achieved by improving the communication between such services and the local healthcare providers. Occupational health services exist to help the workforce. More effective communication with the NHS will improve the contribution that they are able to make.

One simple way of improving such communications would be for the NHS to provide a professional focus for those physicians working in occupational health services in terms of continuing medical education, professional development, peer support and peer review. To this end, professional organisations such as the Faculty of Occupational Medicine have a leadership role to encourage such a development. Geography dictates that a single model will not be the ideal solution in every case. Nevertheless, lack of universality should not be a bar for such progress being made where possible.

References

1   Faculty of Occupational Medicine (1998) *Core Curriculum for Occupational Medicine Training for Undergraduates* (2e). Faculty of Occupational Medicine, London.

2   Philipp R (1996) Conceptual frameworks for setting environmental standards. *International Journal of Occupational Medicine and Environmental Health*. **9**: 201–10.

3   Department of Health (1982) *Occupational Health Services*. HSG (82) 33. DoH, London.

4   Secretary of State for Health (1998) *Our Healthier Nation: a contract for health*. Cmnd 3852. The Stationery Office, London.

5   Whitehead TN (1938) *The Industrial Worker*. Harvard University Press, Cambridge, MA.

CHAPTER TWELVE

Population ageing

John Grimley Evans

The population of Britain is ageing, in that the proportion of people in the older age groups in increasing. This is the result of two processes, changes in the birth rate and increases in survival. The process began with a 'demographic transition' from a pattern of high birth rate and high mortality to one of low birth rate and low mortality. This transition has occurred, or is occurring, in most nations of the world. As national income rises there comes a point when, for reasons that are not always clear and probably differ between nations, infant and child mortality rates fall. There is then a lag, typically of a generation, before fertility and completed family sizes also decline. During this lag a bolus of unprecedented survivors of childhood is released into the population. This transition took place in Britain during the early years of this century, following the fall in child mortality rates which began around 1900. The passage of the resulting large cohort of survivors from Edwardian and Georgian families through old age has been responsible for much of the increase in numbers of older people over the past 20 years. Birth rates in the 1930s were low, and the size of the elderly population will now become more stable for a couple of decades. A new wave of population ageing will come with the arrival in old age of the large cohort of post-war 'baby boomers', peaking in the third and fourth decades of the new millennium. These two waves of ageing can be predicted from the population structure of England and Wales in 1971 (Figure 12.1).

The second cause of ageing of our population has been a fall in mortality rates in middle age and later life. This has been continuous for women since the start of the century, but in men the fall was delayed by various effects, including the epidemic of smoking-related diseases (Figure 12.2). We do not know whether older people in the UK are now living longer because they are fitter or because unfit and chronically ill people are being kept alive longer. These two processes, which may coexist, have very different implications for health and social services. One means of monitoring the needs for (and the success of) services for an ageing population would be by some measure of healthy active life expectancy at later ages.[1,2] At present we have no adequate data on this in the UK. Suggestions[3] that recent increases in total life expectancy in Britain involve prolongation of the average period of disability before death are derived from the General

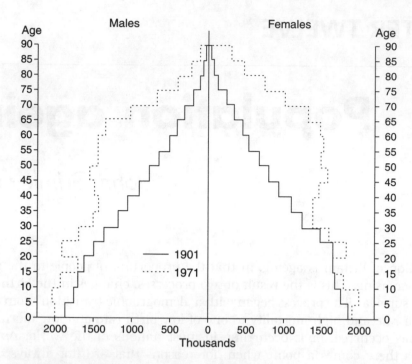

Figure 12.1: England and Wales: age structure of population 1901 and 1971

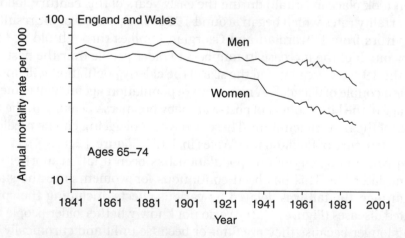

Figure 12.2: Annual mortality rates at ages 65–74 since 1841, England and Wales. Five-year means to 1955, individual years thereafter. Note logarithmic scale of ordinate

Household Survey, which bases estimates of disability on self-report in response to poorly standardised questionnaires and its sampling frame does not include institutionalised people. It will register an increase in disability if improvements in community care enable more unwell older people to live in their own homes rather than having to move into institutions. In the USA, where regular reviews of the health status of large samples of the population are available from the National Health and Nutrition Examination Study, there is encouraging news. It seems that American older people are not only living longer but are fitter and have less need of healthcare.[4] This should not lead to any sense of complacency among the managers of British health services. Although the needs of older individuals in the USA for healthcare are falling, the numbers of older people are growing at such a rate that the total need for healthcare is increasing, albeit to a smaller degree than data from 10 or 15 years ago would have suggested. More importantly, we have no evidence that the same improvements are happening here. A major factor in the improvement of health in older Americans seems to be their adoption of healthier lifestyles and this may well not happen in our poorer, less well-informed and less self-reliant British population. Nonetheless, the changes in the USA are an indication of what could be made to happen here if it were made a matter of national policy.

Where good data on active life expectancy are available, two interesting features emerge. Table 12.1 presents data calculated from a study in Massachusetts over 20 years ago,[5] but recent data from The Netherlands[6] show the same pattern. The partition of total life expectancy into dependent and non-dependent years shows that although women outlive men, their extra years are accounted for entirely by years of dependency. Moreover, women tend to marry men older than themselves and so are likely to bear their heavier burden of disability when widowed and in relative poverty. In the USA this pattern means that while only 1 in 7 of men who attain the age of 65 can expect to spend a year or more in a nursing home before death, for women the figure is 1 in 3.[7] The second feature of interest is that, at least among the women, on whom the major burden of disability falls, the older one is and still independent, the shorter the average period of disability one can expect before death. This makes epidemiological sense in that the fatality of diseases rises with age. The older one is when attacked by a potentially disabling disease such as stroke, the more likely one is to die of it rather than survive with

Table 12.1:   Life expectancy in years: Massachusetts 1970–72. Calculated from data of Katz *et al.*[5]

Age	Total		Active		Dependent[a]	
	Men	Women	Men	Women	Men	Women
65–69	13.1	19.5	9.3	10.6	3.8	8.9
70–74	11.9	15.9	8.2	8.0	3.7	7.9
75–79	9.6	13.2	6.5	7.1	3.1	6.1
80–84	8.2	9.8	4.8	4.8	3.4	5.0
85–	6.5	7.7	3.3	2.8	3.2	4.9

[a] 'Dependent' implies needing personal help with one or more activities of daily living.

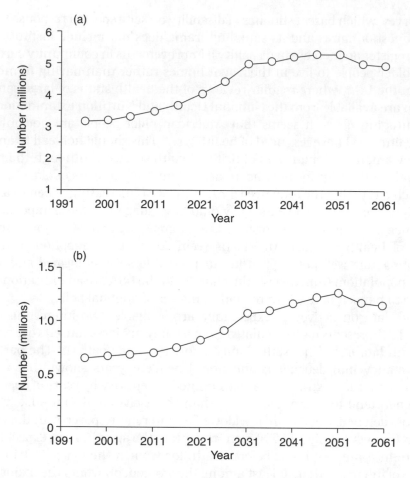

Figure 12.3: (a) Great Britain: projected number of people aged over 65 years with disability of grade 3 or more (likely to require personal help). Based on National Disability Survey[12] and population projections.[26] (b) Great Britain: projected number of people aged over 65 years with dementia. Based on the MRC Cognitive Function and Ageing Study[27] and population projections[26]

a disability. This offers scope for a policy of 'postponement as prevention' in both the clinical and public health approach to human ageing.

The need for some coherent policy towards the health of our ageing population is clear. In the absence of clear indications of how age-associated morbidity is changing, we can only view the future by projecting current patterns of illness and disability and use and costs of services on to future age structures. Figure 12.3 combines data on disability and prevalence of dementia with population projections to estimate the growth in numbers of older people affected over the next decades. Predictions about the costs of healthcare are also worrying. If present levels of disability and costs of care in later life continue, by the year 2030 expenditure on long-term care alone will amount to nearly 11% of the GNP, equivalent at present values to £2000 per head of the population of working age, a rise approaching 50% on 1991 figures.[8]

Government must clarify its policies in terms of the aims of care for older people and in identifying the sources of funding for the increased expenditure that seems inevitable in the early years of the new millennium. Clinicians and public health doctors have two other tasks. We must maximise the efficiency of the services we provide, and we must minimise the need for care by reducing the incidence and prevalence of age-associated disease and disability.

Table 12.2:   The process of geriatric care

Assessment
    health (diagnoses, prognosis)
    function (physical, mental)
    resources (culture, education, social, economic)
Agree objectives of care
    What does the patient want?
    What is feasible?
Specify the management plan
    to close the ecological gap between what the patient can do and what the environment requires:
        therapeutically   improve the patient
        prosthetically – reduce environmental demands
Regular review
    Is progress as expected?
    Does the plan need changing?

Efficiency of services

The importance of assessing the efficiency, in the sense of cost utility, of services rather than merely the efficacy of treatments has been recognised in the growth of health services research (HSR) and health technology assessment as major research domains. The UK developed its system of healthcare for older people pragmatically. Its underpinning lies in ready access of older people who fall ill to a full range of modern medicine informed by specialist geriatric expertise,[9] and embodying the four-stage 'geriatric process' summarised in Table 12.2. None of this has ever been adequately evaluated in the UK, but studies of replications in the USA have shown it to be more cost-effective than conventional care.[10] Whether this reflects the value of geriatric expertise or merely the poor quality of conventional care in the USA is unclear, but American experience does give warning of the consequences if the British NHS were to lose the specialist vision and commitment of geriatric medicine.

For all its faults and lapses, the NHS has achieved wonders over its half-century in providing effective, efficient and compassionate care for older people. We must doubt, however, whether a successful future can lie merely in providing more of the past. A problem for HSR for an ageing population lies in the difficulties in asking radical and strategically important questions. Innovation and research are restricted by rigid professional structures and political control at a time when we might do well to consider even the unthinkable. If patterns of practice and costs remain as at present, the main financial impact of ageing in the UK will fall on the long-term care sector rather than on primary or acute secondary care.[11] The dominance of long-term care in the predictions arises because at present the use of primary and secondary care rises much less steeply with age than does the use of the various forms of long-term care. We do not know whether this pattern is clinically appropriate or economically efficient. It may partly be the product of accountancy, rather than economics, in distorting the apportionment of costs between health and social services budgets. A GP may think it more efficient economically to save money in the health budget by advising an old lady to go into a nursing home, at the expense of the social services department, rather than have her painful hip joint replaced. The cumulative cost to the tax- and rate-payer, however, may be very much higher and the old lady much less happy. Advocates of age-based rationing of health services are too ready to assert that depriving old people of healthcare will necessarily save money. Advances in technology are increasing the applicability of secondary healthcare to older and frailer people but policies aimed merely at capping costs may prevent full economic efficiency, as well as maximal clinical effectiveness, to be attained. In other words, the working of the structure and in-built incentives of health service funding need to come under the scrutiny of HSR, in addition to more tractable, but also more trivial, matters, such as whether anticoagulant clinics are best run by doctors or by nurses.

In the category of the unthinkable, one example must suffice. British general practice enjoys favoured status with politicians because they see it as a throttle point for controlling costs. But we do not know in an evidence-based way that it is necessarily the most efficient means of providing primary healthcare. It is conceivable that in some situations, and for patients such as disabled older people with complex problems, primary healthcare might be better provided from specialist units as part of integrated primary and secondary care systems. We would never be allowed to find out by randomised trials, but we might gain insight from systematic and critical comparisons of health and social services in the other nations, particularly in Europe.

Whether one argues from an individualist or a collectivist standpoint, prevention of disability in later life carries high priority. Individualists do not want older people to have to suffer disability and the dependency it brings, and collectivists do not want to have to pay for the care needed by disabled people. Disability is most usefully conceptualised as arising from an ecological gap between what an environment demands and what an individual is capable of doing. At a clinical level this gap can be closed by therapeutic intervention to improve patients' capabilities and by prosthetic measures to reduce the demands of their environments. At a population level we should seek to make our environment less disabling for an ageing population. Apart from issues of safer cities and more rigorous traffic control, we can enhance the ease of visual perception and cognitive mapping of outdoor and indoor environments. Environments that are safer and pleasanter for older people are safer and pleasanter for us all.

Minimising the need for care

Disability in later life is rarely due to a single disease, and general age-associated processes also contribute. For a strategic approach to reducing the need for services, we need to think about ageing as a whole and not just about specific age-associated diseases. Ageing in the sense of senescence is the loss of adaptability of an organism as time passes. Loss of adaptability at an organismic level is manifest in a rise with age in the risk of dying. In order to understand the evolution of ageing it is important to recognise that even if we did not age we would all still die eventually. Death would come from disease, accident, famine or warfare, but the chance of death would be constant with age or might even fall as natural selection weeded out those less adept at staying alive. In the human species, senescence first becomes manifest around the age of 12 or 13 when the age-specific mortality rates which fall from birth turn upwards. Then after early perturbations, due mostly to violent deaths, age-specific mortality rises close to exponentially throughout adult life. Rates in males are higher at all ages than in females and there is no discontinuity corresponding in later life to provide any biological basis for distinguishing 'the elderly' from the rest of the human race. Death is a rather crude measure of loss of adaptability but the prevalence of disability[12] also shows a continuous and exponential rise through the years of adult life.

Loss of adaptability in ageing is caused by interactions between intrinsic (genetic) factors and extrinsic factors in environment and lifestyle. Extrinsic factors in ageing can be detected by conventional epidemiological methods, seeking differences in the ageing patterns of populations living in different places, different ways or different times. Extrinsic factors have been shown by such means to be relevant to age-associated trends in blood pressure,[13] hearing loss[14] and femoral fractures,[15] as well as the incidence of vascular disease and cancers.

Identification of the period in life when extrinsic factors act is crucial in a search for interventions. Those citizens who will provide the challenge to the health services of 2030 are already among us and already in their thirties. Benefits from enhanced exercise levels, reducing blood pressure and giving up smoking can be seen in middle age and later. For maximal benefit, extrinsic factors may need to be controlled earlier in life. The amount of bone and muscle laid down in childhood and adolescence may be important determinants of disability in old age. Simple lack of muscle strength in elderly women probably accounts for most of the sex difference in disability rates in later life revealed in Table 13.1. Barker has pushed the origins of late age-associated vascular disease back into the uterine environment by linking measures of intrauterine development with hypertension and coronary heart disease in later life.[16] The intrauterine environment can certainly do direct damage to a fetus, as the fetal alcohol syndrome demonstrates, and subtler effects may emerge if the hypothesis of a uterine factor modulating the hereditability of intelligence survives further study.[17] Intelligence evolved because it improves survival; we must expect it to have a similar influence in modern society. Education as an enhancer of intelligence is potentially one of the most important extrinsic influences on the lifelong pattern of age-associated disease and disability.

If the Barker effect is confirmed, it may reflect the existence of a metabolic switch[18] allowing a fetus to adjust its metabolism to the sort of environment it is destined to be born into. Deprived fetuses could do well on average by switching on mechanisms for storing any excess energy as body fat, but conserving resources in the longer term by restricting body size. If such a fetus finds itself in a better environment than foreshadowed it would be at risk of the metabolic consequences of relative overnutrition. These consequences include a high risk of diabetes and vascular disease in middle life. The mechanism is analogous to that proposed for the possessors of the thrifty genes postulated in populations that have been under heavy selection pressure from famine,[19] and which may contribute to health problems of some immigrant groups in the UK.[20] If this is so, we should not regard an infant from a deprived intrauterine environment as inevitably programmed to develop vascular disease but rather as more susceptible than average to the hazards of relative overnutrition and its interactions with other risk factors. The ageing participants in long-term cohort studies[21] may help to identify aspects of adult lifestyle that mitigate the disadvantages of intrauterine and childhood deprivation. These mechanisms are important in the context of social inequalities as well as of ageing. Perhaps in the next millennium we may see individual prescriptions of lifestyles to match individual patterns of metabolism.

So far much of what we know about extrinsic influences on ageing relate to unsurprising matters such as avoiding smoking and excess alcohol, controlling blood pressure, maintaining a sensible diet and body weight, and, perhaps most pervasively, regular, adequate exercise. Observational studies suggest that exercise helps to establish and maintain bone and muscle strength, prevents vascular disease and may have other more general effects on well-being.[22] Randomised controlled trials of lifestyle modifications are unlikely to be widely applicable, although trials have indicated that exercise can reduce falls in later life[23] and produce short-term increases in weight-bearing bone density.[24] Demonstrating that lifestyle changes could be beneficial in improving the pattern of ageing is less difficult than persuading people to adopt them. Health education improves knowledge but has little effect in changing behaviour. We need to know a great deal more about the opportunities and incentives for optimal lifestyles that could inform a public health approach to an ageing society. Again, thinking needs to be radical and strategic. If disability in later life can be reduced by increasing physical exercise at all ages, this might be better achieved not by homilies from GPs but by making urban environments safer and pleasanter for walkers and cyclists.

The future

The public health response to the ageing population is to adjust the environment and lifestyle of the nation to produce the best overall outcome given the genetic propensities of the population. The findings from the National Health and Nutrition Examination Studies in the USA support the view that the aim of lengthening life but shortening disability is attainable by a policy of postponement as prevention. We may even hope that this will also reduce healthcare costs, and again the American data are encouraging.[25] We cannot be sure, however, because the nature of disability, as well as its average duration, may change with age. Care for older people with dementia could be more expensive than for younger people with stroke. So far, little work has been done on predicting the effects of 'substitute morbidity' arising as causes of disability and death change over time.[26] This is a particular concern in relation to research on intrinsic ageing which, if successful, will lengthen maximum life span but will have unpredictable effects on the incidence and duration of disability. We can recognise the difficulties that might arise if lengthening the lives of people, even with a reduction in the average time spent in a disabled state, increased their lifetime costs of healthcare. We must have the courage not to flinch from research that might benefit humanity simply because it might also present politicians with some difficult decisions.

References

1   World Health Organisation Scientific Group on the Epidemiology of Ageing (1984) *The Uses of Epidemiology in the Study of the Elderly*. Technical Report Series No. 706. WHO, Geneva.

2   Grimley Evans J (1993) Healthy active life expectancy (HALE) as an index of effectiveness of health and social services for elderly people. *Age and Ageing*. **22**: 297–301.

3   Dunnell K (1995) Population review: (2) are we healthier? In: *Population Trends 82*, pp. 12–18. HMSO, London.

4   Manton KG, Corder L and Stallard E (1997) Chronic disability trends in elderly United States populations: 1982–1994. *Proceedings of the National Academy of Sciences USA*. **94**: 2593–8.

5   Katz S, Branch LG, Bransom MH *et al.* (1983) Active life expectancy. *New England Journal of Medicine*. **309**: 1218–24.

6   van de Water HPA, Boshuizen HC and Perenboom RJN (1996) Health expectancy in the Netherlands 1983–1990. *European Journal of Public Health*. **6**: 21–8.

7   Kemper P and Murtaugh CM (1991) Lifetime use of nursing home care. *New England Journal of Medicine*. **324**: 595–600.

8   Nuttall SR, Blackwood RJL, Bussell BMH *et al.* (1994) Financing long-term care in Great Britain. *Journal of the Institute of Actuaries*. **121**: 1–53.

9   Grimley Evans J (1981) Hospital care for the elderly. In: REA Shegog (ed.) *The Impending Crisis of Old Age*, pp. 133–46. Nuffield Provincial Hospitals Trust, London.

10   Rubenstein LZ (1990) The efficacy of geriatric assessment programmes. In: RL Kane, J Grimley Evans and D Macfadyen (eds) *Improving the Health of Older People. A World View*, pp. 417–39. Oxford University Press, Oxford.

11   Laing W and Hall M (1991) *Agenda for Health 1991. The Challenges of Ageing*. The Association of the British Pharmaceutical Industry, London.

12   Martin J, Meltzer H and Elliot D (1988) *Office of Population Censuses and Surveys Social Survey Division. OPCS Surveys of Disability in Great Britain Report 1. The Prevalence of Disability Among Adults*. HMSO, London.

13   Prior IAM, Grimley Evans J, Davidson F and Lindsay M (1968) Sodium intake and blood pressure in two Polynesian populations. *New England Journal of Medicine*. **279**: 515–20.

14   Goycoolea MV, Goycoolea HG, Rodrigues LG *et al.* (1986) Effect of life in industrialized societies on hearing in natives of Easter Island. *Laryngoscope*. **96**: 1391–6.

15   Grimley Evans J, Seagroatt V and Goldacre MJ (1997) Secular trends in proximal femoral fracture, Oxford Record Linkage Study area and England 1968–86. *Journal of Epidemiology and Community Health*. **51**: 424–9.

16   Barker DJP (1992) The fetal origins of diseases in old age. *European Journal of Clinical Nutrition*. **46**(Suppl.3): S3–9.

17   Devlin B, Daniels M and Roeder K (1997) The heritability of IQ. *Nature*. **388**: 468–71.

18   Grimley Evans J (1993) Metabolic switches in ageing. *Age and Ageing*. **22**: 79–81.

19   Neel JV (1962) Diabetes mellitus: A 'thrifty' genotype rendered detrimental by progress? *American Journal of Human Genetics*. **14**: 353–61.

20   McKeigue PM, Shah B and Marmott MG (1991) Relation of central obesity and insulin resistance with high diabetes prevalence and cardiovascular risk in South Asians. *Lancet*. **337**: 382–6.

21   Wadsworth MEJ, Cripps HA, Midwinter RA and Colley JRT (1985) Blood pressure at age 36 years and social and familial factors, cigarette smoking and body mass in a national birth cohort. *British Medical Journal*. **291**: 1534–8.

22   Curfman CD (1993) The health benefits of exercise. A critical reappraisal. *New England Journal of Medicine*. **328**: 574–6.

23   Province MA, Hadley EC, Hornbrook MC *et al.* (1995) The effects of exercise on falls in elderly patients. A preplanned meta-analysis of the FICSIT trials. *Journal of the American Medical Association*. **273**: 1341–7.

24   Brooke-Wavell K, Jones PRM and Hardman AE (1996) Brisk walking reduces calcaneal bone loss in post-menopausal women. *Clinical Science*. **92**: 75–80.

25   van de Water HPA, van Vliet HA and Boshuizen HC (1995) *The Impact of 'Substitute Morbidity and Mortality' on Public Health Policy*. Prevention and Health Division Public Health and Prevention, Toegepast Natuurwetenschappelijk Onderzoek, Leiden.

26   Government Actuary (1996) *National Population Projections 1994-based*. HMSO, London.

27   Parker CJ, Morgan K, Dewey ME *et al.* (1997) Physical illness and disability among elderly people in England and Wales: the Medical Research Council cognitive function and ageing study. *Journal of Epidemiology and Community Health*. **51**: 494–501.

CHAPTER THIRTEEN

Genetics

Ron Zimmern

Introduction

The past two decades have seen unprecedented advances in our understanding of the molecular mechanisms of disease and genetic influences, not only for conventional single gene disorders, but also in relation to common diseases such as diabetes, cardiovascular disease, hypertension, cancer, Alzheimers, schizophrenia, asthma and others. Basic medical research has given us the opportunity to understand the pathogenesis of common diseases and to exploit further the potential for both conventional and gene therapy. The genetic revolution now provides investigative and therapeutic potential for every discipline of medicine, and will in the future exert a growing influence on practice in all specialties.[1-3]

The practical application of these technologies, including the use of population screening, has been particularly fruitful in carrier detection and prenatal diagnosis for certain common single gene and/or chromosomal disorders – Down's syndrome, cystic fibrosis, fragile X – although cost-benefit and some other issues remain contentious. In relation to multifactorial disorders, the identification of BRCA1 and BRCA2, for example, has increased the pressure on cancer geneticists, oncologists and gynaecologists to establish detection programmes for breast and ovarian cancers.

Epidemiology

A number of studies have attempted to estimate the birth prevalence or the total load of genetic disease in a population. The reported data show large variations but a figure of around 4 per 1000 live births for single gene disorders and of 2 per 1000 for chromosomal abnormalities was found in one large survey in Canada. The total load of genetic disease before the age of 25 was estimated in that study to be around 50 per 1000 live births, the remaining proportion being due to common disorders with a significant genetic component. Congenital anomalies have multifactorial causes and both genetic and environmental factors play a part. The inclusion of all congenital abnormalities as part of the genetic load would increase the estimate of the figure for birth prevalence to 80 per 1000 live births.[4]

Other studies have shown that in a paediatric hospital one in five admissions is accounted for by a genetic defect or congenital malformation and one in three by a disease with a genetic component.[5] These figures derive from work in the last decade and it is likely that they will turn out to be an underestimate in today's clinical practice.

The ethical, legal and social framework

Great interest is shown in genetics and related matters by the world at large. In almost every newspaper each day there is some material based on genetic or molecular science. Books devoted to genetics, its scientific foundations and social and ethical implications, appear to be in abundance, as do textbooks of molecular medicine and web sites devoted to genetics, whether for clinical geneticists, molecular geneticists or for the lay public. Moral philosophers have found fruitful work in the study of gene ethics, while those involved in the public understanding of science use genetics as a paradigm for their investigations.[6,7] Social scientists in abundance have seen fit to study the sociological implications of the gene, some taking a reasonably positive line abut the benefits of genetic science, others showing concern and antagonism, particularly with regard to the implications of what they regard to be genetic determinism or genetic discrimination.[8,9]

Privacy, confidentiality and informed consent are topics that have rightly been taken seriously be genetic practitioners, and by ethicists and policy makers.[10] A diagnosis of a familial problem raises implications not only for the patient but for her family. Pressures are placed on both the patient and her professional adviser about whether, or how, relatives should be informed about their possible risk of developing a familial disorder. The ethical principles which determine the 'right to know' or the 'right not to know' take on a particular importance in these situations.[11] The potential for accurate prenatal diagnosis in patients and the subsequent decision about the termination of the affected fetus also raises ethical dilemmas, as do the issues of informed consent in children and in people with reduced mental capacity. More recently the issues of cloning have brought forth a huge response from professionals and public alike.[12]

The possibility of genetic discrimination has been considered in the context of insurance, mortgages, pensions and employment. The life and medical insurance industry have, for example, taken a keen interest in the subject. The Association of British Insurers have now published a Code of Practice on Genetic Testing, while the Human Genetics Advisory Commission has set out its own views.[13,14] Although accepting the long-held principle of insurers that they may exercise discretion in setting premiums based on an individual's risk, the Commission concluded that at present the industry did not have the information necessary to make actuarially sound use of specific genetic test results.

In the context of patenting genetic material, an EU Directive on the Legal Protection of Biotechnological Inventions has now been agreed.[15] Some of the issues that have concerned those working in this field are shown in Box 13.1. They have been well summarised recently in a monograph from the Regional Genetics Centre in Cardiff.[16]

Box 13.1:   Ethical, social and legal issues

Privacy and confidentiality
Informed consent
Insurance
Pensions
Employment
Patenting of genetic information
Human cloning

Policy considerations

Policy makers in the UK have begun to address some of these issues, but there has been little to suggest that the NHS has taken into account the implications of developments in genetics and molecular medicine for either service provision or disease prevention. The NHS must now plan strategically for these advances. Developing trends in biotechnology, including the growth in bioengineered pharmaceuticals, the pharmaceutical industry's vision of using an individual's genomic make-up to predict their predisposition to common diseases and their response to tailored pharmacological treatments, are examples of technological development which must sooner or later impinge on the NHS. Health authorities have to date not been instructed to make any strategic assessment of these trends for the development of services in their localities, nor has their been any concerted policy to educate and inform managers and policy makers of the implications of modern genetic and molecular technology.

The two recent reports of the Genetics Advisory Group to the NHS Central R&D Committee highlight the potential of genetic science for medical practice.[17,18] However, these publications have had little practical impact on policy development within the service. This is not to imply that these issues have been entirely neglected. Within the wider DoH the government has involved itself in response to the House of Commons Select Committee Report on Human Genetics by establishing a Human Genetics Advisory Committee under the Chairmanship of Sir Colin Campbell, and an Advisory Committee on Genetics Testing under the Reverend Dr John Polkinghorne.[19] The Human Fertilisation and Embryology Authority was established in 1991 in response to the Human Fertilisation and Embryology Act 1990, and the Gene Therapy Advisory Committee in 1994, following the recommendations of the Clothier Committee on the Ethics of Gene Therapy in 1992.

The potential for public health action is now enormous. The development of standards and guidelines for genetic testing programmes, including the necessary ethical safeguards and the place of counselling, require detailed consideration.[20,21] The evaluation of clinical interventions and of population-based programmes in this field is still in its infancy, while the education of health professionals in a basic understanding of genetic and molecular science and their ethical ramifications has hardly begun.

Simple epidemiological principles such as the distinction between testing and screening are ill understood. Genetic testing is the application of a test in a clinical setting to determine whether or not a patient has a genetic disease or is susceptible (or at increased risk) of developing a disease for which there is a genetic component. In this context, the patient presents to the physician, with or without symptoms, or is sought by the physician because he or she is a member of a family with a known genetic disease. By contrast, genetic screening is the process by which the physician systematically tests a population or sub-population of patients in order to diagnose hidden genetic disease or genetic susceptibility. There are few instances in which genetic screening is justified. Examples include the PKU neonatal screening programme, screening for thalassaemia in Sardinia and for Tay Sachs disease in the Ashkenazy population in a number of states in the USA. In most instances, expert groups have come out against any form of population genetic screening; for example, BRCA1 or BRCA2 in breast cancer, DNA mismatch repair genes in colorectal cancer, or HFE mutations in hereditary haemochromatosis.[22–24]

In the case of genetic testing, when the patient might present to the physician, anxious because of a family history of a disease such as breast cancer or colorectal cancer, the situation is more complicated. Without doubt, a family history confers an increased risk. Using breast cancer as an example, having one first-degree relative with the disease doubles the risk. Does this in itself justify the use of genetic testing in that patient? Almost certainly not. First the chances that the family is a carrier of the BRCA1 mutation is likely to be small. Second, most cases of breast cancer with some family history are likely to be associated with a number of low penetrance susceptibility genes, as yet unidentified, rather than the high penetrance, dominantly inherited BRCA1 or BRCA2. Third, the BRCA1 and BRCA2 genes are huge and over 200 mutations have now been reported. Technology is at present unable to cope with this diversity in any cost-effective way. Unless the mutation has already been identified in a relative with the disease, testing the asymptomatic relative is unlikely to be fruitful. This means that genetic testing for BRCA1 or BRCA2 should be confined to situations where the family history is strong enough to confer at least a 40% chance that a mutation in those genes might be detected in a family member with the disease. Examples include pedigrees with four or more affected relatives on the same side of the family or three affected relatives with an average age at diagnosis of less than 40 or breast/ovarian cancer families with three affected relatives and an average age of diagnosis of less than 60.[22,25]

Another distinction of importance is that between genetic disease and genetic susceptibility. Cystic fibrosis, Duchenne's muscular dystrophy and familial polyposis coli may all be considered genetic diseases. The presence of the appropriate mutation in the gene confers on the individual the manifestations of the disease. A test, even subject to imperfect sensitivity and specificity, is likely to predict with some accuracy the presence or absence of the features of those disorders. By contrast, in other conditions such as ankylosing spondylitis, coronary artery disease or Alzheimers, to be HLA B27 positive, to be a heterozygote for the LDL receptor gene or a carrier of the apoe-4 allele confers only an increased risk for developing those conditions. The presence of the genetic marker is not predictive, and those with it may not develop the disease in question, while those without it may end up with the disease. The situation is thus very much like that of stroke or heart disease in the presence of raised blood pressure or cholesterol levels. The ethical and clinical issues differ greatly depending on whether one is dealing with disease or with susceptibility.

Within the specific context of the NHS, a strategic assessment of the organisation of genetic services, of the nature and structure of regional genetic centres and the organisation of molecular genetic and cyto-genetic laboratories, of training requirements and structures for physicians in all specialities, and of the role of primary care in the future delivery of genetic services will all be required. To take one of these issues in greater detail, one might ask how best to organise molecular genetics services in future years. Is it appropriate that they should be small, research-orientated units, linked to clinical genetic centres, or will a substantial increase in demand for such tests by all clinical specialities in the post-genomic era, and the availability of automated but expensive sequencing technology, determine a service pattern in which such tests are carried out in a few large centralised laboratories for maximum cost-effectiveness?

A public health approach is urgently needed, using epidemiological studies of genetic polymorphisms which predispose to disease and of the environmental factors which interact with them, of the burden of morbidity and mortality, including hospitalisation rates and economic costs, and of the place of and indications for genetic testing and population screening programmes.[26] The R&D programme has as yet hardly considered these issues. Their elucidation will require the skills of fundamental scientific research, linking the molecular to the epidemiological, drawing on medical informatics, biostatistics, social science, health economics, all part of the traditional research base of public health, as well as the skills of health services research.

There is as yet little evidence that genetic and molecular science will directly benefit the health of individuals, but the potential is clearly there, and most informed opinion is of the view that such benefits will materialise.[27] The debate is primarily about timescales rather than the ultimate result. Public health physicians should take action and prepare for the time when the evidence requires us to act and to provide the necessary interventions. They should equally resist public clamour for action and service provision where the evidence of benefit to health does not exist. A good example of how growing knowledge and multidisciplinary discussions with clear epidemiological advice may lead to a better appreciation of the place of and indications for genetic testing is familial breast cancer, discussed in earlier paragraphs.

The next few years will probably require public health practitioners to resist and control demand rather than to push for developments, but as genetic science advances and evidence of benefit accumulates, public health considerations should cause the service to respond in an appropriate manner. The need for this aspect of public health medicine to be evidence-based is as great in genetics as in the other aspects of clinical practice and policy making. These policy issues are all summarised in Box 13.2.

Box 13.2:   Policy issues

Infrastructure
Research
Training and education
Service provision
   • resource implications
   • laboratory services
   • clinical genetics as a speciality
   • counselling
   • genetic associates
   • primary care

The scope for preventive action

The Committee of Inquiry into the Future Development of the Public Health Function (The Acheson Report) in 1988 defined public health as

the science and art of preventing disease, prolonging life and promoting health through organised efforts of society.[28]

This definition clearly envisages the involvement of public health in policy. Some of these were discussed in the section above. The definition also emphasises the importance of an underlying scientific base and its role in preventing disease and promoting health. In this section we discuss the scope for prevention through public health action.

Genetic mechanisms influence the prevalence of disease and ill health, and must be considered in establishing population-based policies and public heath action in much the same way as they have been in the treatment of individual patients. The interaction of gene and environment has been well established at the level of the cell and its bio-chemical pathways; similar interactions take place at the population level, where the differential sensitivities of diverse populations in society to environmental influences are progressively exposed.[29] Evolutionary mechanisms, working through natural selection, rely on the interplay between genetic and environmental factors.[30,31] Biologists are now increasingly aware of the nature of these interactive mechanisms and steer clear of a view which espouses a pure genetic determinism.[32]

These scientific insights now call for an appraisal of the place of genetic influences, and the developing ethical, social and legal framework, in the development of public health policy and the scope for preventing disease. The public health agenda has to date been influenced almost entirely by a consideration of the environmental influences on health.[33,34] These influences remain important, and a continued momentum on health promotional interventions directed at the external environment will be essential for the public health function. Nevertheless, insights generated from molecular biology and genetic studies require that we now attend to and explore the complexities of the interaction between genetic and environmental factors, that we regard the interaction between 'nature' and 'nurture' as complementary rather than competing explanations, and that we attempt to promote health and prevent disease by having regard to how environmental factors and human behaviour might have differential effects on disease risk by virtue of the genetic susceptibility of particular individuals.[35]

It is now possible to implement preventive strategies which do not rely entirely on manipulating the genome or changing the gene pool. To date, genetic disease has been prevented either by advising couples not to reproduce or by a programme of prenatal diagnosis followed by selective termination of the affected fetus. In the future, gene therapy may provide some limited preventive potential. This type of 'genotypic' prevention conjures up in the minds of some the spectre of eugenics.[36] The distaste for fetal destruction and the ethical issues which surround it have led to a different approach, based on developing a much greater understanding of gene–environment interaction and preventive action resulting from selective environmental manipulation for susceptible sub-groups in the population. This approach has been termed 'phenotypic' prevention. It allows us not only to use clinical interventions selectively on individuals with known genetic susceptibilities but also to advise on the degree of risk posed by different environmental determinants, such as diet or tobacco, on populations with particular genetic susceptibilities. These approaches to treatment and prevention will require high-quality genetic services as well as a significant increase in the research effort required for an understanding of genetic and environmental interactions at a cellular level. These two approaches to prevention are outlined in Box 13.3.

Box 13.3:   Approaches to prevention

'Genotypic'
- Contraception
- Selective termination of pregnancy
- Pre-implantation diagnosis and selective destruction of embryo
- Genetic manipulation – gene therapy

'Phenotypic'
- Clinical intervention for susceptible individuals and populations
- Environmental manipulation for susceptible individuals and populations
- Behavioural change in susceptible individuals

Examples of the efficacy of the 'phenotypic' approach are as yet few, but already a great deal of knowledge has been gathered in diseases as diverse as non-insulin dependent diabetes and schizophrenia.[37,38] Genes responsible for the metabolism of drugs and environmental toxins have been known for over 10 years to play a part in determining the risk of cancers and other illnesses. For example, individuals may be shown to be fast or slow metabolisers dependent on the presence of several different mutations in the gene for cytochrome P-450, an enzyme responsible for the oxidation of debrisoquine and other chemicals. Fast metabolisers appear to have an increased lung cancer risk.[39]

The consequence of these developments is that public health practitioners must embrace the new genetics with understanding and enthusiasm and pay greater credence to its impact on preventive activities than hitherto. Public health professionals of all disciplines will require education and updating, while the public will need to be informed about genetic issues. Health service managers must also be alerted to the potential for health gain arising from basic genetic and molecular research and be persuaded to invest in a managed fashion in genetic programmes where benefits can be shown.

Conclusion

Public health genetics is as yet in its infancy. Rapidly advancing science and patient and public expectations require a strategic approach to the assessment, development and implementation of genetic services using all the skills of the public health practitioner. The development of policy for these services must start now, given the pace of genetic science, particularly in view of the need to educate and train a whole cohort of practitioners in the principles of genetics and molecular science. The focus on prevention embraced within the new paradigm of the NHS should seek to use to its best advantage the opportunities embraced by a better understanding of the gene, while holding back those demands of both patients and physicians where evidence is insufficient to justify significant investment. The grasp of both medical and management perspectives available to the public health physician imposes a special responsibility to take up and develop this aspect of public health practice.

References

1   Weatherill DJ (1991) *The New Genetics and Clinical Practice.* Oxford University Press, Oxford.

2   Gelehrter TD, Collins FS and Ginsburg D (1998) *Principles of Medical Genetics.* Williams and Wilkins, Baltimore.

3   Scriver CR, Beaudet AL, Sly WS and Valle D (1995) *The Metabolic and Molecular Basis of Inherited Disease* (7e). McGraw Hill, New York.

4   Baird PA, Anderson TW, Newcombe HB and Lowry RB (1988) Genetic disorders in children and young adults: a population study. *American Journal of Human Genetics.* **42**: 677–93.

5   Rimoin DL, Connor JM and Pyeritz RE (1996) Nature and frequency of genetic disease. In: DL Rimoin, JM Connor and RE Pyeritz (eds) *Principles and Practice of Medical Genetics*. Churchill Livingstone, Edinburgh.

6   Kitcher P (1996) *The Lives to Come: the genetic revolution and human possibilities*. Penguin Books, London.

7   Harris J (1998) *Clones, Genes and Immortality: ethics and the genetic revolution*. Oxford University Press, Oxford.

8   Lewontin RC (1993) *The Doctrine of DNA: biology as ideology*. Penguin Books, London.

9   Marteau T and Richards M (1996) *The Troubled Helix: social and psychological implications of the new human genetics*. Cambridge University Press, Cambridge.

10   Nuffield Council on Bioethics (1993) *Genetic Screening: ethical issues*. Nuffield Council on Bioethics, London.

11   Chadwick R, Levitt M and Shickle D (eds) (1997) *The Right to Know and the Right Not to Know*. Avebury Press, Aldershot.

12   Human Genetics Advisory Commission. (1998) *Cloning Issues in Reproduction, Science and Medicine*. Department of Health, London

13   Association of British Insurers (1997) *Genetic Testing: ABI Code of Practice*. Association of British Insurers, London.

14   Human Genetics Advisory Commission. (1998) *The Implications of Genetic Testing for Life Insurance*. DoH, London

15   European Parliament and the Council of the European Union (1998) *The Legal Protection of Biotechnological Inventions*. Directive 98 of the European Parliament and Council.

16   Harper PS and Clarke AJ (1997) *Genetics, Society and Clinical Practice*. Bios Scientific Publishers, Oxford.

17   Genetics Research Advisory Group. Chairman: Prof Martin Bobrow (1995) *A First Report to the NHS Central Research and Development Committee on the New Genetics*. DoH, London.

18   Genetics Research Advisory Group. Chairman: Prof John Bell (1995) *A Second Report to the NHS Central Research and Development Committee on the New Genetics*. DoH, London

19   Government Response to the Third Report of the House of Commons Select Committee on Science and Technology, 1994–95 Session (1996) *Human Genetics: the science and its consequences*. Cm 3061. HMSO, London.

20   Advisory Committee on Genetic Testing (1997) *Consultation on Genetic Testing for Late Onset Disorders*. Health Departments of the UK, London.

21   Task Force on Genetic Testing of the NIH-DOE Working Group on Ethical, Legal and Social Implications of Human Genome Research. N Holtzman and MS Watson (eds) (1997) *Promoting Safe and Effective Genetic Testing in the United States*. National Institutes of Health, Bethesda.

22   Unit for Public Health Genetics, Cambridge (1998) *Report of a Consensus Meeting on the Management of Women with a Family History of Breast Cancer*. Unpublished.

23   Winnawer SJ, Fletcher RH, Miller L *et al.* (1997) Colorectal cancer screening: clinical guidelines and rationale. *Gastroenterology*. **112**: 594–642.

24   Burke W, Thomson E, Khoury MJ *et al.* (1998) Consensus statement. Hereditary hemochromatosis. Gene discovery and its implications for population-based screening. *JAMA.* **280**: 172–8.

25   Collins FS (Editorial) (1996) BRCA1: Lots of mutations, lots of dilemmas. *New England Journal of Medicine.* **334**: 186–8.

26   Khoury MJ (Editorial) (1996) From genes to public health: the applications of genetic technology in disease prevention. *American Journal of Public Health.* **86**: 1717–22.

27   Weatherall D (1995) *Medicine and the Quiet Art: medical research and patient care.* Oxford University Press, Oxford.

28   The Report of the Committee of Inquiry into the Future Development of the Public Health Function (1988) *Public Health in England.* Cm 289. HMSO, London.

29   Lewin B (1994) *Genes V.* Oxford University Press, Oxford.

30   Darwin C (1859) *The Origin of Species.* Penguin edition (1985). Penguin Books, London.

31   Cavalli-Sforza LL and Cavalli-Sforza F (1995) *The Great Human Diasporas: the history of diversity and evolution.* Addison-Wesley, San Francisco.

32   Rose S (1997) *Lifelines: biology, freedom, determinism.* Allen Lane/The Penguin Press, London.

33   Jacobson B, Smith A and Whitehead M (1991) *The Nation's Health: a strategy for the 1990s.* King Edward's Hospital Fund for London.

34   Department of Health (1998) *Our Healthier Nation: a contract for health. A Consultation Paper.* Cm 3852. DoH, London.

35   Williams RR, Hunt SC, Hopkins PN *et al.* (1997) Practical benefits from understanding the genetics of chronic disease. In: I Day and SE Humphries (eds) *Genetics of Common Diseases.* Bios Scientific Publishers, Oxford.

36   Juengst E (1998) What should we mean by 'prevention' in public health genetics. In: *1st Annual Conference on Genetics and Public Health.* Atlanta, Georgia, May 13–15, 1998.

37   McCarthy M (1997) Approaches to determining the genetic basis of non-insulin-dependent diabetes mellitus. In: I Day and SE Humphries (eds) *Genetics of Common Diseases.* Bios Scientific Publishers, Oxford.

38   Owen MJ and O'Donovan MC (1997) Finding susceptibility genes for schizophrenia. In: I Day and SE Humphries (eds) *Genetics of Common Diseases.* Bios Scientific Publishers, Oxford.

39   Caporaso N, Hayes RB, Dosemeci M *et al.* (1989) Lung cancer risk, occupational exposure and the debrisoquine metabolic phenotype. *Cancer Research.* **49**: 3675–9.

PART 2

Meeting the challenges: practice perspectives

CHAPTER FOURTEEN

Multidisciplinary public health in practice

Ros Levenson, Nikki Joule and Jill Russell

This chapter reflects on public health in practice in the NHS over the past few years, with particular reference to the development of the multidisciplinary contribution to public health. It also looks forward to how the multidisciplinary contribution could be developed and enhanced, and made relevant to the new structures and roles that will follow from recent policy developments including the White Paper *The New NHS: modern, dependable*[1] and the Green Paper, *Our Healthier Nation.*[2]

As is evident from other chapters in this book, public health is by no means the exclusive territory of the NHS. Public health activities also take place in local authorities, in industry, in the voluntary sector and in the wider community. However, the NHS itself remains a key location for an important part of the spectrum of public health activities, and an understanding of public health in the NHS is an essential component of making sense of the wider picture.

The material in this chapter draws extensively on a research project which was commissioned by the NHS Executive and undertaken by Ros Levenson, Nikki Joule and Jill Russell for the King's Fund[3] and considers the findings of that project in the light of foreseeable changes in the NHS. The research was completed before either the White Paper or the Green Paper had been conceived and health authorities were still at a fairly early stage of learning how to develop their commissioning role and how to utilise public health perspectives in doing so. Although we now have a much clearer idea on how both commissioning and public health may develop in the NHS in future, the King's Fund research provides a baseline against which future changes can be understood, as well as providing information about some of the challenges for multidisciplinary public health which are likely to remain relevant to the future.

The King's Fund research project on *Developing public health in the NHS – the multidisciplinary contribution*

The aim of the project was to provide the NHS with knowledge on a range of good practice in relation to multidisciplinary public health, and to help progress the further establishment of good practice in health authorities. Following a seminar in the summer of 1996 to identify the issues and the basis of good practice in multidisciplinary public health in the NHS, a review was carried out to provide information on good practice in developing and integrating the complementary contributions of a range of professions and disciplines in multidisciplinary public health in health authorities and GP purchasing.

The project focused on public health in relation to purchasing, and in particular on what was happening in health authorities. Public health in primary care settings was explored to a lesser extent, and public health in provider settings was examined only briefly.

The project brief gave an indication of what the NHS Executive saw as multidisciplinary, as follows:

> *Multidisciplinary ... refers to public health specialists from the social sciences, natural sciences, clinical sciences, humanities, environmental health and clinical professions (medicine, nursing and professions allied to medicine) etc., who are working in health authorities (but not solely confined to Service Departments of Public Health), GP purchasing practices or are doing work for them, for example, from a university or consulting base.*

However, the research was undoubtedly complicated by the fact that, in practice, many of the key terms in this project (public health, multidisciplinary, purchasing) have a variety of meanings for different people. Differing interpretations of the key words were found amongst those working in the same health authority and amongst those from the same profession.

The variety of working definitions and different formulations of the key issues for the project became increasingly evident in the pilot stages of the research. In view of this it was not practical to impose definitions on the respondents. Rather, in order to capture the richness and diversity of people's perceptions of these key concepts, the research team used the definitions presented by the people in the health authorities and other sites that were studied. As this issue had been anticipated, to some extent, early in the project, respondents were actually asked to provide definitions for some of the key concepts. In other cases these were explored or noted as they arose.

Methodology

The project selected 11 areas for case-study investigation. A two-tiered approach to the identification of cases was adopted. First, cases comprised health authorities and at this level the researchers looked broadly at the relationship between public health and purchasing to examine the context within which multidisciplinary working occurred. Within each health authority, cases of specific initiatives that illustrated multidisciplinary working were identified and examined in detail.

A wide range of professional groups and public health/purchasing roles were covered by this process (health authority Chief Executives, Directors of Public Health, health promotion, finance, health policy, primary care, research and development, nursing, social scientists, town planning, etc.). The range of case studies illustrated examples of multidisciplinary approaches to:

- developing information on local variations
- new frameworks for purchasing for health gain
- priority setting
- strategic inter-agency partnerships
- community development
- multidisciplinary public health work on mental health
- needs assessment in general practice
- GP forums
- community profiles.

Different ways of working

It was evident that there was no single way of working that could provide a blueprint for multidisciplinary public health in all health authorities. Health authorities differed from each other in the models they used, as well as using different models from time to time within the same health authority. Nevertheless, we observed five distinct models of working within the health authorities that we studied.

- **NHS intersectoral partnerships:** staff of health authorities, trusts and primary care practices work across agency boundaries. This may encourage the involvement of different disciplines working together for a common purpose.
- **Inter-agency alliances:** in this model, alliances are formed between the health authority and other agencies, including local authorities and other statutory and voluntary agencies.
- **Cross-directorate co-operation in health authority:** the main characteristic of this model is active co-operation between a public health directorate and other directorates within the health authority, enabling a range of disciplines and skills to be applied to a corporate aim.

- **Resource and research centres:** these centres offer a resource which complements the work done in health authorities
- **Joint work between health authority and primary care practitioners:** in this model, frameworks are developed for involving GPs, nurses, health visitors, etc. in multidisciplinary public health work.

Each of these models provided a framework for pursuing a common or overlapping agenda, between different professionals, different departments or different agencies, and we were unable to conclude that any particular model was superior to any other. Rather, they each flourished in the light of local circumstances, which varied according to many factors, such as the size of the public health department in the health authority, the commitment of individuals, and the range of possible alliances both within and outside the health authority.

Why is multidisciplinary public health a 'good thing'?

Although it is generally seen as axiomatic that multidisciplinary working in public health is desirable, it is actually worth being explicit about the benefits of a multidisciplinary approach to public health. This is particularly so if multidisciplinary working is to survive future changes in the NHS.

In fact, the King's Fund research found that there are a number of difficulties in understanding the specific added value of multidisciplinary work in public health. One is that job titles may give only the scantiest clue as to the nature of an individual's actual job. The second is that what individuals bring to bear on the public health function may reflect current role as much as it reflects the particular background or professional training of that individual.

In some instances, the added value of multidisciplinary work is a result of bringing very particular analyses together in a synergistic manner, and the value of multidisciplinary working does not lie in any particular approach. In other instances, the organisational and corporate need for staff to be flexible makes it more difficult to track what a particular member of staff offers in terms of a particular training or discipline. Multidisciplinary working often seemed to be mostly a question of different roles (or jobs), rather than different skills, except for the specialist skills of some specific posts, such as the Consultant in Communicable Disease Control. However, in spite of these complexities, the research identified a number of benefits that derived from the multidisciplinary contribution to public health.

Multidisciplinary work brings a wider range of perspectives and possible solutions to complex problems

One of the chief advantages of multidisciplinary work in public health is the opportunity that it affords for bringing a range of ideas to bear on complex issues. Different professional backgrounds and skills suggest a range of approaches. This is particularly important where a wider view of public health is taken. It follows that if public health is in itself a broad discipline, then medically qualified personnel can only contribute part of what is required. Multidisciplinary working can be a way of looking for multiple solutions to problems, rather than being one-dimensional. Multiple perspectives may well encourage a commitment to action as well as to analysis. Typical comments from the case-study sites were:

> *A problem has to be defined as broadly as possible to provoke as broad a response as possible.* [Director of Public Health (DPH)]

> *For example, if you sit around a table with a GP, nurse, youth worker, environmental health officer and someone from the chamber of commerce to discuss smoking in young people, you will get a very different picture than if you just involved the public health department. This kind of multidisciplinary input is very important given the new responsibility of health authorities for health (not just health services).* [Public Health Specialist]

In so far as a multidisciplinary approach implies the need to be open to diverse ways of thinking, training in disciplines other than medicine may be particularly beneficial. Some would assert that medical training does not encourage doctors to see problems in a complex and multifaceted way. A multidisciplinary approach can affect dramatically the focus of discussions on what can be achieved and how things can be achieved, and can contribute to discussions of the wide range of determinants of health and diverse models of service delivery.

Sometimes, multidisciplinary work brings necessary differences in emphasis that lead to what is, at its best, a creative tension. Some would argue that within a health authority, public health is based on epidemiology, research evidence and analysis, and tends to be oriented towards a grand plan. Others in the health authority may be driven by shorter-term objectives. These two perspectives need to be brought together, or each will undermine the other.

Change is more likely because of wider ownership of problems and their solutions

Multidisciplinary working tends to mean that the stakeholders of a particular initiative are actively involved and, therefore, more likely to be committed to it. In North Downs

Community Trust, for example, where a range of disciplines contributed to practice profiles, the multidisciplinary aspects of the work were evident not only in the production of practice profiles, but also in the use to which they were put. In fact, the multidisciplinary aspect of the application of the intelligence in the practice profile was larger than the multidisciplinary input into the profile itself, in so far as non-medical and non-nursing people used the material in the profiles to a greater extent than they contributed to it. However, the credibility of the information owed a lot to the fact that many different members of the team contributed to it.

Elsewhere, the development and implementation of the eligibility criteria for continuing care was cited as a good example of multidisciplinary work. It required the input of clinical medical staff, nursing staff, health service managers, and personnel from social services, housing and the nursing homes inspectorate to ensure that all the relevant ground was covered prior to the criteria being developed. In this instance, multidisciplinary working meant that a common goal was identified to which everyone was committed.

In Oxfordshire, the GP public health learning set hoped and expected that the involvement of GPs would cascade through to others, such as the nurses, in the primary health-care team, and present a more uniform front to patients.

A multidisciplinary approach brings in user and community perspectives and is necessary in order to bring in those perspectives

It has been noted that there is a range of implicit and explicit definitions of 'multidisciplinary'. The broader conceptualisation of 'multidisciplinary' encompasses lay views alongside professional views. Many commentators in recent years have argued for the inclusion of user and community perspectives in public health analysis. Davison *et al.*, for example, identify the potential for health professionals to learn from a sophisticated 'lay epidemiology',[4] and Williams and Popay[5] argue that:

> If public health research is to develop more robust and holistic explanations for patterns of health and illness in contemporary society, and contribute to more effective preventive policies, then it must utilise and build on lay knowledge – that is the meanings illness, risk, disability and so on have for people.

If one takes the view that involving lay people and hearing their views is important, then it is necessary to consider how best to have the necessary dialogues. It seems that specific training in public health medicine does not necessarily equip someone with service review skills or community engagement skills, and a wide range of disciplinary backgrounds is, therefore, useful. As one person commented: 'Doctors could talk to groups in the community, but it is not likely they would do it very well.'

Williams and Popay[5] argue not only for the pivotal role of lay knowledge in contributing to the public health agenda, but also the recognition that this knowledge requires social science methods in order to make it visible and accessible.

Multidisciplinary public health work opens the health authority's purchasing to a wider range of professional groups

The role of nursing in public health has already been recognised,[6] though it undoubtedly has further development potential. Multidisciplinary working can help to open up the health authority to other professional groups, such as nurses, professions allied to medicine and many others. This means that those professional groups perceive the health authority as more accessible and it brings the purchasing function nearer to them.

In addition, multidisciplinary work can include a much greater variety of professionals. For example, directors of finance play a key role in health authorities, and their contribution can be valuable to the public health function.

Multidisciplinary work in public health leads to better value for money

Although several respondents in the King's Fund study claimed that multidisciplinary public health helped health authorities get value for money, they mostly referred to the role of the public health function in debates about effectiveness and evidence-based practice, rather than making out a specific case for the multidisciplinary aspects of the public health function in relation to cost effectiveness. Thus, for example, one health authority had altered health visitor staffing on the basis of caseload weighting, effectiveness and needs. In this health authority, public health had had a large role in debates about rationing, and had 'withstood onslaughts', such as demands for prostate cancer screening and population-based dual energy X-ray absorptiometry (DEXA) scanning for bone density, all on effectiveness grounds. In another health authority, the DPH led the Priorities Forum, which determined, among other things, what the health authority would not purchase.

A further aspect of value for money is that, arguably, the broad range of skills that public health specialists bring are, indeed, cost effective. Naturally, it is important that value for money, rather than simple cost is taken into account. It is equally important that where doctors are needed for their particular skills, then they must be utilised, rather than a possibly cheaper but less appropriate alternative.

Multidisciplinary public health can facilitate non-healthcare interventions for health gain

An important aspect of multidisciplinary work in public health is the building of alliances with people outside the health authority, and the encouragement of collaborative and co-operative initiatives to increase health gain.

For example, in Sheffield, public health worked closely with the local authority traffic unit. Traffic-calming areas were introduced and in 2 years there were no accidents in these areas, which were previously bad spots for accidents. In Brent and Harrow, work on coronary heart disease prevention included discouraging people from using cars. This was seen as being as important as making contracts for cardiac surgery. The DPH referred to the need for 'indirect commissioning' – providing alliances and support for others. In North Staffordshire, the health authority led healthy alliances which supported community development programmes.

These approaches raise the issue of whether health authorities should spend money on non-healthcare interventions. On the one hand, it is a powerful way to spend money if the determinants of health lie outside the health service. On the other hand, only health authorities have a budget for healthcare whereas others can spend on non-healthcare.

Multidisciplinary public health can facilitate a considered response to political imperatives

While public health focuses on health in the wider sense, and not just healthcare, the rest of the health authority may have more of an operational (and centrally driven) focus. It would follow from this that if there is a greater degree of multidisciplinary work, there will be a greater ability to respond to short-term imperatives in the context of a steady public health strategy to which the whole health authority can subscribe. At the very least, the multidisciplinary commitment to strategy can bring health authorities back on course when they are blown in other directions by political, fiscal or other urgent forces. Having multidisciplinary public health values underpinning the work helps, because it allows the health authority to make a more considered response to these imperatives. As one public health specialist stated: 'The stronger the health strategy and policies, the more the rest fits into place'.

Taking multidisciplinary public health forward

In order to build on the various advantages of a multidisciplinary approach to public health, much remains to be done. The research looked in detail at the factors that facilitated and obstructed multidisciplinary public health and identified a number of issues that need to be developed or resolved.

Sometimes it was hard to separate factors that facilitated multidisciplinary public health from those that facilitated the health authority to move towards becoming a public health organisation. This fact, in itself, suggests that there is some validity in the assumption that a broader multidisciplinary conception of the public health function would better facilitate health authorities to be public health organisations. While this issue was explored in depth in the research report, it is not discussed fully here, not least because the changing face of commissioning in the light of the White Paper will fundamentally alter the ways in which health authorities function.[1] However, the factors that facilitate or encourage multidisciplinary public health remain relevant, whatever the commissioning body.

Hierarchies and tribalism

The breakdown of unnecessary professional hierarchies and the culture of tribalism within organisations is essential to improving multidisciplinary public health. In particular, the medical profession and the medical model still tend to dominate public health. At the heart of the issue, there are often power differentials that may undermine multidisciplinary work.

Formal and informal structures

For a considerable time, waves of organisational change have been very challenging, and it has become necessary to work in spite of formal structures, as well as through them. Sometimes, informal networks and ad hoc working relationships across agency boundaries later became integrated into organisational structures and provided the basis for collaborative projects, such as the South Bristol Health Park. Overall, the research found that informal structures were at least as significant as formal structures, and no one formal structure or organisational model held a monopoly of good multidisciplinary practice.

Communications

Communication was frequently identified as an area where there is room for improvement. There were, however, varied views on the relative merits of electronic or personal communication. Some based their hopes on technology, while one person ruefully observed: 'People will e-mail each other or ring, but won't walk up the stairs [to another directorate or section].'

Good communications networks for sharing and learning across disciplines, such as the Four Counties Public Health Network (Oxfordshire, Buckinghamshire, Berkshire and Northamptonshire), were of proven value.

Leadership and commitment from the top

While hierarchy, *per se,* was seen as obstructive, leadership from a committed individual was seen as very positive. Leadership on effective multidisciplinary public health could and did come from a variety of sources, be it the Chief Executive, DPH or elsewhere: 'You need this push from the Chief Executive, but also from others such as the Finance Directorate,' commented a Chief Executive.

The active support of a committed Chief Executive seemed to be very important, though in some instances support was more hands-on than in others. It was striking how frequently the leadership came from a senior woman in the organisation.

On the perennial issue of whether the public health function needed to be led by a doctor, the King's Fund study found a range of views:

> There are issues of credibility, and also the experience of being a doctor: 'We don't swallow the bullshit they [doctors] give us.' The experience of being a doctor alters our attitudes; it is not just a matter of clinical skills. [DPH]

> No. The leader does not need to be a doctor. Here, the Directorate is led by a doctor, but that is down to personal attributes rather than discipline/qualification. [Chief Executive]

> Theoretically no, in practice, yes. The profession would rebel. [Chief Executive]

> You would not need to be a doctor to be DPH, but you would have to give status to a clinical person to do the clinical interface. [DPH]

For a more detailed discussion of this issue, see Levenson *et al.*[7]

Personalities, individual relationships and team working

Possibly because informal networks were significant, human relationships mattered very much in ensuring multidisciplinary public health. Many people ascribed success to the chemistry of individuals, or trust between colleagues:

> Things start with individuals then you try to get it embedded into the culture. [Director of Public Health Nursing]

One DPH spoke of the implications of the significance of personal 'chemistry' and felt that recruitment processes had to give opportunities for people to interact to see if they could work together. A Chief Executive also felt that multidisciplinary public health was 'down to individuals'.

Trust between individuals was important. The GPs in the Oxfordshire public health learning set agreed with that, and observed that it helped to know the people in the public health department. A harmonious and positive relationship with the previous FHSA, and the continuity of that relationship, vested in the public health specialist was helpful. A Chief Executive stressed the importance of accepting that the whole is greater than the parts and felt that corporate attitudes were important, more than structures. He also mentioned 'personality' and leadership and charisma as important. His colleague, the DPH, also took the view that people's agendas, styles, inability to share, inability to see the broader picture or to co-operate would obstruct multidisciplinary working.

A senior manager spoke of the need to be part of a 'public health family'. Her Chief Executive spoke of the need to be a team player. An Assistant Director in that health authority favoured judging performance on team objectives rather than personal contributions only.

A Chief Executive said that those working in public health should be willing to share skills and the 'name' of public health. Her DPH colleague felt that effective multidisciplinary public health working occurred when there was recognition from the Chief Executive that public health is not a threat, but a contribution.

While most people might, in reality, aspire to, rather than achieve, this sublime mixture of human relationship skills, combining individual responsibility with teamwork and sharing, it is clear that the human dimension of multidisciplinary work is very important. While such relationships can thrive in a variety of contexts, stability, trust, respect and sharing are all essential to effective work, and at the very least, structures that do not undermine such attributes are essential.

Education, training and career development opportunities

People who worked in public health in non-medical disciplines perceived themselves as having much poorer opportunities for training and consequent career development. Their views are supported by a recent report on public health training and development,[8] which found that:

- the current situation with regard to the career progression of non-medical staff is chaotic and ad hoc
- the inequitable system between medical and non-medical personnel in public health acted as a barrier to joint working
- full membership of the Faculty of Public Health Medicine is still not open to non-medical staff
- training opportunities for non-medical public health staff are also ad hoc, but are improving, with several cited examples of good practice.

The continuing existence of different pay scales and career pathways for public health doctors and other public health disciplines also presented many difficulties to a truly multidisciplinary approach. The issue of differential status is closely linked to issues of training and career opportunity, and remains an obstacle.

Status of non-medically qualified people working in public health

The issue of status is closely linked to issues of training and career opportunity, and it was keenly felt by some respondents. One DPH was eloquent on this matter:

> *Historically, health promotion and other disciplines in public health defined themselves in opposition to medicine. The trick is to avoid defining yourself by opposition to medicine. There are two ways to define identity. If identity is defined as distinctiveness to 'the other', then the relationship between two groups can either be opposing, or 'I feel fully part of my professional identity, but only part of the world, and others are equally important and valid'. It is this latter view that means that we can work towards making the whole more than the sum of the parts. To take this position individuals need confidence and to recognise the value of the other. Us and themism is the most destructive element of public health, as it perhaps is of human life! [In this health authority] we are trying to work towards putting this theory into practice, in an evolutionary way. I respect the non-medical disciplines I work with as much as I do the medical and they respect me.*

A broad view of what constitutes good information and evidence in public health

While it is probable that doctors in public health tend to have a broader outlook than clinical doctors, even doctors trained in public health still have an overreliance on quantitative work and can be dismissive of qualitative work. Effective multidisciplinary public health depends on no one professional group claiming that its analysis and its perspective are more valuable than others. In particular, qualitative work needs to be fully valued alongside quantitative work.

Resource constraints – time and money

While more time and greater financial resources may not, in themselves, solve problems, resource constraints are generally obstructive features. There is evidence in recent literature that there is a difference in the extent of innovation between health authorities that are experiencing growth as a result of changes to weighted capitation, and those that are experiencing losses. As Watt and Freemantle[9] explain:

> *Purchasing authorities which experienced growth were often using the increased funds innovatively, and were attempting to purchase for health gain... Where there was no new*

money, ... ideas on how to improve the health of the local population were often subsumed to the overall aim of containing costs... In the authorities experiencing little or no growth, the role of departments of public health in facilitating change and helping to obtain improvements was often limited.

Pragmatism and political imperatives

People working in public health tend to have a keen awareness of the constant compromises that are made between idealism and pragmatism. Nevertheless, a public health approach can be unduly blown off course by the urgent demands of the day, or by national imperatives, particularly if those imperatives are developed in isolation from each other. A short-term perspective in performance management which does not take into account the nature of public health can also undermine attempts at a more strategic approach to public health. Multidisciplinary public health tends to result in a focus on health and not just healthcare, while central priorities can pull in the opposite direction, towards acute hospital issues in particular.

The future – life after the White Paper and the Green Paper

While the King's Fund research was conducted well before the 1997 White Paper, *The New NHS: modern, dependable*, and the 1998 Green Paper, *Our Healthier Nation*, many of the issues that have underpinned public health in health authorities to date still apply, though possibly with a new emphasis. The big issues of multidisciplinary working, and the considerable cultural and organisational issues that can impede it, are unlikely to be resolved by ministerial edict. Nor will the real barriers that hold back public health specialists who have the benefit of professional training in disciplines other than in medicine disappear unless the protectionism and defensiveness that have impeded a truly multidisciplinary approach to education, training and career development are tackled with a new determination at local, regional and national levels.

While the White Paper offers many exciting prospects to make commissioning at a local level a reality, it is also possible that opportunities to pursue a multidisciplinary approach could be reduced by the relatively small population to be covered by Primary Care Groups (PCGs), and it may be necessary to evaluate a range of creative options to address this potential problem.

As we have seen, different disciplines working together can produce different solutions and creative, synergistic approaches. Commissioning by local GPs and nurses may bring many benefits, particularly in terms of making the NHS more genuinely focused on primary care than has previously been the case. However, unless other disciplines, including epidemiologists, social scientists, community development workers, professions allied to medicine and others, are involved in genuine partnerships within PCGs, it is difficult to see how their perspectives will be drawn in and their skills utilised in a consistent way. It is also very important to ensure that local communities are actively involved alongside the range of multidisciplinary professionals.

Much depends on how health authorities manage the transition into their new, more strategic roles. In some respects, in the long term, they may be better able to offer a real public health perspective, without having to worry about the day-to-day minutiae of commissioning, and without the burden of the excessive bureaucratic demands of the old internal market. However, it is equally possible that in spite of their strategic role, they may lose influence precisely because they will be at one remove from many of the day-to-day commissioning activities.

We saw from the King's Fund research that there was no one model in which effective public health could be guaranteed, nor did any one model hold a monopoly of wisdom. This may provide cause for optimism, as PCGs may themselves vary considerably as they reflect local circumstances and local needs. If they can rise above the enormity of their urgent commissioning tasks, and look towards a critical and creative approach to drawing on public health intelligence from a variety of sources, they may yet reap the benefits of a multidisciplinary approach more fully than 'old' health authorities were ever able to do.

It has long been a truism that public health is not just a matter for the NHS, and of course, local government has an honourable past as well as aspirations for the future in this regard. Future approaches to public health must be not only multidisciplinary, but also fully multi-agency, with all the challenges that that implies. The statutory duty of partnership placed on local NHS bodies to work together for the common good is welcome news indeed, particularly since this will extend to local authorities.

HIMPs, as described in the White and Green Papers, could be a vehicle for real and sustained improvements to health and healthcare. Then again, they could turn out to be just so much rhetoric. Only a huge amount of commitment at a local level, backed up by an unstinting determination from central government, will make improvements to the public health achievable. What is certain is that no one professional group and no one NHS or local government agency can deliver the goods alone.

The message that public health must be the concern of both the NHS and others is strongly reinforced in the Green Paper *Our Healthier Nation*, which describes a national contract for better health, in which the government, local communities and individuals all have a part to play in partnership. The new duty on local authorities to promote the economic, social and environmental well being of their areas should give a clear steer to the kind of inter-agency alliances that we found in some case-study sites in the King's Fund research. It is possible that within this broader approach to public health, the perspectives of lay people, as patients and carers, may also be valued more highly, alongside multidisciplinary professional expertise.

The fundamental perspective of *Our Healthier Nation* is that in addition to a healthcare system to treat those who fall ill, there is a need to recognise that the causes of ill health are complex and require collaboration to tackle the diverse factors that contribute to ill health and health inequalities. In identifying a range of determinants of health, including genetic factors, lifestyle and socio-economic issues, the Green Paper implicitly lends support to a multidisciplinary approach to public health. In proposing a national contract for better health, the Government makes the need for multi-agency work explicit. The need for a truly multidisciplinary approach must surely be part of that vision.

However, the Green Paper has rightly been criticised for a lack of appropriate, measurable targets and for falling short of hopes of additional funding for the new responsibilities of health and local authorities.[10] If public health is to be multidisciplinary in future, it is important that new ways of working between disciplines and across agencies should not be weakened by a lack of available funds to invest in genuine partnerships.

Finally, while both the White Paper and the Green Paper provide a context in which multidisciplinary public health might do better in future than in the past, it should not be assumed that overcoming professional and institutional barriers and a historical legacy of the predominance of a largely medical model will vanish overnight. A public health perspective, dedicated to reducing avoidable health inequalities, should be the cornerstone of a progressive NHS. This will only happen if the knowledge, skills, perspectives and experiences of a wide range of contributors from different disciplines and professional backgrounds are valued and encouraged. As we have seen, there are a number of lessons to be learned from the past in making a genuine multidisciplinary approach succeed in the future, and the challenge of abandoning narrow, monodisciplinary perspectives in favour of symbiotic, multidisciplinary co-operation is a prerequisite for making real progress in improving the health of the public.

References

1   Secretary of State for Health (1997) *The New NHS: modern, dependable.* Cm. 3807. HMSO, London.

2   Secretary of State for Health (1998) *Our Healthier Nation: a contract for health.* Cm. 3852. HMSO, London

3   Levenson R, Joule N and Russell J (1997) *Developing Public Health in the NHS – the multidisciplinary contribution.* King's Fund, London.

4   Davison C, Davey Smith G and Frankel S (1991) Lay epidemiology and the prevention paradox. *Sociology of Health and Illness.* **13**(1): 1–19.

5   Williams G and Popay J (1997) Social science and public health: issues of method, knowledge and power. *Critical Public Health.* **7**(1,2): 61–72.

6   Department of Health (1995) *Making it Happen – Public Health – The Contribution, Role and Development of Nurses, Midwives and Health Visitors.* Report of the Standing Nursing and Midwifery Advisory Committee.

7   Levenson R, Joule N and Russell J (1997) Leading questions. *Health Service Journal.* 9 October: 24–5.

8   Somervaille L and Griffiths R (1995) *The Training and Career Development Needs of Public Health Professionals. Report of Postal Survey and Discussion Workshops.* Institute of Public and Environmental Health, University of Birmingham.

9   Watt I and Freemantle N (1994) Purchasing and public health: the state of the union. *Journal of Management in Medicine.* **8**(1): 6–11.

10 Chadda D and Limb M (1998) Anger as Green Paper falls short on inequalities and funding pledges. *Health Service Journal.* 12 February: 9.

CHAPTER FIFTEEN

Public health practice in health authorities

Tony Jewell

Introduction

Responsibility for local health strategies lies with health authorities who need to work in partnership with local government and others to produce a health improvement programme. Health authorities are also where Directors of Public Health (DPH) for the defined local population are based, with responsibilities that include needs assessment, alliance working, strategy development, developing clinical and cost-effective healthcare services, and ensuring the surveillance and control of communicable disease. The DPH is a statutory appointment and the combination of such a post within health authorities makes this setting important for public health practice.

This chapter will briefly outline the political changes that have led us to the current position and still influence us, describe the public health functions expected of a health authority, comment on some of the tensions that exist and look to the future in the context of *Our Healthier Nation* and the consequences of the 1997 White Paper *The NHS: modern, dependable*.

History

Over the 150 years of the modern public health movement there have been some landmark events and many of these historic changes still shape current practice. For example, the 1848 Public Health Act is such a watershed and was associated with the development of the first MOH, who were based in local government with responsibilities for controlling the new notifiable diseases and promoting the hygiene and sanitation movement. Later these Medical Officers of Health (MOH), forebears of DPH, became involved in the development of preventive public health programmes for mothers and children, immunisation, the school health service and social services. These became known as community health services. Although the independent family doctors (GPs), dentists, ophthalmic practitioners and pharmacists were not their responsibility, the MOH were often involved in the management of municipal hospitals. However, the teaching and voluntary hospitals stood apart from the municipal hospitals, which were often associated with the old Poor Law institutions.

The Ministry of Health was established in 1919, formalising the state's role in health. There then followed nearly three decades when the political case for State Health Services was argued, the experience during the war of the Emergency Medical Services and Public Health Laboratory Services was noted, and the 1942 Beveridge Report was broadly accepted. The creation of the NHS in 1948 combined the three sectors – the local government public health and community health services, the independent contractors and the hospital services – under one umbrella. The 50 years of the NHS since 1948 have seen the gradual structural, if not functional, unification of these three sectors.

The local public health function was, for the first 25 years of the NHS, predominantly within local government. In 1974 the public health and community health services were brought into the NHS, separating personal social services from other community health services and placing MOH as Area or District Medical Officers within newly established Area and District Health Authorities, covering populations of about 750 000 and 250 000, respectively. These new community physicians remain linked to local government as Medical Officers of Environmental Health but this relationship was unclear and many of the organisational links atrophied. The 1974 reform was a massive change and many experienced MOH left the service prematurely, leaving the field to relatively few people who had not been trained for their new role, who became distanced from local government and faced confusion of role and responsibilities within the NHS.

By the early 1980s, the 1974 reforms were subjected to Roy Griffiths's review of NHS management, which was critical of consensus management in health authorities. The inquiries into the Stanley Royd Hospital salmonella outbreak and an outbreak of Legionnaire's disease at Stafford during the same period exposed weaknesses in the function of Medical Officers of Environmental Health. The Acheson inquiry into public health was called in the wake of these outbreaks and a wider concern about the role and responsibilities of community medicine. The report on public health in England was published in 1988 and laid the template for the development of Directorates of Public Health, based in local and regional health authorities as part of a national framework.[1] This report remains a key text in the understanding of modern public health. Its proposals have been robust and subject to counter-pressures from other changes in the NHS and wider environment. The history of public health still finds expression in everyday practice in understanding sensitivities with local government colleagues, clinicians in hospitals, and primary care and general management.

The Acheson Report on public health in England outlined the need for health authorities to have an explicit responsibility for public health, and to have the functions listed below.

- To review regularly the health of the population for which they are responsible and identify problems. To define objectives and set targets to deal with the problems in the light of national and regional guidelines.
- To relate the decisions that they take about the investment of resources to their impact on the health problems and objectives identified.
- To make arrangements for the surveillance, prevention, treatment and control of communicable disease and infection.
- To give advice to and seek co-operation with other agencies and organisations in their locality to promote health.

The report recommended that one person in a health authority be responsible and accountable for this function on behalf of the authority and its general manager. The new person – a DPH – would have responsibilities for:

- providing epidemiological advice on the setting of priorities, planning of services and evaluation of outcomes
- developing and evaluating policy on prevention, health promotion and health education involving all those working in the field
- undertaking the surveillance of disease and co-ordinating the control of communicable disease
- acting as chief medical adviser to the authority and as spokesperson on public health matters
- preparing an annual report on the health of the population
- providing public health medical advice to local authorities, family practitioner committees and other sectors.

Not long after these recommendations were accepted and circulated to the service (HC(88)64) the 1990 Working for Patients reforms were unleashed on the NHS and public health's role in the new purchasing authorities was revisited by an expert committee.

The 1993 Abrams Committee broadly endorsed[2] the Acheson Report's findings and reaffirmed the public health responsibilities of health authorities as:

- monitoring the health of the population
- ensuring that public health drives the authorities' purchasing and commissioning activities
- monitoring health outcomes
- improving the effectiveness and value for money of clinical and non-clinical interventions
- developing local health strategies and alliances necessary to implement these
- developing and sustaining effective relationships with local clinicians, including those working in primary and community-based programmes
- collaborating with local authorities and other agencies to monitor, control and prevent communicable disease and non-communicable environmental exposures
- informing the public about health and what can be done to improve it; involving the community in discussion about health needs and service provision

- ensuring that local GP fundholders and all providers of primary, hospital and community care, including those in private and voluntary sectors, have access to adequate and appropriate public health advice.

The recommendations also identified a need for a strong public health function in each district, led by the DPH as a senior member of the corporate team. It remarked that a close working relationship between the DPH and Chief Executive was essential and that the DPH should be the focus for all public health advice. The new public health responsibilities outlined by Abrams were clinical and cost effectiveness, primary care and the need for public involvement. However, the main locus for public health, despite some innovative joint appointments with hospital trusts and GP purchasers, became the health authority and therefore within the purchasing function.

The 1974 reforms unified the hospital and community health services and their respective budgets. The changes that occurred in the mid-1990s brought health authorities and independent contractors, family health services authorities, together as new unified health authorities. These reforms laid the foundation for the unification of the independent contractor family health services budgets and hospital and community health services budgets within new local health authorities (Figure 15.1). The next stage of the NHS reforms will unify the budgets through PCGs which is perceived as a risk to GPs who have enjoyed some parts of their budget not being cash-limited by government.

The 1974 reforms separated health and personal social services, which had been part of the MOH's department. This division lies at the heart of the health/social divide between health authorities and local government social services departments. There is now an opportunity to unify these budgets at the level of PCGs, but there are substantial problems to overcome in managing both free and means-tested services from one budget.

This brief historical resume provides insight into the source of some of the current tensions felt by public health practitioners in health authorities, as shown in Table 15.1.

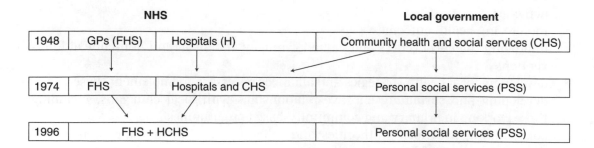

Figure 15.1:   Unification of family health services, hospital and community health services budgets within the NHS, separation from local government personal social services.

Table 15.1: Tensions felt by public health practitioners in health authorities

Local government	⟷	Health authority
Professional independence	⟷	Managerial corporacy
Public health doctors	⟷	Clinicians
Strategic	⟷	Operational
Health	⟷	Health services
Doctors	⟷	Multidisciplinary public health

Tensions

Local government and health authority

The historical background that I have described shows that contemporary District DPH developed from MOH, who were employed by, and based in, local government. These MOH managed relatively large departments, providing community health and social services. Their departure has been filled in recent years by Directors of Social Services and Chief Environmental Health Officers. Consultants in Communicable Disease Control still work closely with environmental health, and this is symbolised by the 'proper officer' status accorded to them for some residual statutory local government functions. Their other public health consultant colleagues share the communicable disease control rota for 24-hour medical cover and remain part of the medical team in support of environmental health.

Many people in local government believe that it is their organisations, rather than health authorities, that are public health authorities. Health authorities and local government manage their shared health and social care agenda through joint planning groups. Apart from rare examples, this is often difficult territory where different organisational cultures and imperatives meet and where usually the public health improvement agenda has been absent. Joint finance budgets are being used to pump-prime joint health and social services provision. There are now some examples of joint appointments of DPH between health authorities co-terminous with unitary local authorities. Such appointments are designed to overcome tensions and facilitate joint working.

General manager and professional

The Acheson Report on public health in England was influenced by the Griffiths Report on general management[3] and the ensuing period ensured that general management replaced a largely administered NHS system. The burden of the Griffiths Report was that personal identifiable management responsibility is critical to ensure that speedy action is taken and that the effectiveness and efficiency of such action is kept under constant review. Importantly, the DPH was identified as leader of the public health function. In addition, and more contentious, was the managerial accountability to the general manager of the authority, and professional accountability to the authority itself. In practice, professional accountability has also been exercised through the Regional DPH, although this has been less clear with the advent of regional offices in 1996 rather than the former statutory regional health authorities. DPH have individual performance reviews undertaken by Chief Executives, who are also involved in recommendations to health authorities about pay enhancements such as discretionary points.

This relationship between the DPH and general manager (more recently, the Chief Executive) is crucial and difficult to get right. Professional freedoms and accountability are to professional peers and are judged by the General Medical Council, for example, who identify the duties of doctors and register doctors. This is qualitatively different from employer–employee relationships and similar tensions are observed within hospital management. In public health terms, there are professional duties reminiscent of the supremacy of duties to patients. For a public health doctor 'the health of the people is the highest order'.[4] For example, a DPH may act as advocate on behalf of a particular disadvantaged group in great health need where he or she considers the health of the people is the highest order, and sees 'cabinet responsibility' of the health authority executive team and management relationships with the Chief Executive as being subordinate. There are times when this can mean appealing directly to the Health Authority Board in the independent Chief Officer role or to other appropriate higher authorities at regional or national levels, depending on the issue. There may also rarely be the recourse to resignation.

This undeniable and often productive tension between the independent role of a DPH and corporate health authority responsibilities is exercised through the Chief Executive. Sometimes the difficulties of managing the rising demands and needs within a cash-limited NHS has meant that the public health agenda has been squeezed by apparently more important health service crises. The voice of the DPH, as advocate on behalf of unmet health needs and health improvement, can seem to managerial colleagues as being uncorporate behaviour. Recent political NHS objectives during the internal market period, such as the efficiency index, Patient's Charter and private finance initiatives, seemed to be a diversion from health objectives and yet consumed a disproportionate amount of NHS managerial resources.

The DPH's annual report is meant to be an independent professional report by the director on the health of the local population. The contents of such reports can seem to be at odds with executive director corporate responsibilities within a health authority executive team. Many NHS management priorities are short term, while typically public health goals are longer term and usually involve inter-agency work. The DPH has other responsibilities to local government as a civic authority and to the public at large, which make the position different to other executive director colleagues. The advantage of being an executive director of a health authority, on the other hand, is that DPH are part of the executive team and are able to influence and shape policy from within. If they were outside this executive team, then the distribution of NHS resources would be outside direct public health influence. The objective, of course, is for health authorities to become public health organisations.

Public health physicians working within health authorities have provided a useful vehicle for decisively and appropriately shaping health policy. Many managers feel uneasy when dealing with the medical profession. Even managers committed to debunking and demystifying the skills, knowledge and status of doctors at one level can feel uncomfortable having to do without any medical input when making decisions about healthcare. Where these skills are coupled with managerial ones, the effect can be very powerful.[5]

Clinicians and public health doctors

The Chinese walls that emerged during the annual contracting rounds of the internal market made it more difficult for public health doctors to engage with hospital clinicians in service reviews and act as 'honest brokers'. The finite and comparatively scarce resources allocated to the NHS have led to difficult negotiations with NHS providers, and inevitably tense relationships. This made the Abrams recommendation to develop and sustain relationships with clinicians and the local community more difficult. It also perpetuated the distance of public health doctors from primary care, which was new territory for public health even from MOH days when community clinics were commonly quite separate from GP surgeries. This legacy is still visible in the community, where community clinics often stand apart from GP surgeries and where modern purpose-built multidisciplinary health centres are rarely found. Primary care has always been the basis of the NHS, and the underdeveloped public health presence in this setting has been to the detriment of both parties. GPs have too often been reactive clinicians, slow to develop an anticipatory population approach, working with extended primary care teams. Public health doctors have been slow to realise the potential for systematic population approaches through primary care and the power of a targeted personal practice approach for non-attenders and vulnerable groups.[6]

The tension between individual patient care and the utilitarian population/public health perspective has not facilitated close relationships between public health practitioners and clinical colleagues. Priority setting and rationing of services creates tensions between a population-based approach, and the clinician's principal responsibility to meet the needs of an individual patient. The GP's advocacy role is important and there is value in determining overall priority-setting policies away from the doctor–patient encounter.

Strategic and operational

One of the responsibilities of public health within health authorities is to develop strategies that promote health and help implement them. Sometimes this has led to the development of strategies in isolation from practitioners, who then fail to own them sufficiently well to assist in implementation. One of the problems with the health market was that the purchasing side was comparatively weak, which allowed providers to drive the changes. An example in the drive towards evidence-based medicine is the so-called 'evaluation bypass', which has occurred frequently despite exhortations from public health for more appraisal of clinical and cost effectiveness before introducing service changes. In practice, public health practitioners often find themselves shutting the stable door after the horse has bolted! Reactive rather than anticipatory public health. As health-care is becoming increasingly specialised and technical, public health practitioners need to develop specialist knowledge and skills to better influence clinical practice towards improving clinical and cost effectiveness and shaping service configuration. Getting greater congruence between the strategic and operational policy is a priority.

Health and health services

One of the key questions and the cause of tensions between health and health services is whether health authorities are responsible for improving the health of the population or simply for providing health services. The 1919 Ministry of Health Act imposed on Ministers the responsibility 'to take all such steps as may be desirable to secure the preparation, effective carrying out and co-ordination of measures conducive to the health of the people'. The 1977 NHS Act charged the Secretary of State 'to continue the promotion of a comprehensive health service designed to secure improvement in the physical and mental health of the people and in the prevention, diagnosis and treatment of illness'. The immediate and pressing needs of the NHS, with easily measureable indicators such as waiting lists, has often led to health promotion and health improvement being marginalised. The Acheson Report on public health comments that these aspects tended to be in the policy background.

It has only been comparatively recently that the *Health of the Nation* strategy (1992), and *Our Healthier Nation*[7] which will replace it, has explicitly stated that health improvement, as embodied in the new HIMPs, is a statutory responsibility of health authorities. The practice has been that health promotion and the influencing of the wider determinants of health has not been a health authority priority when these compete with policy pressures on activity, waiting lists or patient charter standards.

Doctors and multidisciplinary public health

The Acheson Report, which proposed the creation of DPH, recommended that they be medical practitioners with special training in epidemiology and those environmental, social and behavioural factors that affect the balance between health and disease. Although there have been some exceptions, in practice this has meant consultants in public health medicine. Public health doctors are employed on the same salary scales and terms and conditions as other consultants, and this has many advantages in helping public health physicians relate to clinical colleagues. However, it has also opened up a gap with their non-medical public health specialist colleagues, and has been seen as restricting access by other professionals to the top jobs in NHS public health.

The public health function is delivered by a much wider professional group, which includes clinicians and others trained in epidemiology, statistics, geography, sociology and economics. Indeed, as we move towards health authorities becoming public health organisations, managers need to see themselves as public health practitioners too. The definition of public health promulgated by the Acheson Report[1] describes it as the science and art of preventing disease, prolonging life and promoting health through organised efforts of society. The WHO definition of the new public health adds the fostering of social equity within a framework of sustainable development to the development of healthy public policies. Public health management is concerned with mobilising society's re-sources, including the specific resources of the health service sector, to improve the health of the population.[8] General managers armed with basic knowledge of public health principles working alongside public health specialists can be highly effective agents of change in delivering the organisation's public health objectives and those that the population needs most. Mutual respect of skills and roles with a shared vision is crucial. A joined-up approach avoids marginalising public health and adds value to achieving the corporate health agenda. This description of the public health role and of general managers' corporate public health goals is reminiscent of Virchow's description of politics as medicine writ large!

There is certainly a tension between the self-evident contribution of multidisciplinary public health practitioners to public health and the current leadership role within health authorities of DPH (medicine). In the academic field, non-doctors head departments, and many key public health organisations, such as the Office for National Statistics, also have non-doctor leadership. Within local government, too, the lead usually comes from managers with environmental health professional backgrounds. Certainly, public health physicians will continue to have a critical role in change management within the NHS because of doctor-to-doctor communication. Tribes reform better from within, but whether the role and responsibilities of a DPH require the person to be a doctor is less certain. The recent CMO's review on the need to strengthen the public health function in the light of *Our Healthier Nation*[7] sees the need for a network of public health practitioners based in international and national government levels, the regions, local health authorities and primary care. Outside the NHS, public health practice occurs in national organisations such as the Office for National Statistics, the universities and institutes, as well as in agencies such as the proposed Food Standards Agency, Centre for Communicable Disease Surveillance and Control, and the private sector. The important message in the review is that the public health function needs to be strengthened to deliver the ambitious new agenda and that better networking of existing resources will add value. This is part of joined-up thinking by sharing the strategic vision and mutual responsibilities.

The future

The historical background to modern public health practice has a habit of continuing to influence contemporary practice in both positive and negative ways. This is exhibited by the current divide between the NHS and local government, the relatively weak links between public health practitioners and clinicians, the greater focus on commissioning and priority setting, and strategic rather than operational inputs. The CMO's review on strengthening the public health function has identified the network of public health skills that are scattered around the country within and outside the NHS. Certainly, linking academic public health, developing public health skills in primary care, steering the research agenda and developing relationships with local government are key areas. The public health function needs to be multidisciplinary and spread throughout the healthcare system and influencing all relevant policies.

The New NHS: modern, dependable[9] describes the role of health authorities as:

- assessing the health needs of the local population
- drawing up a strategy for meeting those needs in the form of a HIMP developed in partnership
- deciding on the range and location of healthcare services
- determining local targets and standards to drive quality and efficiency in the light of national priorities and guidance
- developing PCGs, allocating resources to them and holding PCGs to account.

These responsibilities of health authorities and their DPH are wholly consistent with the public health functions described by the Acheson and Abrams reports and provide real continuity rather than the sea of change that market forces and privatisation had represented.

PCGs will have responsibility for registered populations of about 100 000. This size has been chosen because it has some epidemiological stability for health service planning and cost containment, yet it is small enough to allow peer pressure to influence primary care development. The needs assessments, which will be carried out within GP practices and across the PCG, should be informed by local public health practitioners who will need to cover the PCG and, ideally, the co-terminous local government organisation. Whether this requires a return to a District DPH linked to local government and an Area DPH in the health authority remains to be seen. Certainly, for DPH to develop a corporate role in local government as well as in the equivalent NHS structure, more practitioners at this level will be required. Some health authorities already relate to six unitary authorities, which are impossible for one DPH to cover if part of the role for the director is to have a personal corporate relationship with local government. This is an opportunity for new DPH roles aligned to local government and involved in their corporate agenda and accessible to non-medical public health specialists.

PCGs will need to work within the local HIMP which will have been developed in partnership with them, the local health authority, local government, the public and

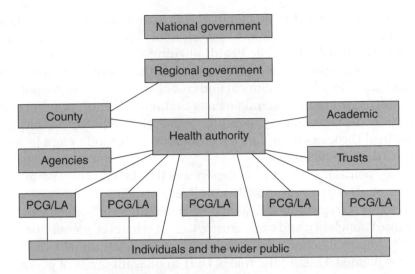

Figure 15.2:   Hub-and-spoke model for public health. PCG/LA, primary care groups and co-terminous local government authority, assume 6–10 per health authority. Populations: 5–10 million per region; 500 000–1 million per health authority; and 100 000 per primary care group

other agencies. The HIMP is arguably the *raison d'être* of the new health authorities, who need to lead in its production through a multiagency process, and who will be required to performance manage its implementation by trusts, PCGs and other agencies. In addition, clinical effectiveness and audit will need to be developed in primary care as part of the clinical governance agenda. All these activities need to be influenced by public health practitioners who may be based in local health authorities but linked to PCGs or employed by them. There is a risk that public health capacity will be divided and isolated if each PCG wants to own its own person rather than be part of a hub-and-spoke model (Figure 15.2). Single-handed public health physicians in PCGs risk being isolated and unable to deliver the complex public health agenda, which requires multidisciplinary team working.

Public health practitioners will need to sustain academic links, allowing development of specialist skills, and will be responsible for HIMPs for coronary heart disease and stroke, specific cancers, mental health and injuries. Such comprehensive programmes will be within national strategic frameworks and incorporate health promotion, disease prevention, assessment and diagnosis, treatment, rehabilitation and continuing care. Other practitioners might be attached to NHS trusts, to contribute to clinical governance and specialist public health work in these settings. Larger trusts may wish to employ their own public health specialists working as, or with, medical or nurse directors.

In addition, *Our Healthier Nation*[7] emphasises the statutory responsibility for health improvement and equivalent responsibilities for local government to protect health by safeguarding the social economic, environmental well-being of their populations. The annual report of the DPH needs to be developed for local government populations and

Our Healthier Nation expects the development of closer working relationships between health authority public health and local government. This will drive changes in public health practice which will see public health aligning staff with PCGs and the relevant local government organisation, as well as training others and spreading public health knowledge and skills. In addition, clinical and cost effectiveness and support responsibilities for the clinical governance agenda means that public health practitioners will also need to get closer to clinicians in hospitals. Again the employment of public health doctors as Medical Directors or as part of the medical directorate team in hospitals and PCGs is likely to develop further.

One of the key points in the Acheson Report was that for each population group there needs to be a named leading person with overall responsibility for the public's health, e.g. locally a District DPH, regionally a Regional DPH and nationally the CMO. In the future we must not lose that clarity and must ensure that at whatever population we choose to organise public health functions (local government, health authority or PCG), the lead responsibility is defined. Linking the role of DPH to relevant levels of governance would make sense at local, regional and national levels, and would offer a more direct link with democratically accountable bodies. The requirement for the DPH to undertake an annual report on the health of the defined local population must be supported as a vehicle for inter-agency collaboration and partnership working. This lead responsibility must also be supported by well-staffed, multidisciplinary, public health departments, that can rise to the challenge of developing HIMPs and meeting the twin challenges of *Our Healthier Nation:* to reduce health inequalities, and add years to life and life to years.

References

1   DoH (1988) *Committee of Inquiry into the Future Development of the Public Health Function. Public Health in England.* Cmd 289. HMSO, London.

2   DoH (1993) *Public Health in England. Roles and Responsibilities of the Department of Health and the NHS.* HMSO, London.

3   Griffiths R (1983) *Report of NHS Management Inquiry.* HMSO, London.

4   Cicero *De Legibus,* III, iii. Inscription in Southwark Council, London.

5   Richardson A, Duggan M and Hunter D (1994) *Adapting to New Tasks. The Role of Public Health Physicians in Purchasing Health Care.* Nuffield Institute for Health, Leeds.

6   DoH (1998) *Shared Contributions, Shared Benefits: the report of the Working Group on Public Health and Primary Care.* HMSO, London.

7   Secretary of State for Health (1998) *Our Healthier Nation: a contract for health.* Cm 3852. HMSO, London.

8   Hunter D (1993) Public health management: implications for training. *Health for All 2000 News,* No. 23 (Summer): 6.

9   Secretary of State for Health (1997) *The New NHS: modern, dependable.* Cm 3807. HMSO, London.

CHAPTER SIXTEEN

Annual public health reports

Anne Davies

One of the key recommendations in the government's White Paper[1] is for the introduction of HIMPs in every health authority area; they will provide the local strategy for improving health and healthcare, and will be the means to deliver national targets locally. Furthermore, the White Paper states:

> *The independent annual report by their Director of Public Health will inform the decisions of both the Health Authority and its partners. It will be the starting point for the Health Improvement Programme.*

Recognition of the value of annual public health reports, and of their essential independence, makes it all the more important to clarify their purpose and to upgrade their overall standard. Hitherto, while many reports have been ambitious and progressive documents, for many DPH they are still the 'annual chore of questionable value', the 'statistical exercise which diverts resources from other work', which the Acheson Committee warned against in 1988.[2]

The publication of an annual report on the health of the local population is one of the duties inherited by the DPH as successor to the MOH. Following the transfer of the public health function from local councils to health authorities in 1974, the annual public health report was allowed to lapse until it was reinstated by ministerial directive which implemented the recommendations of the Acheson Report, in 1988.[3] Thus, the appointment of Dr William Henry Duncan as the first MOH by the City of Liverpool in 1847 could be commemorated 150 years later in the annual report of the DPH for that city.

The longevity of the practice demonstrates the continuing need for publicly accessible information about the health of local communities, based on sound epidemiological evidence, objectively interpreted by an independent expert. The annual publication of public health reports has survived seismic changes for over a century, including the advent of the NHS, the transfer of public health from local government to health authority, and the repeated redrawing of boundaries as district, area and regional health authorities have been set up and, later, abolished. Today, although the public health function has become an integral part of health service commissioning, the DPH must, once a year, step back from corporate duties as an executive member of the health authority and, acting in an individual capacity, deliver an independent report. It can be a difficult balancing act to perform.

The value of regular public health reports may be summarised in terms of six broad principles:

- it provides the knowledge base for health action
- information about the health of a democratic society may be interpreted as a social or political right
- the annual report embodies the public health function, which is not only to survey the health of the population, but also, as defined by the Acheson Committee, to evaluate existing health services; hence the need for independence from health authorities
- without a regular health survey, there can be no adequate understanding of the needs of the whole population and services could become biased in favour of those able to articulate demand
- regular reports are the means of measuring progress towards agreed targets
- agreement about what is measured and reported enables comparisons to be made with other areas.

Since the new Labour Government took office in May 1997, a new agenda for public health has emerged, its increased importance borne out by the appointment of the first Minister for Public Health. New policies, including a strategy to address inequalities in health[4] and to introduce HIMPs and experimental HAZs, have been promised. The commissioning of services will pass to PCGs. These changes will present new challenges for public health professionals,[5] and indicate a different role for annual public health reports.

Issues

A recent analysis of the subject, commissioned by the Institute For Public Policy Research[6] has pointed to the incoherence surrounding the purpose of annual public health reports. The few attempts at evaluation have had little success, failing to find criteria whereby annual reports could be evaluated or compared, and confounding the expectation of the Acheson Committee that annual reports would enable comparisons between districts to be made.[2] The Institute for Public Policy Research report identified three key issues:

- erosion of the independent authorship which is the *sine qua non* of the reports' status
- widely varying interpretations by DPH as to the purpose of their annual reports

- a widespread failure to make use of the reports as agenda-setting or strategic documents.

Since the creation, in 1990, of health authorities to purchase or contract health services within the 'internal market', a tension has existed between the role of the DPH as author of an independent annual report and as an 'Executive Director' of the health authority. The private-sector manager model has supplanted the professional individual. Until 1974, the MOH was employed within local government specifically to give independent professional advice. His annual report was presented to the local council and debated in an open meeting in the presence of the press and public. While many DPH today do not perceive a conflict of interest, even when producing their annual report, anecdotal evidence from others suggests that the erosion of independence may be insidious,[6] but is nonetheless real. A more overt example is provided by the merging of at least one annual public health report with the annual report of the health authority.[7] In this case, independence was explicitly abandoned on the grounds that 'the main aim of both the Health Authority and the Public Health Directorate is to improve the health of the local population', a somewhat disingenuous, if irrefutable, claim, which cannot justify deviation from the historic interpretation of the task, or current DoH guidance on the subject.

Annual public health reports vary widely, from the descriptive 'health profile' type, to the prescriptive report encompassing not only analysis of health needs but also criticism of relevant policies and recommendations for action. There are variations in terms of target audience, contents, format and style.

If there is no simple agreement as to the purpose of annual reports, a more productive line of enquiry might focus on their impact: what use is made of them? Contrary to what Acheson envisaged, neither the Regional Offices of the NHS Executive nor the DoH use annual public health reports as a source of statistical information. Since 1989, the *Public Health Common Data Set* has been produced, specifically to act as a source of such information for DPH in making their reports. While this avoids unnecessary duplication and provides a valuable central resource, it has effectively changed the function of the annual report. Public health data are no longer obtained from them, but, conversely, is disaggregated for them, from the *Common Data Set*. The importance of the annual reports is thus in the relaying and interpretation of statistics for a local readership, and in the qualitative material they contain – the reporting of local initiatives to improve health, identification of need, reviews of policy impact and recommendations for action.

The Acheson Committee envisaged that district-level reports (and their health authority's response to them) would contribute to 'the information base upon which strategic plans and short term programmes are drawn up' at the regional level. A regional public health report would draw together information from the district reports and assess the implications for regional specialist services and education. The regional reports would, in turn, inform ministerial reviews of the RHAs. RHAs have since been abolished, to be replaced by regional offices of the NHS Executive, and although they retain the services of Regional DPH, they may no longer produce a regional public health report (and they are no longer independent). The impact of annual public reports is thus confined to the local or district level.

Some DPH make strenuous efforts to disseminate their reports, presenting them at public meetings, to local councils and their relevant committees, and to local schools and neighbourhoods. Their reports are carefully written and designed, with imaginative use of graphics and accessible language. Their contents will include ideas and recommendations for action by the individual, the health authority, local authorities and other agencies whose remit has a bearing on health; progress on implementing recommendations in previous reports will be reviewed. The whole thrust of these reports is to provide further impetus for health improvement.

Other reports have evidently fallen victim to the torpor that Acheson warned against, and appear as a turgid presentation of statistical information, the compliance with a duty that has clearly lost its purpose.

Despite these variations in practice, the case for continuing to publish annual public health reports, and indeed, for exploiting them more fully, can be made in terms of the six principles already outlined. Nothing but insignificant financial savings would be gained by their demise – the costs involved are small (an approximate average is £10 000 annually for direct production costs, excluding staff time[6]) – and much would be lost, not only in terms of detailed local knowledge but as a lever for change of, as yet unrealised, potential. New policy proposals, specifically the health inequalities strategy and the renewed emphasis on partnership between health and local authorities, already imply an enlarged role for Directorates of Public Health (which have been exempt from prospective management cuts).

Options for change

Responding to these challenges, the aim should now be to make the annual health report a more influential document. Anticipating the initiative to tackle health inequalities, the duty to produce annual reports could be redefined in terms of the following four objectives:

- to provide the public with an independent assessment of the local population's health in the context of related demographic and socio-economic data
- to provide a knowledge base for action to redress inequalities in health, both within and between districts
- to include in the report a minimum data set to allow comparisons with other similar areas for publication as national audits of specific policy initiatives
- to review the proposed HIMPs or health strategies set by the health authorities by providing annual 'snapshots' and recommendations for change or adjustment.

A renewed emphasis on the independence, or at least the arm's length distance, that should exist between the health authority and the Public Health Directorate would enable them to act as facilitators in the proposed partnerships between health and local authorities. Many DPH already see this as an important part of their remit (a similar role was proposed in the Abram's Report). Taken a stage further, DPH could be designated lead agents in developing partnerships with local authorities, and in the production of local strategies to tackle health inequalities.

Following the Conservative Government's policy to emphasise the corporate role of the DPH within the health authority, it would now be appropriate to play up the role of the Public Health Directorate (being multidisciplinary), as distinct from the wider health authority. This would have the benefit of increasing public awareness of the difference between the responsibility for health services, which lies with the health authority, and the responsibility for health, which must cross institutional boundaries. Directorates of Public Health must operate at arm's length from health authorities in order to protect the advocacy role, which is widely perceived to have been impaired by their involvement in commissioning health services.

For annual public health reports to have credence, it must be evident to the public that they come from the Directorate of Public Health, that DPH have duties of advocacy which are distinct from those of other health authority members, and that their reports are independent. One way to affirm that independence would be to target specific funds to be controlled by the Minister for Public Health for administration by DPH to cover production, publication and dissemination.

The content of the health authority's annual report, which is a record of that institution's activity and expenditure over the year, should be redefined in relation to the annual public health report, so as to present a clear distinction between the two. Both reports should be published within a cycle, rather than simultaneously, an analogy being the Parliamentary Select Committee Report followed by the appropriate departmental response. A duty to respond publicly to recommendations in the public health report could be imposed on the health and local authorities concerned. Formal response should be required at open meetings or in publicly available documents.

Public health reports could usefully include an assessment of the impact of any 'rationing' policies of the health authority. This would help to raise the level of public debate by informing the public about the need for priorities and the availability of resources, leaving the health authority to explain and justify its rationing decisions in its own annual report. If a clash of interests between independence and corporacy roles of DPH renders this impracticable, it merely illustrates the need for revision of the role and status of the DPH in relation to health authorities. The need for public support for rationing decisions, which will continue to vary between authorities, will grow and require regular review and debate.

Local sovereignty in producing annual reports should continue, but with important modifications. The freedom to select different topics and invite contributions from key local people allows the DPH the opportunity to exploit local surveys and other data on the health impact of any policies (see, for example, the Newcastle and North Tyneside Annual Report of the DPH 1995–96,[8] which focused on mental health services). However, if useful comparisons between areas covered by health authorities are to be made on the basis of annual public health reports, as the Acheson Committee anticipated, consideration might be given to reviving the pre-1974 practice of an annual ministerial directive on the content of annual reports. This could achieve a degree of standardisation of content and, possibly, format. DPH would remain free to include other additional issues of local importance (local targets being emphasised in *Our Healthier Nation*[4]).

Comparisons can, however, be invidious and misleading. While it is important to present the big picture and show how a local population compares with that of all other health authorities, the most meaningful measurements of health improvement are in comparison between those authorities that share demographic and socio-economic characteristics (see, for example, the Dorset Public Health Report (1996)[9] which provides comparisons with 11 like authorities classified as 'resort and retirement' by the Office for National Statistics).

For example, the pace of progress towards any national targets for reducing health inequalities could be monitored in annual public health reports by grouping local and health authorities on the basis of the Office for National Statistics classification,[10] using clusters, groups or families. DPH would select a minimum number from a range of benchmarks for equity appropriate to their grouping, as specified by the minister, and would be free to add any others as they saw fit.

Public health reports in each grouping might be published simultaneously. The Minister for Public Health would then be in a position to publish some sort of national overview of the various groupings of authorities, to compare progress and describe successful initiatives. This kind of selective comparison would enhance popular understanding of public health, rather than rely on crude nationwide 'league-table' information, which does not compare like with like. It would also address specific questions raised in *Our Healthier Nation*, i.e. how progress on local targets, including local inequality targets, can be monitored nationally and whether progress on similar problems in different localities can be aggregated nationally. This is not simply a matter of comparing progress in terms of statistics, but of sharing experience of what works – which again accords nicely with proposed policy:

> *We will also need to consider ways of monitoring and evaluating local processes to build and share knowledge on the effectiveness of different strategies, techniques and activities.*[4]

Annual public health reports could be required to make policy recommendations in terms of effective interventions, using the four policy levels from the Dahlgren model, and providing evidence of their effectiveness. A good example of this approach is provided in the 1995 annual report for Birmingham.[11] Policy recommendations can be directed not only at health authorities, but at local authorities and other relevant agencies. They are more likely to be effective if they include recommendations for disinvestment or redistribution of resources.

As part of the proposed health inequalities strategy, DPH would have a duty, in their report, to present a lay readership with information linking health with socio-economic factors, such as levels of deprivation, using both Jarman 8 and Townsend scores. Many annual reports, like that for Birmingham, already do this in map format, with differences in health between wards made strikingly evident.

Local alliances to develop triennial HIPs are proposed in *Our Healthier Nation*, and a new duty of partnership will be imposed on local authorities as well as NHS bodies. Local authorities will also have a new duty to promote the social and environmental well being of their residents.[1] DPH could be required, in their reports, to audit progress towards working in partnership, to identify barriers and report on successful initiatives. The Institute for Public Policy Research report recommended that annual public health reports be based on the populations of local authorities rather than those of the health authority. A proposal to this effect is included in *Our Healthier Nation: a contract for health*, together with several policy changes to enhance the role of local authorities in public health. Any increase in workload (where health authority areas span several local authorities) could be balanced by lengthening the publication intervals.

Alternatively, a more independent framework for the joint commissioning of annual public health reports[6] could be provided by the establishment of local Public Health Commissions or Forums, being a partnership between health authorities, local government, community health councils and local people. They would jointly commission from DPH annual health reports, which would monitor progress towards the proposed HIMPs – not unlike the City Health Plan which is reviewed in Liverpool's annual public health report 1996–97.

A formal duty to produce such a plan could be imposed on these commissions, in much the same way as local authorities have a duty to produce a Community Care Plan, and to work with health authorities and the voluntary sector through Joint Consultative Committees. Such a duty could operate in conjunction with the new duties of partnership being proposed by the Government.

Further options, which exceed the remit here, might include 'shared posts' or the joint appointment of specific public health officers by health and local authorities. The development of the proposed PCGs is likely to produce a whole range of modifications to the way Public Health Directorates work. Until these unfold, radical change in the role of the DPH is unlikely, notwithstanding the Government's current review of the whole public health function. Even so, simply by redefining the duty to produce an annual public health report in some of the ways outlined, the new HIMPs would be subject to regular audit, which would ensure the necessary modifications to stay on course.

If annual reports were revitalised as a specific component of new health inequalities strategy, they would provide information for comparisons between similar areas, to both the government and the public. This would provide another evolutionary development within the historic, reforming tradition of public health. Without a restatement of their purpose, annual public health reports will continue to atrophy and, whether cause or effect, DPH may find themselves with a correspondingly diminished role.

References

1   DoH (1997) *The New NHS: modern, dependable.* Cm 3807. HMSO, London.
2   Acheson D (1988) *Public Health in England.* HMSO, London.

3   DoH (1988) *Health of the Population: responsibility of health authorities.* HC88 (64). HMSO, London.

4   DoH (1998) *Our Healthier Nation: a contract for health.* Consultation Paper. Cm 3852. HMSO, London.

5   DoH (1998) *Chief Medical Officer's Project To Strengthen The Public Health Function In England: a report of emerging findings.* HMSO, London.

6   Davies A (1997) *Reporting The Public Health.* Institute for Public Policy Research, London.

7   Redbridge and Waltham Forest (1995–96).

8   Director of Public Health for Newcastle and North Tyneside (1995–96) *With Health in Mind: working together for health in Newcastle and North Tyneside.* Annual Report.

9   Dorset Public Health Report (1996) *Priorities For Improving Health In Dorset.*

10 Office for National Statistics (1996) *The ONS Classification of Local and Health Authorities of Great Britain.* HMSO, London.

11 Birmingham Public Health Report (1995) *Closing the Gap: ten benchmarks for equity and quality in health.*

CHAPTER SEVENTEEN

Primary care perspectives

David Colin-Thomé

Primary healthcare, with its long tradition of effectiveness and uniquely longitudinal care[1] coupled with the general practice-registered population, has a wonderful opportunity to deliver both the public health and the patient-focused imperatives of current government policy.

Primary care has many connotations, from the holistic WHO definition[2,3] to the narrow usage in the UK, meaning general medical practice only. With the advent of a government that clearly states a public health vision to improve health and reduce inequalities, and concomitantly stresses the importance of primary care, there must be an opportunity, if not an imperative, to deliver a broader, more holistic health agenda through primary care.

What can primary care do to deliver this public health vision? Ideas have been around for some time[4-6] and lend themselves well to a strategy that encompasses the following:

- health needs assessment
- anticipatory care
- inter-agency working
- community development
- clinical governance.

Some of the strategic development in general practice began with the previous government's policies, which spawned fundholding variants, total purchasing, commissioning and (a specific policy retained by this government) the primary care pilots, enabling new approaches to primary healthcare provision but, in particular, GP provision.

Health needs assessment

Health needs assessment in general practice, over the past few years, has, with increasing enthusiasm, been both undertaken and written about.[7,8] Useful, practical contributions are an excellent *Needs Assessment in Primary Care: a rough guide*[9] and an equally excellent primary care team-building workbook.[10]

On a slightly precautionary note, health needs assessment, as it becomes more in vogue in general practice, suffers from the potential problem of becoming simply a bureaucratic exercise carried out to fulfil a somewhat mechanistic agenda, rather than being the prerequisite to managerial action. If needs are identified, primary care teams have a duty to address them, directly or indirectly.

Anticipatory care

Primary anticipatory care

This involves health promotion and health education approaches. Many primary healthcare teams were enthusiastic supporters of practice-based health promotion, much influenced by the seminal work of Julian Tudor-Hart in his practice in Glyncorrwg,[5] but found difficulty in inducing change in behaviour or often interest in such health promotion by a sufficient number of patients. It was, of course, an approach that simply colonised health via a biomedical vehicle without fully realising the significance of the socio-economic environment and culture. Moreover, it did not heed the voices of sceptics such as Professor James McCormick,[11] who were predicting the uselessness of engaging clinicians in work they were not suitably trained to undertake. A recent analysis of such work[12] demonstrated minimal return for such major effort and resource usage.

All is not completely lost as Julian Tudor-Hart's work did seem to influence health gain, and this needs to be revisited, and there is evidence that brief interventions[13] during a consultation are a more effective health promotion approach for clinicians than any other. The Stott–Davis consultation model for GPs[14] still holds good. It also goes without saying that vaccination and immunisation remain a major piece of prevention that primary care delivers, helped by incentives contained in the much-maligned 1990 GP contract. That contract demonstrates the effectiveness of offering incentives to primary care. Other members of the primary healthcare team, in particular nurses, also need to adopt the brief intervention approach, but health visitors and school nurses have an opportunity to be more proactive by combining reactive care with health promotion. Health visitors in particular are an integral member of the core primary healthcare team and have a multifaceted role, but more of this later. Primary healthcare teams need to move on from a narrow model of health promotion,[15] be more community-focused and be part of approaches similar to that demonstrated in Karelia, North Finland, described as 'primordial' prevention of cardiovascular disease.[16]

Secondary anticipatory care

This involves screening, to which, for efficacy, the new framework for screening must be applied. Examples of screening in primary care are:

Cervical cytology

Uptake has increased following the incentives contained within the 1990 GP contract. The instance of death from the disease has recently fallen, although evidence demonstrating direct causality with the increased uptake of screening has not been produced. It is also a depressing fact that some two-thirds of the women who die of this cancer have never had any sort of cervical smear test. Are we, in fact, regularly screening only the women who are at lowest risk?

Breast cancer screening

Breast cancer screening through breast mammography has not been linked to incentives at the GP level and the uptake around the country varies widely.

Opportunistic screening

The consultation offers an excellent opportunity for opportunistic screening as well as the other facets of good general practice.[14] Other primary healthcare team members have a similar opportunity, often not grasped. The proportion of patients consulting their GP in 1 year is 70%, rising progressively to 97% having consulted over 7 years[17] and, together with sufficient assiduity on the part of all professionals, at least a similar number of patients could have their blood pressure screened as well as their body mass index measured, together with smoking, alcohol and exercise status as well as relevant family history.

Tertiary anticipatory care

This concerns the improvement of outcomes in chronic disease management. Such disease management probably offers the best opportunity for primary healthcare clinicians to demonstrate their effectiveness. The hallmark of good chronic disease management is a systems approach where patients are called and recalled, failed appointments identified, patients encouraged to attend, and regular tests and treatment undertaken according to guidelines. An example of good-quality guideline production is the SIGN[18] guideline development (Scottish Inter-Collegiate Guideline Network) which, as its name implies, involves all the royal colleges and recommends actions that are evidence-based. Furthermore, the evidence base is classified according to its validity as defined by the American task force on preventive healthcare.[19]

However, guidelines are like health needs assessment activity, good if they lead to action but often become an end in themselves. We need more research-based evidence but, more importantly, a clear dissemination and development programme to ensure that such guidelines are in use to improve care. The performance framework and, in particular, the emphasis on clinical governance in current government policy[20] may well be a useful catalyst for action.

Chronic disease management programmes need to be systems-based, multidisciplinary, co-ordinated, with a long-known key role for nursing.[21] Furthermore, such programmes lend themselves well to at least achieving good intermediate outcomes, e.g. the measurement of glycosolated haemoglobin in diabetes mellitus and peak expiratory flow rate in asthma, rather than the traditional measurement of inputs, e.g. the numbers seen.

Inter-agency working

In order to fulfil the public health agenda, the primary healthcare team, as well as other local public service organisations such as schools, need to act as a resource for their communities.[22] Being the fulcrum of inter-agency working is one manifestation of being such a resource. The NHS White Paper[20] strongly emphasises the need for primary medical care and for the hospital services to work closer together to develop a health systems approach to care. Tools and vehicles for such workings include shared guidelines, care pathways, interchange of staff and, probably more effectively, staff as co-ordinators. Examples of such co-ordination are the diabetic liaison nurse and the asthma nurse or physiotherapist working in both primary and secondary care. Mental health schemes further enhance inter-agency working as there is usually a parallel local Social Services Mental Health Organisation.

There are currently an increasing number of examples of good primary care and social services collaboration,[23] which address historical misapprehensions.[24] The primary care/social services interface, understandably due to the volume of work between the two organisations, attracts most attention but other inter-agency work is essential to deliver more holistic services for the community. Relevant local government departments are:

- Housing: a department every primary healthcare team worker has experience of through their involvement in potential housing moves for their patients. Such involvement could be more systematic and better focused so as to ensure a better advocacy role for the primary care team.

- Leisure: there are many existing examples of primary care teams prescribing exercise for health via local leisure facilities.
- Youth services: a relatively unexplored interface but one such interface is described later in the Castlefields case study.
- Environmental health services: another unexplored connection but together the environmental health officer, health visitor and school nurse could become an influential, local public health triumvirate to develop primary care.
- Education: schools are traditionally reasonably well connected to the primary healthcare team, through the work of health visitors and school nurses. American evidence from the 1960s Head Start programmes[25] demonstrates the striking health gains produced from quality pre-school education. Investment in this area seems of paramount importance, and primary care could aid this investment mainly through focusing existing health visitor and school nurse work to develop family education, for instance, within the Healthy Schools Initiative. The sharing of such resources is also an excellent opportunity for the development of Healthy Living Centres, which should be a community resource run by the community and utilising existing physical resources that are often underutilised. Primary healthcare teams could work through Healthy Living Centres in their quest to be a resource for their community. These Living Centres and the Healthy Schools Initiative are part of current government policy thinking,[26] but if delivered mechanistically could just become a new building programme.

Other local government departments, such as transport, with its relevance to access, and planning, with its relevance to the siting, for instance, of leisure facilities and shopping, have great importance in deprived, socially excluded communities. The healthy food options within such shops are, of course, an area in which the primary healthcare team, in particular, can become involved. Such teams, if they identify a key worker with guaranteed time, can become more active in influencing local government decisions, partly through working with local councillors, as well as providing the evidence to influence local government decisions. Joint health service/local government appointments at local community level is another initiative worth pursuing. The whereabouts of resources available for such public health work is discussed later.

Of course, inter-agency working involves wider relationships than simply with local government but, as with local government, these are often unexplored due to lack of primary care vision, but also lack of primary care resources to fund such work. Other relevant organisations to work with include voluntary agencies, welfare rights workers and local industry.

The need for welfare rights workers is particularly important to ensure that rightful monies come into deprived communities. The siting of such workers in primary care buildings aids access to such resources for socially excluded communities.

Community development

This is potentially the action most beneficial for the health of communities but the one that induces most scepticism in biomedical primary healthcare team workers. This role is well described for health visitors,[27] but primary care could further identify resources to fund community development workers to work in communities with significant social deprivation. Hopefully, such community development would increase the locus of control over their surroundings of people suffering from deprivation[28] which, in turn, should produce health gain. Community audit would ensure that such community development would be shown to be in response to need and thus validate such activity. This is an unavoidably short paragraph despite the importance of the task, and contains an imperative to search for, and carry out research of the relationship with and the validity of, community development within the NHS in general and primary care in particular. GPs, in particular, argue that their role is that of patient's advocate, but it is often a narrow concept of advocacy, more to do with access to national health services than to advocating health-gain interventions. Armed with a health needs assessment which involves the community, and undertaking the activities described, the primary healthcare team can become true advocates *vis-à-vis* other organisations such as local government, but also by enabling increased locus of control within their community of patients.

Health visitors

As already described, health visitors, school nurses and environmental health officers have the opportunity to work together as locally based public health workers, helping to lead, educate and train the primary healthcare team and other local public service organisations to develop a public health focus. Health visitors, as core primary healthcare team workers, have many key roles that a health visiting team could undertake:

- aiding health needs assessment, although ultimately this should be a team responsibility and involve the community
- a reactive role, responding to people and families in need
- a health promotion, health education role around healthy lifestyles.
- a potential care-management approach for a functional group, such as, but not exclusively, for children under 5 and their families, to enable co-ordination of their care and services
- a community development role.[29,30]

Health visiting thereby could, and should, have the key public health role within the primary healthcare team in meeting the wider health agenda, but needs to ensure that the work is both evidence-based where possible and certainly audited to demonstrate effectiveness – reflective activities not enough in evidence in health visiting practice.

Clinical governance and clinical resource management

Much has been written about evidence-based medicine, particularly of late, and the combination of research-based evidence, clinical audit, and managerial action centred on effectiveness and quality offer three clear opportunities.

- To ensure better and less-variable clinical quality.
- To identify inappropriateness, as this will protect patients from unnecessary and potentially harmful interventions. Many clinicians seem oblivious to harmful effects of even everyday interventions such as X-rays, and yet the National Radiological Board suggest otherwise.[31]
- Resource release. If inappropriate care is challenged, there are potentially large resources to be released from current clinical activity. Professor Michael Peckham, the former director of the DoH R&D Programme, was quoted as estimating that £1 billion could be released, whereas the organisation formally known as the Anti-Rationing Group suggests that 20% of NHS activity is inappropriate.[32]

Primary care, at its various levels, from individual practitioner through to the practice and to the new White Paper intermediate organisations, such as primary care groups, local healthcare cooperatives and primary care trusts, has a significant part to play. Primary care clinicians as providers need to challenge their own activity, whether as providers or referrers, which to some effect, fundholding accomplished. What primary care needs to focus on further, is what happens to the clinical care of their patients when they are treated elsewhere. Primary care clinicians undertake inappropriate care as much as anyone else, but the consequences of their actions, in mitigation, are at least cheaper than hospital inappropriateness. The task for current primary care is to ensure good-quality, appropriate provision, but, through either the media referrals to hospitals, in commissioning for secondary care, or in redesigning secondary care, primary care needs to ensure that the three opportunities described above are achieved. The monies released, of necessity over time so as to phase the redesign of hospital care, could be spent on funding activities that aid health gain rather than fostering biomedical vested interests. Achieving these three clinical aims could be the initial criteria for success for what could be called the New Primary Care, combining the new public health with the new public management as well as the facets of good primary care.

Castlefields case study

The Castlefields practice in Runcorn, situated in an area of considerable social deprivation, was a first-wave fundholding practice and one of the originators of total purchasing. It has, for some time, been imbued by a public health ethos and adopted the budget-holding initiatives so as to free up resources and address the public health activities previously described.

Health needs assessment

This was undertaken, led by a public health nurse working to a 2-year project.[33,34] The final practice health needs assessment covered information management, patient participation, public health development and social care.[35] This assessment has recently been refreshed, utilising the primary care team-building workbook.[10]

Anticipatory care

Given the already-described poor returns from health promotion initiatives in primary care, the practice concentrated its efforts on brief interventions and opportunistic screening, and at the same time has continued an antismoking programme, issuing free nicotine patches as well as offering a comprehensive health visiting service. As part of the assessment of their chronic disease programme, the practice experimented with aggregated intermediate outcomes, such as peak expiratory flow rate, to measure improvements to the client group as well as to the individual.

Inter-agency working

The practice adopted *inter alia* a care-management approach to inter-agency working, in particular developing two models.

- The community psychiatric nurse, hospital-employed but working as a care manager for the practice's mentally ill patients, to enhance co-ordination of care as well as being an educational resource for the primary healthcare team.
- A jointly funded social care manager, who has access to social care and primary care resources for the over-65s registered practice population. The outcome of this work has been partially evaluated and demonstrates better co-ordinated care packages for this group of clients, as well as keeping within the healthcare and social care budget and, furthermore, lessening the need for inpatient hospital care.

The practice has funded a welfare rights worker who attends weekly and has also worked closely with local youth services, one of the many community activities generated by the work of the public health nurse. The Youth Project entailed the practice bringing together many organisations, as well as members of the local community, to pool ideas and resources to meet the identified needs of the young people, who are either registered with the practice and/or attend the local Youth Centre.[36] This involvement was a significant development for the primary healthcare team, a role that the local council wished to spread out to other areas, not necessarily led by primary healthcare teams but by organisations, either statutory or otherwise, who had the wish and capacity to undertake this task – a model of community commissioning through local government.

Community development

The work of the public health nurse[33] produced many community initiatives, some self-sustaining (such as an Exercise Cooperative), others one-off activities (such as the Healthy Eating Initiative), whereas the Youth Service interface involved the practice. Currently, release of resources has funded the part-time deployment of one of the community nursing team to continue community initiatives, including the revivification of the Patient Participation Group.

Clinical governance/clinical resource management

The most notable practice successes have been in the strong clinical audit culture and the release of resources from inappropriate clinical care. Further significant potential releases from the hospital sector have been identified through both questioning clinical practice which was not evidence-based, and questioning hospital utilisation management. Monies were released through fundholding, but the potential release of resources through total purchasing never materialised due to the NHS's traditional reluctance to challenge hospital funding, however inappropriately applied.

Social exclusion

The government's Social Exclusion Agenda, concerned with the wider determinants of health, is a further opportunity for primary healthcare to demonstrate its connectedness with the broader health agenda. The primary healthcare team can engage the socially excluded of their patients by addressing:

- attitudinal issues of the primary healthcare team
- welfare benefits uptake (described elsewhere)
- targeting of services
- employment opportunities
- community development/facilitation (described elsewhere)
- educational opportunities.

The socially excluded, for various reasons, present a difficult challenge to primary healthcare as currently delivered. The level of empathy, knowledge or understanding by primary health workers to the socially excluded can best be addressed educationally. The training handbook for health and welfare practitioners[37] who work with families in poverty offers further opportunity to use public health issues for team building.

The effective targeting of services to the socially deprived population is well described[38] and is considerably aided by computer records. Interrogating such systems can identify morbidities related to geography and, in more sophisticated systems, to housing type and employment. Information management is, furthermore, an excellent tool for auditing effective targeting.

General practice, by engaging and paying volunteers, for example, in running crèches and poster displays, offers an opportunity to the unemployed to earn money and gain self-confidence and esteem, so as to enable their further participation in social activity and enhance their employment prospects.

The government's recent Education Green Paper[39] highlights the UK's problem of paucity of broadly based educational opportunities. The British education system tends to offer further educational opportunities to the already educated, thus leaving the UK with the unenviable record amongst countries in the Organisation for Economic Co-operation and Development of having some of the highest figures for functional illiteracy and innumeracy. As good education facilitates good health, the NHS in general, and the primary healthcare team in particular, given the right resources, could offer education opportunities to the many low-paid workers in the NHS who have not benefited from further educational activity, thereby benefiting themselves and their communities. Companies such as Ford and Rover, albeit largely to obtain better productivity from their workers, offer such educational programmes to their workforce, unrelated to the workers' direct job needs. Where such car makers have led the way, could not the public-financed, health-orientated NHS follow?

Summary

- Public health action in primary care needs to infuse all levels, whether the individual primary healthcare team workers, the practice or the new primary care intermediate organisations (PCGs, local healthcare co-operatives, primary care trusts).
- Health needs assessment needs to lead to action and can be undertaken as a primary healthcare team-building exercise.
- Anticipatory care, as for clinical activity, should be evidence-based.
- Inter-agency working can be aided by link workers and jointly managed budgets.
- Community development also needs to be evidence-based and audited, although primary healthcare workers need to accept social science as a valid evidence base.
- Health gain is largely outside the remit of traditional NHS care, but can be funded or facilitated by the NHS and in particular primary care.
- Clinical governance and resource management can lead to significant resource release.
- The primary healthcare team, with its frequent longitudinal contacts and registered population, is in a unique position to deliver both personal and population-based activities.

- Health authorities should commission primary care in response to the needs of communities. The holistic approach described in this chapter could be achieved by some primary care teams. Where primary healthcare teams wish to address only the biomedical agenda, the wider public health agenda should be addressed by health authorities commissioning through other organisations.

Conclusion

Only when both personal and population approaches are delivered effectively, through primary care, will the health service be truly primary care led. The potential is there in primary care to deliver this agenda if nurtured, although there is a dearth of developmental skills within the health service. Primary healthcare needs to develop its public health skills to ensure health gain, as current NHS organisations have been unwilling, or unable, to undertake this work. If we in primary care and the NHS at large fail in this, then the minimalist position we should aim for is to ensure the maximum cost effectiveness of NHS resources, and any consequent release of resources should be used by others, such as a quality education service, to ensure the betterment of the public's health. The potential is to be more than minimalist. Julian Tudor-Hart wrote that 'GPs cannot defend territory they have failed to occupy'.[5] This is no doubt true, but primary healthcare teams, with a wider health agenda, can occupy such territory.

References

1   Starfield B (1993) Primary Care. *Journal of Ambulatory Care Management.* **16**(4): 27–37.

2   World Health Organisation (1978) *Alma Ata 1977. Primary Health Care.* WHO UNICEF, Geneva.

3   Vuori H (1984) Primary health care in Europe – problems and solutions. *Community Medicine.* **6**: 221–31.

4   Kark SL (1981) *The Practices of Community Orientated Primary Health Care.* Appleton, Century, Crofts, New York.

5   Tudor-Hart J (1988) *A New Kind of Doctor.* Merlin Press, London.

6   Ashton J (1990) Public health and primary care: towards a common agenda. *Public Health.* **104**: 387–98.

7   Murray S and Gillam AM (1996) *Needs Assessment in General Practice.* Royal College of General Practitioners, Exeter.

8   Harris A (ed.) (1997) *Need to Know: a guide to needs assessment for primary care.* Churchill Livingston, London.

9   Cavanagh J (1998) *Needs Assessment in Primary Care: a rough guide.* SNAP (Scottish Needs Assessment Programme), Glasgow.

10 Rowe A, Mitchinson S, Morgan M and Carey I (1997) *Health Profiling – all you need to know.* John Moores University, Liverpool and Premier Health NHS Trust, Burton-on-Trent.

11 McCormick J (1989) Follies and fallacies in medicine. *Physician.* **8**(2): 104–8.

12 Association of Primary Care Facilitators (1994) Critique of Oxcheck and Family Heart Study. In: *King's Fund Centre, Cardiovascular Prevention in Primary Care: the way forward.* King's Fund, London.

13 Sheldon T, Long A, Freemantle N *et al.* (1993) *Effective Health Care.* November: No. 7. Nuffield Institute for Health, University of Leeds; Centre for Health Economics, University of York and The Research Unit of the Royal College of Physicians, Leeds.

14 Stott NCH and Davis RH (1979) The exceptional potential in each primary care consultation. *Journal of the Royal College of General Practitioners.* **29**: 201–5.

15 Cowley S with Buttigieg M (1994) In: *King's Fund Centre, Cardiovascular Prevention in Primary Care: the way forward.* King's Fund, London.

16 Davis B (ed) (1998) *Health Bulletin.* **56**(5): 785.

17 Kessel N and Shepherd M Original papers (*circa* 1962) The health and attitudes of people who seldom consult a doctor. Journal unidentified.

18 Scottish Inter-Collegiate Guideline Network. Royal College of Physicians, Edinburgh.

19 US Preventive Services Task Force (1989) *Guide to Clinical Preventive Services. An Assessment of the Effectiveness of 160 Interventions.* Report of the US Preventive Services Taskforce, Williams and Wilkins, Baltimore.

20 Secretary of State for Health (1997) *The New NHS: modern, dependable.* HMSO, London.

21 McLaughlin FE, Cesa T, Johnson H *et al.* (1979) Nurses' and physicians' performance on clinical simulation test: hypertension. *Research in Nursing and Health.* **2**: 61–72.

22 Colin-Thomé D (1996) *The Return of the Local.* Demos, London. Issue 9, pp. 46–7.

23 Thistlethwaite P (ed.) (1997) *Impressions of Links between GP Fundholders and 5 Social Services Departments in England.* ACC Publications, London.

24 Huntington J (1981) *Social Work and General Medical Practice.* Allen and Unwin, London.

25 Schorr L (1988) *Within our Reach.* Anchor Press/Doubleday Books, New York.

26 Secretary of State for Health (1998) *Our Healthier Nation: a contract for health.* Cm 3852. HMSO, London.

27 Luker K and Orr J (eds) (1985) *Health Visiting.* Blackwell Scientific Publications, London.

28 Everson S, Kaplan G, Goldberg D *et al.* (1997) Hopelessness and four years progression of carotid atherosclerosis. *Arteriosclerosis, Thrombosis and Vascular Biology.* **17**(8).

29 Dalziel Y (1994) Integrating a community development approach with mainstream health visiting. *Health Visitor.* **67**(11): 355–6.

30 Craig P (1996) Community development health visiting. *Health Visitor.* **69**(11): 459–61.

31 Royal College of Radiologists (1993) *Making the Best Use of a Department of Clinical Radiology.* The Royal College of Radiologists, London.

32 Roberts C, Crosby D, Dunn R *et al.* (1995) Rationing is a desperate measure. *Health Service Journal.* **12**: 15.

33 Colin-Thomé D (1993) The public health nurse: a new model for health visiting? *Primary Care Management.* **3**(5): 4–6.

34 Cernick K and Wearne M (1994) Promoting the integration of primary care and public health. *Nursing Times.* **90**(43): 44–5.

35 Colin-Thomé D (1994) Practice population commissioning. In: R Sheaf, V Peel and J Higgins (eds) *Best Practice in Health Care Commissioning.* Longman, Harlow, Essex.

36 Colin-Thomé D (1996) Care of young people. *Practice Nurse.* **11**(6): 389–92.

37 Blackburn C (ed.) (1992) *Improving Health and Welfare Work with Families in Poverty.* Open University Press, Buckingham.

38 March GN and Channing DM (1988) Narrowing the health gap between a deprived and an endowed community. *British Medical Journal.* **296**: 173–6.

39 Department of Education and Employment (1998) *The Learning Age.* HMSO, London.

CHAPTER EIGHTEEN

Public health and local government

Tony Elson

These are unsettling times for those of us in local authorities who have maintained an interest in the health of our communities. On the surface there are, for the first time in a generation, new opportunities to redefine the strong links between the duties devolved to local government and the mission set for our NHS. However, this new dawn poses a new set of challenges to our thinking which may prove every bit as daunting as those that have gone before. Instead of playing out the role of evangelists preaching the public health message to the seasoned practitioners and policy makers of local government, we now find ourselves searching for a new language that will allow us to spread the gospel of local government amongst the non-believers in the health sector.

No one should underestimate the size of the task before us, nor the potential benefits to be gained from a successful conclusion. A closer integration of the means of delivering those social policies designed to address social exclusion holds out the prospect of real progress towards the goal of more sustainable communities. Now that it is possible to recognise the links between poverty and ill health, we can start to build new approaches that exploit opportunities to maximise health gain through broader social and economic regeneration initiatives.

This chapter seeks to offer some thoughts about the way in which progress might be achieved. It provides ideas that may help to lay the basis for more effective communication between people from various disciplines, who claim to share common language and objectives but who frequently display through their actions little understanding of each other's worlds. It is written from a local government perspective, but the messages contained are as relevant to people on either side of the border.

First the context. There can be no assumption that people in local government automatically identify health issues as ones that are central to their interests and responsibilities. At a time when we are celebrating the fiftieth anniversary of the NHS, it is perhaps easier to understand the reasons why many councillors are still in a mindset that defines health as the province of a national government agency.

Radio and television documentaries and newspaper articles have shown the failings of pre-war health provision based on private and voluntary practice, with the main socially funded services coming from the local government sector. In a very real sense, the quality and length of your life depended upon where you happened to live, unless you had sufficient money to buy healthcare.

Given this background it becomes easier to understand the strength of public opinion that still supports the value of a system of healthcare managed nationally and operating to centrally prescribed standards. It is hard to imagine any political party that seeks electoral success arguing for a return to a system of locally provided healthcare with locally determined priorities and funding, and it is probably relevant to remember that in local government there is a strong age bias amongst councillors, which means that a substantial proportion will have first-hand memories of the birth of the NHS and what went before.

This estrangement between the NHS and local government, started in 1948, has been further emphasised over the years, both in structural terms with subsequent transfers of health-related services from local government to health and by the removal of local council nominees from NHS management boards. Meanwhile, professionals and managers have spent so much effort in futile but determined attempts to define precise and tidy boundaries between health and social care responsibilities. The energy spent in debating the distinctions between a social and a medical bath or the level of nursing or care skill required to administer eye drops must qualify as one of the more absurd activities of the public sector this century.

So the starting point for the rapprochement between health and local government demonstrates the need to overcome half a century of emphasis on difference and separation, in what has become two traditions. Only in recent years, as local government has started to open itself up to influences from elsewhere in the world, has the modern generation of local government officer started to conceive that health issues can form part of a local government agenda.

For those with an interest in health, the task has been to raise awareness about the links between traditional local government services and health. A common feature of those linkages has been the focus on the prevention of ill health. Whether it is traffic calming and accident reduction, the prescription of exercise rather than drugs, or healthy lifestyle education in schools, the kind of project-based initiatives advanced by local government have a creditable record set alongside the relatively low investment in health promotion funded by the NHS.

Perhaps it should not be so surprising that a national service which came into being to resolve the problems experienced by people who could not afford access to health services when they were ill, has been so dominated by treatment-based approaches at the expense of prevention-based strategies. Add to this a strong ideological belief in central government over the past two decades that health inequalities could be explained either by chance or in terms of people's chosen lifestyles rather than through social factors, and we can perhaps understand the strength of the underlying value systems in the health service which continually lean towards redefining national public health strategies in terms of illness reduction rather than the promotion of good health.

There is also real danger that the new commitment to move towards evidence-based investment in health will be used to justify the continued bias in investment. Relatively little research has been carried out into ways of influencing the social determinants of health. How could the NHS justify research in this area when politicians had decided there was no linkage between poor social conditions and ill health? Meanwhile local government could hardly justify expenditure on public health research when it fell outside its legislative responsibilities.

It is indeed easy to forget the constraints on local government's powers to operate outside specific legislative authority. Powers of general competence, which would allow a local authority wide-ranging rights to act in the interest of its communities, do not exist in British law. The new Government's declared intention to impose a general duty on local government to promote the economic, social and environmental well being of their areas makes no specific reference to health, but will allow for a more holistic interpretation of the regeneration agenda to include health gains as major contributors to economic and social sustainability. The more specific duty to co-operate in the preparation of HIMPs and HAZs opens up direct and substantial opportunities for progress.

The speed with which these new powers are embraced will depend very much on the extent to which local government and health establish a common agenda. From a local government perspective, new responsibilities in public health sit alongside a wide range of other new initiatives. For example, there are specific commitments to the improvement of education, new duties for community safety and for aspects of central government's approach to crime and disorder, and an increased role in integrated transport strategies. These are relatively well-defined changes, which have substantial resource implications but are reasonably discrete areas of work with clear goals and measurable outcomes.

More challenging is the whole programme of democratic renewal which is dominating a lot of the creative energy within local government. The redefinition of the relationship between local government and the people it serves, which concentrates the focus on the processes of policy development and service delivery and fundamentally questions the extent to which individuals and communities are involved in decision making, has the potential to dominate work programmes for several years. Not least, it requires a programme to change the very culture of the political and administrative structures of local government.

A pessimist could easily conclude that given these changes the chance of bringing health issues from the shadows to centre stage is remote. However, an equally credible interpretation can be made. Radical change, which affects the very way in which local government officers and councillors think through their relationship and responsibilities to the community, may be just the quantum change necessary to achieve the re-evaluation of local government's role in health. In particular, a reaffirmation of local government's representational role, acting as both advocate and community conscience, could help to address matters that affect the quality of life in local communities, and may provide the impetus necessary to help those in the health service charged with the responsibility to move the emphasis in public policy more towards the promotion of good health and away from the professional dominance of the medical profession, who are trained to be experts in illness rather than experts in health.

To make this more optimistic assessment a reality requires a new approach from both within and outside local government. The ground has moved in a way that has significant implications. Whereas the health lobby within local government was satisfied by an emphasis on identifying the health impact of council activities on health in an attempt to bend local government spending in small ways to support local health strategies, we now have to make a case for a far more substantial commitment of effort and resources. Given the other priorities that are referred to earlier, such an effort will only be successful if it can be justified in terms of the contribution this work makes to mainstream local government programmes. Quite simply, we have to present a convincing argument that improvements in health are an essential precondition for the achievement of some of the primary objectives of local government.

Practical examples always help to put meaning into argument which may otherwise seem somewhat theoretical. In my local authority we are fortunate to have many committed staff who have embraced the health agenda and have worked hard to develop projects that demonstrate the positive role we can take in promoting better health for local people.

One such project was designed to explore the way in which chronic asthma in children could be reduced by intervention in their living conditions. With sponsorship from a vacuum cleaner manufacturer, the project team undertook extensive home cleaning, using steam cleaning equipment where appropriate and providing dust-mite-proof bedding. The results were extremely encouraging, but what is most relevant here is the way we can present the story.

The traditional approach we adopted was to present it both within the council and to our health colleagues as an initiative we were undertaking to demonstrate our commitment to help the local health service achieve one of its primary targets, the reduction of childhood asthma. The success criteria we set related to positive changes in peak lung capacity, reduced incidence of hospital admissions and lower prescribing levels, which will generate budget savings for the health service. Health gain for these children was seen as an end in itself and, while we were happy to assist with this project, we saw our role as secondary to that of the health service. If the project was successful, we would be looking to them to take on responsibility for extending the initiative.

Exactly the same project could easily be repackaged to tell a very different story. This time we would talk of an initiative that is designed to tackle some of the health factors that are preventing the local authority from achieving its key policy objectives. The critical success factors now become the measured reduction in sickness absence from school, the improvements in literacy and numeracy in this group of children, and improvements in household income as carers are able to become more actively involved in employment. Financial savings can be measured over time through the reduction in additional special educational support. If these key performance measures are achieved, then it may become possible to make a sound business argument for the council to expand the project.

None of the facts have changed. The same project can be presented in ways that hit the right targets in each agency and, of course, it is clear that the most effective way of presenting the project to stimulate partnership working is to demonstrate clearly the mutual gain that can be achieved through an initiative like this. The interrelationship between health and social outcomes moves us away from divisive relationships to a new partnership model.

So my central message is that the DoH's new agenda, which requires a stronger local government involvement in health strategy, also requires a more involved commitment from health in the new local government agenda that is being promoted by the Department of the Environment, Transportation and Regions. The accident of history that has given us two separate central government departments running health and local government has meant that this two-way interdependency is poorly understood at a national level, and the practical implications in terms of co-ordination of the development of the health and local government agendas is visible more by its absence than its presence.

Yet the opportunity does exist to achieve greater synergy at this point in time. The underlying model proposed in *Our Healthier Nation* of a three-way partnership between central government, local agencies and the community has direct parallels in the democratic renewal agenda, which emphasises the need for local government to develop an effective and responsible partnership with its local communities and other local agencies in order to justify the powers and responsibilities devolved to it from national government. In practical terms, the debate is about the right of central government to set consistent minimum standards of service and conduct across the country, while allowing for local responses that are sensitive to locally defined needs and expectations. It will clearly be helpful if similar approaches are adopted across different Departments of State.

It would be unfair not to recognise that there is an awareness by national government of the problems of integration of public policy across departmental divides. The creation of the Social Exclusion Unit is perhaps the most visible illustration of a commitment to tackle some of these difficulties. A more significant step forward may come potentially through the review of public spending. Changes to allow greater flexibility in the use of budgets across agency boundaries may open the way to new and more creative responses which will not be so easily achieved through traditional departmental policy initiatives.

Whatever the difficulties created by the lack of coherence at a national level, the opportunity exists for effective progress at a local level. This is not to underestimate the magnitude of the changes and the huge amount of work that has to be done to implement a very challenging work programme for every part of the public sector. In fact, this pressure may provide a stimulus to more joint working in order to make the most of scarce resources.

The pilot New Commitment to Regeneration programme sponsored jointly by the Local Government Association and the Department of the Environment, Transportation and Regions will be seeking to establish new approaches to regeneration which encompass local health strategies as an integral part of a comprehensive approach to public service provision and the tackling of social exclusion at a local level. Rather than waiting for national frameworks to be handed down from above, local partnerships can drive the agenda forward. If they are to do so successfully, they will have to learn more about each other's individual objectives and establish sufficient common ground to create a shared work programme.

Those involved from both disciplines will need to listen more to each other, and try to see situations from each other's perspective. They will need to recognise that the change we seek does require substantial cultural change in the mindsets of people at every level of our respective organisations. This will not happen without conscious effort, and is a long-term project requiring substantial leadership at a professional and managerial level as well as at the political level. The goals that are there to be achieved are so important for the future stability and success of our society that the effort is well worthwhile. Those of us who work within local communities are perhaps best positioned to see the value of this mission, and perhaps should accept responsibility for providing the stimulus necessary to turn these ideas into reality.

CHAPTER NINETEEN

Environmental health perspectives

Graham Jukes

At the UN Conference on Environment and Development in 1992 in Rio de Janeiro, 175 nations, including the UK, signed an action plan for the 21st century which became known as *Agenda 21*. It is a comprehensive document which sets out a blueprint for sustainable development. Principle 1 of Agenda 21 states that 'Human beings are at the centre of concerns for sustainable development. They are entitled to a healthy and productive life style in harmony with nature'. Sustainable development recognises that we must meet the needs of people today without compromising the ability of future generations to meet theirs and has subsequently become the cornerstone of international, national and local policies.

One of the main thrusts of Agenda 21 is a call for action at a local level. This has become known as Local Agenda 21 and is driven by local people and local communities. It is well recognised that a balance must exist between strategic and local action if sustainable development is going to be achieved.

It is against this background that perspectives on the attainment of environmental health should be viewed.

In July 1997, the Environmental Health Commission, a body conceived by the Chartered Institute of Environmental Health, published their report following 14 months of deliberations. They were tasked with:

> ... *considering the principles of environmental health and their application to the health of individuals and the pursuit of sustainable development of communities; examining the relationship between environmental health and relevant socio-economic factors; and recommending a framework for action in the United Kingdom to reinforce and take forward the principles of environmental health with the involvement of the whole community.*[1]

It proved to be a challenging task, to break out from the constraints of existing understanding of the term 'environmental health' and to assign a more meaningful and modern approach to it.

The Public Health Act 1848 created the foundation for the administrative and bureaucratic interventions that we in the UK recognise as environmental health today. It is a narrow understanding and the local authority service in the UK is seen as being an enforcement-orientated regulatory tool on specified environmental problems affecting health. The training of environmental health officers is geared to that approach and to ensuring competence in the exercise of that function. The traditional areas of work are environmental protection (air quality, noise control, water quality, contaminated land, nuisance, pest control, animal welfare); food safety and control (food hygiene in commercial and factory premises, fitness of food for human consumption); health and safety at work; housing (fitness, repair and rehabilitation of the housing stock); and communicable disease control. There are over 200 separate items of legislation enforced by the environmental health service on behalf of local government.

The foundations of environmental health were created in a different era, within a vastly different cultural and socio-economic climate. A climate where the gross public health issues of the time were being addressed by political and social reformers and benevolent industrialists; where information and civic involvement were the privilege of the rich. The keys to resolving the gross public health issues were strategic infrastructure development and their maintenance, i.e. sanitation, water supply, waste management and housing. Regulatory interventions on factory emissions to the atmosphere, for wholesome unadulterated food and on dangerous working conditions ensured that improvements to health were maintained. The bureaucratic models set in train 150 years ago have evolved and so, too, has scientific knowledge and with it the social and economic climate.

In examining the current model of administration, the Environmental Health Commission found that the traditional model of environmental health in the UK was now 'well past its use-by date' and that 'environmental health having invented itself in the 19th century, needs to re-invent itself at the start of the 21st'. The evolution of the service could no longer be expected to deliver the wider environmental health agenda, given the complexities of modern life and understanding.

The government's *UK National Environmental Health Action Plan* (NEHAP), published in 1996, reiterated the traditional view and functions of environmental health, but for the first time, mapped out the wide number of actors who contribute to the achievement of it.[2] The UK was one of six countries who agreed to pilot a NEHAP at the Second Conference on Environment and Health in Helsinki in 1994. NEHAPs have now been developed by 46 of the 51 member states and provide a necessary link between environment and health, which are still different fields of activity in some countries. The UK will publish an update reflecting current thinking in time for the Third European Conference to be held in London in June 1999. The theme of this conference is 'action in partnership' and will set the agenda for environment and health across Europe at the start of the 21st century.

Environmental health can be interpreted in two different ways:

1   the collective term for the administrative and regulatory functions carried out by the environmental health service in local authorities in the UK

2   the development of a wide understanding of the links and trade-offs between the
    environmental, social and economic factors that affect human health and the inter-
    ventions needed to improve it. This was the interpretation of environmental health
    assigned to it by the Environmental Health Commission.

It is this second, and far wider, interpretation of environmental health that enables
the links to sustainable development and the traditional public health functions to be
made. It offers the best opportunities for restructuring environmental health so that it
becomcs a meaningful, effective way of considering and tackling the problems that today's
communities will face well into the 21st century.

What are these problems? Traditionally, they were poor housing, lack of sanitation,
adulteration of and unfit food and water supplies, unhealthy working conditions, infectious disease and poor air quality. There is now a real danger that the problems of our
past are fast becoming those of the future for some countries, particularly in Central
and Eastern Europe; problems which are characterised and measurable by gross health
indicator statistics with limited sophistication.

Today's problems in the UK are the maintenance and evolution of existing control
systems; the re-emergence of key infectious diseases and the identification and control of
new ones; inequalities in health; decline and lack of investment in infrastructure; poor
nutrition; and the synergistic effects on health of exposure to a variety of poor environmental and associated socio-economic conditions. These conditions are characterised by
the lack of clear cause-and-effect health indicators despite the sophistication of scientific
methods used today.

Tomorrow's environmental health profession will require a different range of skills
and competencies to address these issues, working within different administrative and
operational frameworks. There will still be a need for the regulator and the regulated.
Many of the improvements to environmental health have been hard fought for and
maintained by seldom seen vigilance. It is only when failures in existing systems come to
light, for example the *E. coli* O157 outbreak in Lanarkshire in 1997, that the effectiveness of regulation and the systems operated are questioned and re-evaluated.

Over the past 20 years, local government has been in a constant state of flux. Resource
pressures and the sheer complexities of the issues that are dealt with have forced local
government to adopt ever-changing management and organisational structures to
address the needs and expectations of their communities. The information revolution has
only fuelled the speed of change that has occurred. From rigid, predictable departmental
and professional frameworks to multidisciplinary, dynamic, corporate management
structures in two decades is change indeed, and there is more to come. Recent political
innovations to encourage salaried mayors, coupled with changes in civic engagement
brought about by the information revolution, will ensure that the shape of local government is constantly being re-formed.

Environmental health officers are now required to be specialists in so many fields that
the training they receive is not necessarily specifically designed for the roles they are
expected to fulfil. Where that training and skill is most appropriate and valuable is in

managing and planning corporate strategies for improvements for environment and health and ensuring that the basic regulatory function is maintained. With the growth of central agencies, many are now beginning to question whether the regulatory role is best carried out at local level or whether the future role of environmental health professionals is destined for regional-level activity.

This subtle change from principal regulator to corporate manager and strategist has benefited from the need for local governments to take a wider, more cohesive look at their policies and practices to ensure that sustainable development and 'best value' are at the heart of what they do.

The Environmental Health Commission identified eight agendas that are affecting the prospects for wider environmental health and the future:

• quality of life
• inequality
• lifestyle
• sustainability
• globalisation
• democracy
• information
• integration.

The interrelationship of these agendas will shape the development of new environmental health professionals for the future. The Commission challenged the Chartered Institute of Environmental Health to review the education and training of environmental health professionals in order to address the needs of the future, and that challenge has been accepted. Others also recognise that there are shortcomings in the training of people who will deliver solutions to the agendas set. The former CMO, Sir Kenneth Calman, commenced a wide-ranging review of public health. A review of training for public health professionals is one of the key outcomes.

The two approaches, while sharing the same roots 150 years ago, are clearly separated today, as the public health professional will inherently focus on those who are manifestly ill, while the environmental health professional is seeking to prevent illness from occurring. However, a common understanding and a working link between the two disciplines must be achieved.

Sustainable development was the starting point in looking at environmental health perspectives. It is currently an extremely potent concept that is driving much of the policy and practice in achieving effective environmental health solutions to problems.

The agendas for future change have been identified and professionals who work within the framework must be properly equipped and trained to tackle the tasks demanded of them. Therein lies the challenge: to anticipate far enough in advance the evolutionary socio-economic and political changes taking place in society to enable effective recruitment and training to take place which will allow and enable sustainable solutions to be achieved.

References

1   Chartered Institute of Environmental Health (1997) *Agendas for Change.* Report of the Environmental Health Commission. Chartered Institute of Environmental Health, London.

2   DoH/Dept of the Environment (1996) *The UK National Environmental Health Action Plan.* HMSO, London.

Further reading

Chartered Institute of Environmental Health (1998) 150 Years of Public Health. *Environmental Health Journal,* Commemorative Issue (June).

Laffin M and Young K (1990) *Professionalism in Local Government.* Longmans, London.

Laffin M (1996) Beyond Bureaucracy – Understanding Recent Change in the Public Sector Professions. Unpublished draft.

Local Government Management Board (1995) *Local Agenda 21, Principles and Process – A Step by Step Guide.* LGMB, London.

Rayner S and Malone E (1998) *Human Choice and Climate Change – 10 Suggestions for Policy Makers.* Battelle Memorial Institute, Battelle Press, Ohio.

World Health Organisation (1997) *Health and Environment in Sustainable Development – 5 Years after the Earth Summit.* WHO, Geneva.

CHAPTER TWENTY

Public health and health promotion

Charlotte Black

Introduction

In any discussions about public health it is important to explore the role and contribution of health promotion. There are two aspects to this discussion: health promotion as a process and health promotion as a specialist activity. In order to understand some of the current issues and influences on health promotion, it is necessary to trace its origins and the theoretical base that has been developed. This provides the backdrop to understanding the current and potential role of health promotion in public health and some of the dilemmas that this complex area presents.

History and theory

Health promotion is an integral part of public health. It has often been described as the implementation arm of public health. However, it is far more than a series of practical strategies. It is a broad aim that includes a diverse range of activities and approaches, all of which are concerned with public health.

As a term, health promotion means many different things to different people and there is no easy consensus as to what it includes.[1] The origins of health promotion theory can be found in the WHO's Alma Alta declaration in 1946, that 'health is not merely the absence of disease but a state of complete physical, mental and social well being'.[2] This definition has been criticised as being utopian and unattainable, but it provides a useful contradiction to the medical definition of health that predominates healthcare in the Western world.

The health promotion movement in the UK grew out of health education, which began with the information-giving role of MOH[3] and later resulted in the establishment of the Health Education Council in 1968, a non-governmental organisation established to run population-based health-education campaigns. *Health for all by the Year 2000*[4] proposed a wider agenda that took into account the determinants of health and the factors that influenced health choices and were outside of individual control. Gradually, the need for social and political change to improve health came to the fore in health promotion theory and practice.[1] Consequently, from the 1980s onwards, there is evidence of increased emphasis upon reducing inequalities and building healthy public policy and collaborative work between sectors.

In 1985 the WHO set 38 targets, revised in 1991,[5] for health improvement in the European region, resulting in the Healthy Cities movement. Thirty cities were identified around the world as demonstration sites and intersectoral action plans were developed and local targets set for health improvement.

The health promotion movement in the UK is built upon the *Ottawa Charter for Health Promotion*[6] which sets out the following activities as the main components of health promotion.

- **Build healthy public policy** – putting health on the agenda of policy makers in all sectors and at all levels, directing them to be aware of the health consequences of their decisions and to accept their responsibilities for health.
- **Create supportive environments** – systematic assessment of the health impact of a rapidly changing environment is essential. The protection of the natural and built environment and the conservation of natural resources must be addressed in any health promotion strategy.
- **Strengthen community action** – health promotion works through concrete and effective community action in setting priorities, making decisions, planning strategies and implementing them to achieve better health. At the heart of this process is the empowerment of communities.
- **Develop personal skills** – health promotion supports personal and social development through providing information, education for health and enhancing life skills.
- **Reorient health services** – the role of the health sector must move increasingly in a health promotion direction, beyond its responsibility for providing clinical and curative services.

This list of activities has been criticised for being too all-encompassing to help organisations identify and fulfil their own discrete role in the promotion of health. However the Ottawa Charter has provided a useful backdrop to the development of health promotion theory and practice in the UK. The Society of Health Promotion Education and Promotion Specialists (SHEPS) draws upon the WHO *Health for All* strategy, the Ottawa Charter and Agenda 21,[7] and defines health promotion as:

> *... any activity that promotes health. Health promotion is achieved through activity focused on the social, economic and environmental determinants of health.*

The desire to develop a firm theoretical base for such a complex subject has resulted in the proliferation of a series of models of health promotion. It is not within the scope of this

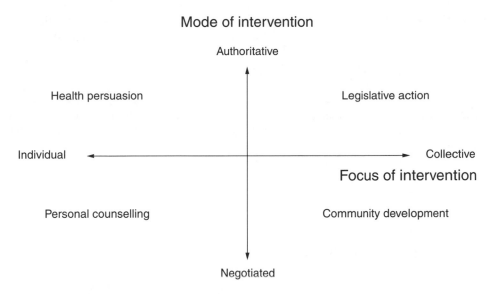

Figure 20.1:   Beattie's conceptual map model of health promotion

chapter to describe them all and further reading is recommended. The most commonly used is Ewles and Simnett's five approaches to health promotion developed in 1985 and refined in 1992 and 1995.[8] Their five approaches are: medical, behaviour change, educational, client-centred and societal change. The weakness of this classification of health promotion activity is that it does not reflect the dynamic nature of health promotion nor the relative value of the different approaches.

Readers can turn to many other models, such as those of French and Adams,[9] Tones and Tilford,[10] and Downie, Fyfe and Tannahill.[11] Beattie[12] created a conceptual map which differentiates as to whether the intervention has been imposed or negotiated, and whether the focus of the intervention is on the collective or the individual. This provides a useful social and political perspective and invites the reader to explore how health promotion activities have been initiated and the subsequent impact they may have (Figure 20.1). This model sets out four main strategies for health promotion:

- health persuasion – interventions directed at individuals and led by professionals, e.g. a community nurse or midwife encouraging a pregnant woman to stop smoking
- legislative action – interventions that are decided by professionals or expert bodies that are intended to protect the health of the community, e.g. lobbying for legislation for compulsory fluoridation by water companies
- personal counselling – interventions that are client-led and focus on personal development and facilitating individuals to make their own choices, e.g. helping a young person identify their own health concerns and working with them to develop their own confidence and skills

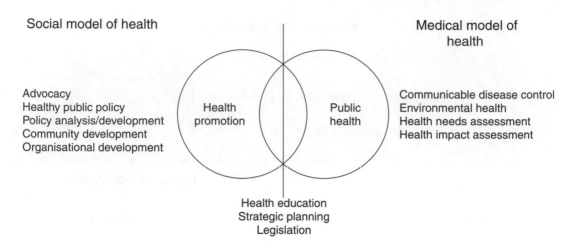

Figure 20.2:   Scott Samuel's model of public health and health promotion

- community development – work that takes place within a defined community. Local priorities for health are identified and the community concerned is supported and facilitated to take action on those local priorities and concerns, e.g. residents on a housing estate setting up a food co-op or credit union.

There is a need to describe health promotion in the broader context of public health, rather than as a separate entity. The model shown in Figure 20.2 was recently proposed by Alex Scott Samuel as part of a review of the health promotion function being carried out by the Health Education Authority.[13] It demonstrates the overlapping spheres of public health and health promotion, and the difficulty of labelling a specific activity as public health or health promotion. If a broad interpretation of health promotion is applied, it is difficult to distinguish the two. It provides a useful basis for discussion as the position of some of these elements is contestable and dependent on interpretation, such as the difference between community development and needs assessment, and whether healthy public policy can be described as health promotion or public health.

Health promotion and public policy

Public policy is an essential component of public health and health promotion. International, national and local policy decisions provide a framework for health promotion action and have a profound impact upon health. Public policy can also influence the funding and organisational position of specialist health promotion services. The reason for concentrating on it here is that public policy can be one of the most powerful approaches to health promotion and is often least evident in practice.[14] Health promoters in all sectors, at national and local level, can work to influence public policy and use policy making and enactment to secure change.[15]

The attempt to influence policy can take place directly or through local community and pressure groups. Public awareness of the health impact of policy decisions can be raised through the media and community networks, and evidence of need and local health problems can be brought to the attention of local politicians. This is particularly effective when a number of organisations work in partnership through their various networks, offering different perspectives, with a view to achieving the same ends.

Policy development is not an adequate strategy on its own and does have some inherent dangers. Health promoters seeking to influence public policy need to consider on whose behalf they are acting and whether they have a legitimate right to do so. Critics of policy making as an approach to health promotion see it as a form of social control, taking the power out of the hands of the individual and making decisions on their behalf.[16] When deciding to embark on work concerned with public policy, those involved need to consider whether it is the most effective approach, whether their goals are realistic, and to ensure that strategies are in place to involve and inform local people. It is unlikely that changes in public policy will not have adverse consequences for some sectors of the population.

Mention has already been made of the impact of international policy, such as *Health for All* and related WHO initiatives that the UK has signed up to. UK involvement in international policy work on the environment and sustainable development, such as Agenda 21[17] (Earth Summit 1992), also has direct implications for health promotion. Supportive environments for health can be created by specific legislation, regulation and the creation of voluntary codes of practice. The most commonly cited example of successful health promotion legislation at national level is seat-belt legislation for front-seat passengers in 1981. This resulted in a 30% reduction in accidents in that year and compliance levels of around 95%.[18] There are many current examples of health promotion policy that are surrounded by controversy, such as tobacco advertising, drink–drive limits and food safety. Many other areas of central government policy, such as transport, education and welfare, are of equal if not greater significance to health.

DoH policy also has a direct and indirect impact on health promotion. Major policy landmarks have been: the publication of *Prevention and Health: everybody's business*[19] and, in 1992, *The Health of the Nation: a strategy for health in England*.[20] A series of national and local targets were set in five key areas of coronary heart disease and stroke, accidents, cancer, mental illness, and HIV/AIDS and sexual health. Equivalent strategies were produced for health in Wales, Scotland and Northern Ireland. *The Health of the Nation* has been subject to much criticism for its narrow, disease-based focus and the inappropriate focus on lifestyle and individual behaviour change, which limited its impact on organisations outside the NHS that have a health promotion function. An additional key area was added on 'variations in health',[21] in recognition of the increasing body of evidence on inequalities in health.

The NHS and Community Care Act of 1991 divided the NHS into purchasing and providing functions. In the absence of any national guidance on where specialist health promotion departments belonged, decisions were taken on a local basis. Individual staff or whole departments were either maintained in the health authority or became part of a trust or a stand-alone agency. There are many examples around the country of departments being moved from purchaser to provider, or vice versa, as circumstances have changed and the realities of the internal market have developed.[22] In some instances there have been advantages and the health promotion units and specialists affected have adapted well, but the costs of constant change have been great. In some instances the budget for the specialist health promotion department has been significantly reduced, whereas in others it has grown as alternative sources of funding have been secured.

These reforms also meant that the health promotion activities of NHS providers had to be considered as part of the commissioning and contracting process. It became more difficult to develop the role of NHS organisations and professionals without having money attached to any suggested development.

The White Paper on *The New NHS* and the Green Paper on public health, *Our Healthier Nation*, that will replace *The Health of the Nation* has been published recently.[23,24] *Our Healthier Nation* demonstrates a much clearer understanding by government of the true determinants of health and the role of government policy in promoting public health. However, despite that major shift in thinking, it proposes a set of narrow priorities that are very similar to those of *The Health of the Nation*: mental health, accidents, cancer, and heart disease and stroke. This fairly traditional way of describing public health priorities may not facilitate the process of engaging non-NHS organisations in the health promotion agenda.

Our Healthier Nation does not distinguish between health promotion and public health, although the CMO's report on strengthening the public health function in England[25] recommends that more work is needed to examine the role of the specialist health promotion function as part of the local public health function. The implications of the White Paper for health promotion are discussed at the end of this chapter as we look to the future.

Health promotion in general practice has also been subject to a considerable amount of policy change. By 1990, health promotion had become part of the national contract for general practice. Between 1990 and 1996 the contract had been reformed twice, and health promotion was rapidly losing favour in general practice as further changes were imposed. In 1996, the General Medical Services Committee renegotiated the contract to a professionally led approach. Practices are now asked to submit their proposals for health promotion activity and these are approved by a local Health Promotion Committee consisting of GP and health authority representatives. Although some practices have found innovative and effective ways of promoting health through these changes, there is widespread feeling that there is much ground to be made up on health promotion and general practice. The proposals in the White Paper[23] for the establishment of PCGs states that health promotion will be one of their functions. This presents both challenges and opportunities for health promoters to develop the role of the primary care team in health promotion.

Who is responsible for health promotion?

The wide variety of influences on health means that health promotion is the responsibility of a diverse range of organisations and individuals. The challenge for those working in the field has always been to develop the skills and capacity of others, and to integrate health promotion into their work in a way that will result in sustained change.

At national level the Health Education Authority secures income through bidding for contracts from the DoH and other purchasers. The DoH and NHS Executive provide the strategic framework for the NHS, but other government departments are also critical to the creation of change at a national level, hence the appointment of a Minister for Public Health to work across government departments.

Although the NHS, and in particular health authorities, are expected to take the lead on local action to promote health, local authorities are key players. A survey carried out by the Health Education Authority and the Local Government Management Board in 1996[26] revealed that almost 80% of respondents recognised health promotion as a specific area of activity, and 25% indicated that they had a corporate health strategy. Health promotion is traditionally associated with Environmental Health Officers, but departments of transport, housing, planning, leisure, education and social services are also taking a more active role in recognition of the wider determinants of health.

Health promotion specialists are core members of the multidisciplinary public health team. They are usually employed within the NHS or local authorities, with responsibility for developing strategy and stimulating and co-ordinating activities to promote health. Specialist health promotion units vary in size, funding and approach, and much depends upon where they are placed within the NHS, in trusts, health authorities or as stand-alone agencies. Those based in health authorities generally have a more strategic role in planning public health strategy, commissioning other organisations to deliver health promotion and providing input to the development of local health services. However, the pattern across the country varies and it is impossible to generalise, as several units do not distinguish between their purchaser and provider functions, which many feel has created a false dichotomy.

Health professionals and others who make up the primary care team are an essential part of the health promotion, and therefore public health, resource. Health promotion is a core function for professional groups such as practice nurses, health visitors and school nurses. The relationships they establish with local people and communities mean they are well placed to provide one-to-one support and advice. There are also examples of community nurses taking on a public health role through direct involvement in developing neighbourhood strategies and community development work.

Health promotion activity in the NHS is not limited to primary care and community services. Health Promoting Hospitals is an example of an initiative that has been implemented in some acute and combined trusts, as a way of taking an organisational development approach to health promotion.[27] A similar organisational development model has also been applied to the development of health promotion settings such as schools and workplaces.[28]

The local voluntary sector has an important part to play in health promotion. Volunteers are often commissioned to provide outreach services to community groups and deliver community-based projects, having established strong local networks with their client group. The voluntary sector can advocate on behalf of local people and is an important partner in community development work.

Finally, we should not forget the contribution the commercial sector can make to health promotion. This can be as an employer, alliance partner, funder or as a producer. If the energies and commitment of the commercial sector can be harnessed, in a way that does not compromise the objectives and principles of health promotion, this can bring considerable benefit to local health promotion work and to the organisation concerned. The same applies to the national and local media. Health promotion is not their core business, but health promoters can develop partnerships with the media which will benefit the health of local people.

The most important point to make is that health promotion is not the domain of one professional group or organisation. Throughout the country examples can be found of formalised partnership arrangements that have been set up to harness the energy and co-ordinate the action of these various organisation. These often result in joint funding of initiatives to promote health and a shared approach to policy making and stimulating community action through community development.

Current issues and dilemmas in health promotion

Health promotion is a political issue. It is an exciting and dynamic area of work, which raises some fundamental ethical dilemmas, and consequently attracts both controversy and debate. In common with public health, health promotion is besieged with problems around funding, outcomes, priorities and effectiveness.

A major issue for those working in health promotion is how to target limited resources. There are many different ways of setting priorities, such as settings, client groups or topic areas, and many health promotion professionals will use a combination for the way they plan and present their work. However, the more fundamental question is whether health promotion should concentrate on disadvantaged groups and communities, in order to reduce inequalities in health. Community development is generally the approach to health promotion that is regarded as more effective and appropriate in communities experiencing disadvantage.

The discussion on public policy earlier in the chapter raised questions about the legitimacy of health promoters working to influence public policy on behalf of local people. The same question could be raised about targeting. Attempts by an organisation to target a local community and work with them to identify health issues and take action accordingly, can be viewed as worthy but intrusive. Community development requires considerable skill and expertise for that reason, and it also requires a realistic timescale to build a dialogue with a community.

The questions that health promoters have to consider are what impact is their work having? and do the means justify the ends? Is it doing good rather than harm, and who decided what was 'good'? The term 'victim blaming' grew out of a concern about the negative effects of lifestyle campaigns and individual advice to change behaviour, without consideration of individual circumstances. The importance of being able to quantify the impact of health promotion cannot go without mention. Historically there has been an emphasis in health service research on quantitative methods and the randomised control trial as the gold standard. This presents problems for health promotion where changes in health status are not immediate, and the influences on health are so diverse that it is rarely possible to attribute change to one intervention. In addition, there is the question of how 'success' is measured. There is a need to identify appropriate methodologies for the future, with a view to measuring the effects of health promotion and target future efforts. A series of effectiveness bulletins have been published on specific issues which have been put to good use in the field, although the scope of the reviews is limited to studies that fall into very specific criteria of having carried out a randomised control trial. There is an immediate need to establish a robust evidence base for health promotion using a broader research base, including studies that measure the impact of interventions on systems and organisational development as well as change in individual behaviour.[28]

Limited funding for health promotion has always been a constraint. An inquiry into the cost effectiveness of the *Health of the Nation* strategy[29] showed that in 1996 £3 million was spent on the strategy, £45 million on the HEA, £73 million on health promotion payments for general practice and £90 million on NHS Specialist Health Promotion Units. This represents less than 1% of the total annual budget for the NHS. In some parts of the country, investment in health promotion has been increased in recognition of the need for health authorities to look to the future,[30] but many have reduced their investment. In order for health promotion to make its full contribution to public health, sustainable investment plans need to be developed. Many health promoters have been successful in attracting new money from external sources with local partners, such as the EEC and Single Regeneration. Possible future sources are lottery funding for Healthy Living Centres and central government funding for HAZs to encourage partnership work.

The future

Health promotion will be an important element of an emerging wider public health agenda, as set out in *Our Healthier Nation* and in the NHS White Paper. Health promotion and collaborative work with local authorities and voluntary and commercial sectors will become an increasingly important part of the role of health authorities as commissioning responsibilities are devolved to primary care. HIMPs should provide the main vehicle for setting local priorities for health promotion and setting out the arrangements for joint working and the responsibilities for each partner organisation. It will become increasingly difficult to distinguish between health promotion and public health as health improvement becomes a shared aim. Success will be more likely if organisations such as health authorities, local authorities, and PCGs and trusts have sufficient organisational capacity and commitment to put health improvement at the centre of their organisation. It is also hoped that increased action by central government at a policy level will create a climate of change and new possibilities, which will enhance local action by involvement of a number of different agencies and individuals.

References

1   Jones L (1997) The rise of health promotion. In: J Katz and A Peberby (eds) *Promoting Health Knowledge and Practice*. The Open University, Buckingham.

2   World Health Organisation (1946) *Constitution*. WHO, Geneva.

3   Naidoo J and Wills J (1994) *Health Promotion Foundations for Practice*. Ballière Tindall, London.

4   World Health Organisation (1977) *Health for All by the Year 2000*. WHO, Geneva.

5   World Health Organisation (1991) *Revised Targets for Health for All in Europe*. WHO, Copenhagen.

6   World Health Organisation (1986) *Ottawa Charter for Health Promotion*. WHO, Geneva.

7   Society of Health Education and Promotion Specialists (1997) *Principles of Practice and the Code of Conduct*. SHEPS.

8   Ewles L and Simnett I (1985) *Promoting Health* (3e). Scutari Press, Chichester.

9   French J and Adams L (1986) From analysis to synthesis: theories of health education. *Health Education Journal*. **45**(2): 7–14.

10 Tones BK and Tilford S (1994) *Health Education: effectiveness, efficiency and equity*. Chapman & Hall, London.

11 Downie RS, Fyfe C and Tannahill A (1990) *Health Promotion: models and values*. Oxford Medical Publications, Oxford.

12 Beattie A (1991) Knowledge and control in health promotion: a rest case for social theory. In: J Gabe, M Calnan and M Bury (eds) *The Sociology of the Health Service*. Oxford Medical Publications, Oxford.

13 Scott Samuel A (1998) Submission to working group on the 'current function of health promotion' as part of HEAs Review of the Health Promotion Function.

14 Chapman S and Lupton D (1994) *The Fight for Public Health: principles and practice of media advocacy*. BMJ Publishing Group, London.

15 Jones L (1997) Making and changing public policy. In: L Jones and M Sidell (eds) *The Challenge of Promoting Health Exploration and Action*. The Open University, Buckingham.

16 Jones L, from a first draft by Adams L (1997) The politics of health promotion. In: L Jones and M Sidell (eds) *The Challenge of Promoting Health*. The Open University, Buckingham.

17 Earth Summit (1993) *Agenda 21*. New York, United Nations.

18 Ashton SJ *et al.* (1985) *The Effects of Mandatory Seat Belt Use in Great Britain*. The 10th Annual Conference of Experimental Safety Vehicles, July, Transport Road Research Laboratory.

19 Department of Health and Social Security (1976) *Prevention and Health; Everybody's Business*. HMSO, London.

20 Department of Health (1992) *The Health of the Nation: a strategy for health in England*. HMSO, London.

21 Department of Health (1995) *Variations in Health, What can the Department of Health and the NHS do?* Report of the Variations Sub Group of the Chief Medical Officer, Health of the Nation Working Group. HMSO, London.

22 French J (1997) The current position of health promotion services in the UK. *SHEPS Debate*. **1**(4): 15–19.

23 Department of Health (1997) *The New NHS: modern, dependable*. HMSO, London.

24 Department of Health (1998) *Our Healthier Nation: a contract for health*. A Consultation Paper. Cm 3852. HMSO, London.

25 Department of Health (1998) *Chief Medical Officer's Project to Strengthen the Public Health Function in England*. A report of emerging findings. HMSO, London.

26 Moran G (1996) *Promoting Health and Local Government* A report prepared for the Health Education Authority and Local Government Management Board. Health Education Authority, London.

27 Grossman R and Sceala K (1993) *Health Promotion and Organisational Development: developing settings for health*. WHO, Vienna.

28 Speller V, Learmouth A and Harrison D (1997) The search for evidence of effective health promotion. *British Medical Journal*. **315**: 361–3.

29 Limb L (1996) *Health of the Nation* under scrutiny. *Health Services Journal*. **106**: 8.

30 Cambridge and Huntingdon Health Authority (1997) Draft annual plan 1998/99.

CHAPTER TWENTY-ONE

The practice of public health medicine: past, present, future

June Crown

The past: public health to community medicine

Before 1974, the practice of public health medicine was the domain of the MOH, who was a respected and influential person in each community with considerable powers as a senior local authority officer. The position goes back to 1847, when the first MOH, Dr William Henry Duncan, was appointed in Liverpool (*see* Chapter 3). The best of the MOH fully understood the breadth of their task. They ensured that their localities had safe water supplies and sewage systems; they pressed their authorities to replace slum housing; and they influenced education departments and introduced preventive and school health programmes. Each MOH was required to present an annual report to the council, and many of these were forthright, soundly scientifically and epidemiologically based, and elegantly written documents which still make compelling reading. The MOH's responsibility to set out plainly the health problems of the community was recognised by his or her protection from dismissal. The MOH was expected to propose change even if the action needed to tackle the problems was expensive for the council, and was expected to draw attention to continuing problems even if they were a result of wilful and embarrassing inactivity or neglect by the council.

At this time, local authorities, advised by the MOH, provided community-based health services, such as family planning, home nursing, health visiting, maternal and child health, and vaccination and immunisation programmes. The MOH, working with the environmental health officers, was also responsible for the control of communicable disease by preventive measures, surveillance programmes and the management of outbreaks. In addition, local authorities were also responsible for the provision of personal social services, environmental services, education and housing. The potential impact of local authority activities on public health was therefore enormous, since they controlled major determinants of health as well as providing the key preventive and health promotion services.

Meanwhile, from the inauguration of the NHS in 1948, the hospital-based treatment services were separately planned and administered. The majority of hospitals came under the control of Regional Hospital Boards, which were advised by their senior administrative medical officers. The teaching hospitals and London-based postgraduate hospitals had Boards of Governors, responsible directly to the Department of Health and Social Security. Few hospitals were influenced by public health professionals, save in relation to statutory matters such as the control of infectious disease.

The other arm of treatment services, general practice, was provided by doctors who, while part of the NHS, were employed as independent contractors, with no obligation to collaborate with, or even acknowledge, the activities of either local authorities or hospital services.

Research and education in public health medicine was largely undertaken in university and medical school departments, most often called 'social medicine'. These departments were engaged in a wide range of epidemiologically based studies which established the scientific basis for some of the most important health promotion programmes of this century. Sir Richard Doll demonstrated the links between smoking and cancer, and Professor JN (Jerry) Morris identified the relationships between physical activity and health.

These four important strands – local authority-based public health, hospital services, general practice and academic social medicine – remained relatively isolated until the 1970s. In 1972, three documents were published which were to bring about major changes in public health practice and in health services in the UK. The most important was the White Paper, *National Health Service Reorganisation: England*,[1] which set out arrangements for the first major reorganisation of the NHS since its inception in 1948, and which took place in 1974. The aim was to improve patient care by better integration of services. In a prescriptive structure of regions, areas and districts, the community health and preventive services of local authorities joined the hospital services (except the London postgraduate hospitals). Similar arrangements, but without the regional tier, were introduced in Scotland, Wales and Northern Ireland. Significantly, local authorities retained responsibility for social services (except in Northern Ireland) and environmental health services. GPs retained their independent contractor status, although they were represented on the management groups at each level.

The duties of the new 'community medicine specialists' were identified as:

assessing need for health services, evaluating the effectiveness of existing services and planning the best use of health resources. Equally, they will concern themselves with developing preventive health services, with the links between health and the local authority personal social, public health and education services.[1]

The *Report of the Working Party on Medical Administrators* (the Hunter Report)[2] developed the concept of 'community medicine' (as opposed to medical administration) and set out the proposed roles of 'Community Medicine Specialists' at regional, area and district levels. This again was a prescriptive document which proposed the expected number and areas of expertise of doctors in each department. It also made recommendations about the training and career structures in the new speciality and established the important principle of equivalence between community medicine specialists and clinical consultants.

The *Second Report of the Joint Working Party on the Organisation of Medical Work in Hospitals*, chaired by Sir George Godber (the Cogwheel Report),[3] provided a blueprint for medical advisory structures which, although focused on hospital practice, encouraged the establishment of 'Divisions of community medicine and general practice'. It also stated that 'the help of the Community Physician will be needed to enable hospital doctors to play their part in the management of a fully integrated health service', thus reasserting the public health doctors' role as a bridge between clinicians and managers.

These reports formed the background to the establishment of the Faculty of Community Medicine, in 1972.[4] The Faculty is the body responsible for standards of professional practice and training in the speciality. It was founded following discussions between the Society of Medical Officers of Health, the group of Senior Administrative Medical Officers, the Scottish Association of Medical Administrators and the Society for Social Medicine. It brought together in its foundation membership and fellowship representatives of service practitioners from local authority and Regional Hospital Board backgrounds, the Defence Medical Services and academics from the university departments of social medicine, under the presidency of Professor Archie Cochrane. The final draft of the proposal to form the Faculty of Community Medicine (1970) states:

> At a later date, and by agreement with the Royal Colleges, consideration would be given to the eligibility of non-medical colleagues practising, teaching or conducting research in the field of Community Medicine.

From past to present: community medicine to public health medicine

The new NHS community medicine departments were established in 1974, staffed according to DoH guidance with Regional Medical Officers, Area Medical Officers and Specialists in Community Medicine in the regions and areas, and with District Community Physicians. Most of these consultants, from former local authority or regional board backgrounds, undertook special courses to prepare them for their new roles.

The prescribed staffing arrangements were matched by a centralist approach to the work. Energy was largely centred on the organisation of healthcare. An early priority for many was the integration of community-based services, which had previously been run by local authorities, into the NHS. Each area or district had a 'Joint Care Planning Team' for children, mental health and services for the elderly, with hospital, community, primary care and local authority membership. Although some modest allocations of money were available for these services, they frequently continued to suffer the fate of the designated 'priorities', in falling behind the acute, hospital-based services in the attention paid to them and in the resources secured for them.

The central-planning, rationalist approach also applied to hospital services. National guidelines set out the number of hospital beds required per 1000 population, though these were more often based on historic patterns of supply rather than on assessments of need. Staffing levels were similarly calculated on a normative basis, with little expectation of changes in patterns of care between professions and between disciplines.

The concept of equity of access to healthcare was implicit in this planning approach. The implementation of change therefore required the problem of historically diverse resource allocation across the NHS to be addressed. This was done by the Resource Allocation Working Party (RAWP),[5] which produced a formula for the population-based allocation of funds. Although it included weightings for demography, social disadvantage and other variables, it was a relatively crude approach. The government's response to the vociferously expressed concerns of influential 'RAWP losers' was to initiate a system whereby increases in NHS funds were to be given to the 'poorest' areas, until such a time as they caught up with the 'rich' areas, and equity was achieved. Although there were arguments about the pace of change, this approach was fine in principle while the economy was expanding and there was a real growth, year on year, in the health service. However, this situation changed following the 1970s oil crisis, and the RAWP was less able to cope with the distribution of cuts. The search for a genuinely equitable formula for resource allocation, based on need, continues still.

Although the community physicians based in the NHS in the 1970s were preoccupied with inequalities in health services, inequalities in health were not forgotten. Sir Douglas Black chaired a DoH research working group on 'Inequalities in health'[6] which concluded that socio-economic differences in health existed and had been increasing since 1951. The report achieved considerable publicity because of political efforts to suppress it. The Government did not accept its conclusions and rejected the recommendation, which included shifting NHS resources from hospital to primary care and preventive services, and increasing social security benefits, because they were too expensive.

The enthusiasm for broadly based public health action which the Black Report generated was diminished not only by government rejection of the report, but also by a further reorganisation of the NHS in 1981, when areas were abolished, leaving just regions and districts. Community physicians who had not taken early retirement in 1974 and had competed for posts in the integrated NHS now found themselves involved in a further round of centrally organised competition, often for the post they currently occupied. The complex arrangements meant that friends and colleagues found themselves on the opposite sides of interview panels on consecutive days, followed by periods of matching of employing authority and consultant preferences, before they knew which job in the new structure had been offered to them. Unsurprisingly, a further tranche of consultants retired, many of them older colleagues with wide general public health experience.

Although the emphasis of public health work in the NHS following the 1981 reorganisation remained on health service provision, a wider agenda began to emerge. The WHO published the *Health for All* strategy and the European Region set out 38 targets to be achieved by the year 2000, which were endorsed by all member states.[7] The application of this strategy to urban health resulted in the Healthy Cities movement[8] and many district community medicine departments grasped this opportunity to widen their activities and invest energy in the promotion of health, the reduction of inequalities and the associated reorientation of health services.

This thrust was assisted by the publication of Sir Donald Acheson's report on his inquiry into the public health function.[9] The inquiry had been set up because of concern about standards of practice, particularly in relation to the control of communicable disease. There was unease that expertise in this field had been lost following the reorganisations and that its importance was not adequately recognised in either practice or training in community medicine. The Acheson Report, however, addressed the public health function more broadly. It recommended the appointment of a Consultant in Communicable Disease Control in every district, but also went on to assess the other public health functions of health authorities and the resources needed to provide them. It concluded that there should be 15.8 public health consultants per million population (a number still not yet achieved across the UK). It proposed that each health authority should have a DPH as an executive member of the management team. It also proposed the reinstatement of the Annual Health Report – discontinued in 1974 – to be produced by the DPH as a public document. Acheson further suggested that the name 'community medicine' should be dropped in favour of 'public health medicine', which led to a change of name of the Faculty, following a vote, to the Faculty of Public Health Medicine.

The turbulence of the 1980s continued for public health physicians in the NHS with the introduction of general management, which left some departments flourishing, though others experienced considerable difficulties in maintaining their resources and their influence in their authorities, and there was yet another wave of early retirements. This was followed in 1990 by a more fundamental reform affecting the whole NHS,[10,11] in which health authorities (and in some circumstances GPs) were given responsibility for the assessment of the health needs of the population and for purchasing services through contracts to meet those needs. The services were to be provided in hospitals or the community sector, managed by NHS trusts. Public health departments were largely placed in health authorities, which were expected to provide the epidemiological expertise for needs assessment and service monitoring and the medical advice on purchasing decisions. The language of this reform at the outset was combative. The concept of the market was assumed to require distance, or even 'Chinese walls', between purchasers and providers. This often affected relationships between public health physicians and their clinical colleagues, who may have worked closely together on service developments in the past, but were now meant to confront each other during contract negotiations. Although it was later recognised that the efficient working of the market requires collaboration between purchasers and providers, in some places the working relationships took time to repair.

The 1990 NHS reform had more significant effects on public health practice. The 'Health for All' focus in the late 1980s and the many innovative areas of work springing from it were overwhelmed by the sheer volume of activity required to deal with the purchasing function and the annual renewal of contracts. Once again, public health physicians were occupied largely with the issues of healthcare and unable to pay sufficient attention to broader public health priorities.

Some assistance came with the publication of a national strategy for health, *The Health of the Nation* in 1992,[11,12] which set targets in five priority areas (heart disease and stroke, cancer, sexual health, accidents and mental health). Although health authorities were expected to establish programmes aimed at achieving these targets, it was clear that the political priority, and the NHS performance management, was still focused mainly on health services and issues such as the 'Patient's Charter' and waiting lists. This was also seen in *The National Health Service: a service with ambitions*,[13] which emphasised the commitment to a primary care-led NHS confirmed in *Primary Care: delivering the future*[14] and *Choice and Opportunity: primary care: the future*.[15]

Meanwhile, within the medical profession, there was concern about undergraduate education in public health, and the General Medical Council document *Tomorrow's Doctors*[16] asked for a change of emphasis in the curriculum, which has been addressed, but not yet achieved, by all medical schools.

From present to future: public health medicine to public health

Public health departments in the NHS and in the universities have always been multi-disciplinary. Consultants in public health medicine have worked alongside statisticians, geographers, economists and others. Trainees in public health medicine have been taught by experts from a wide range of backgrounds. However, the NHS has never identified appropriate grades for these staff; their training has been poorly supported; and their career paths have been uncertain. In spite of the expectations of its founding fathers, there were no moves for the Faculty of Public Health Medicine to extend membership for non-medically qualified public health practitioners beyond a small number of 'Honorary Members' until 1994. A vote was taken in 1995 in which the proposal to extend membership by examination was rejected. This resulted in dismay and hurt for many public health practitioners who not only felt disadvantaged financially and in career opportunities, but were also disappointed at what seemed a failure to recognise their scientific expertise and an unwillingness to accord them professional esteem. The Multidisciplinary Public Health Forum was established in 1995 to represent the interests of public health practitioners from all specialities. The Forum is now (1998) working with other bodies, including the Faculty, to develop training and recognition of its members and to strengthen public health advocacy more generally.

Further progress has now been made by the Faculty of Public Health Medicine. At its Annual General Meeting in 1998, a proposal to introduce a new category of Diplomate Membership open to all professional groups, by examination, was unanimously approved. It has been agreed that there will be one set of examinations for the Diploma and for Part I of the Faculty Membership (at present only open to medical practitioners), demonstrating equivalence of achievement for all candidates.

This strengthening and broadening of public health practice comes at a crucial time. Following the 1997 general election, the first ever Minister of Public Health was appointed in the UK. Although located within the DoH, it is explicitly accepted that the influence of the new minister must extend to all government departments, for all their policies will have an impact on the health of the population. It is recognised that the NHS makes only a modest contribution to overall public health status. Real improvements will depend on reducing socio-economic inequalities and tackling poverty.

The government's strategy has been set out in a White Paper, *The New NHS: modern, dependable*[17] and in a Green Paper, *Our Healthier Nation.*[18] These documents are complementary. Their implementation will lead to major changes in the role of NHS public health departments. Much of the burden of commissioning healthcare will pass to PCGs, which will have to assess the health needs of their population. Contracts will no longer have to be renewed annually, so longer-term service planning and development will be facilitated. Health authorities will take the lead in developing HIMPs, in collaboration with local authorities, voluntary agencies and commercial organisations. Within NHS provider trusts, 'clinical governance' will be introduced, with an emphasis on clinical quality and evidence-based, effective professional practice.

All of these changes will require public health skills, if they are to be successful. The CMO's report on the public health function[19] draws attention to the need to improve and extend all aspects of training and practice in public health, if we are to achieve the capacity that the present national agenda demands.

So the future of public health practice looks busy, exhilarating and fulfilling. The external environment in which we are working is supportive. The recognition of the breadth of issues that affect health should encourage an even wider public health family to join forces to achieve common goals.

We cannot, however, face the future with credibility if we plan only to offer 'more of the same'. Public health professionals, like all others, must be constantly moving forwards and aiming to anticipate, rather than just to react to, the important issues of the day.

Although in the UK, the main health problems are not likely to change in the next few years, some of the approaches to health and prevention will change. There are many contemporary examples.

- Our understanding of genetics is advancing rapidly, and will change significantly our capacity for risk assessment as well as opportunities for treatment. The public health, ethical, moral and resource implications all require careful attention now.
- We have been unsuccessful in tackling some problems, in spite of major efforts over many years. For example, young people, especially girls, continue to take up smoking.

Should we be seeking and testing new ways of helping this important group to protect their health? Which partners will be able to develop the societal and personal programmes that may succeed?

- The public health connections with food and nutrition were well recognised by the earliest MOH. The problems now are of obesity rather than malnutrition, and are increasing, especially among some vulnerable groups. The MOH laid down standards of hygiene but could not have anticipated BSE or the development of antibiotic-resistant bacteria, partly due to animal husbandry practices.
- The increasing public interest in the physical environment and its impact on health is welcome, although in some instances the assumed connections with disease have still to be demonstrated. Nevertheless, action at local and global levels to achieve sustainable environmental improvement is essential. The health impact of the social and economic environment is less publicised but equally important, and issues such as Third World debt also require urgent discussion and action.

In many areas, we do not need more scientific knowledge, but better understanding of how to bring about change. In other areas, improved methodologies are needed for more sophisticated monitoring and surveillance of health. Elsewhere, research is still required into new and persistent public health problems.

Public health medicine has an important contribution to make to this extensive array of activities. It is clear, however, that progress will come from more effective and extensive partnerships and from many different leaders, all of whom are recognised and valued for their contributions to public health.

References

1   Department of Health and Social Security (1972) *National Health Service Reorganisation: England*. HMSO, London.

2   Department of Health and Social Security (1972) *Report on the Working Party on Medical Administrators* (Hunter Report). HMSO, London.

3   Department of Health and Social Security (1972) *Second Report of the Joint Working Party on the Organisation of Medical Work in Hospitals* ('Cogwheel Report'). HMSO, London.

4   Warren MD (1997) *The Genesis of the Faculty of Public Health Medicine*. University of Kent at Canterbury.

5   Department of Health and Social Security (1976) *Sharing Resources for Health in England*. HMSO, London.

6   Black, Sir Douglas (1980) *Inequalities in Health. Report of a Research Working Group*. Department of Health and Social Security, London.

7   World Health Organisation (1985) *Targets for Health for All – Targets in Support of the European Regional Strategy for Health for All*. WHO, Copenhagen.

8   Ashton J (1986) Healthy Cities. *Health Promotion*. **1**(2): 319–42.

9   Department of Health and Social Security (1988) *Public Health in England* (Acheson Report). HMSO, London.

10   Department of Health (1989) *Working for Patients*. HMSO, London.

11   NHS and Community Care Act 1990. HMSO, London.

12   Department of Health (1992) *The Health of the Nation: a strategy for health in England*. HMSO, London.

13   Department of Health (1996) *The National Health Service: a service with ambitions*. HMSO, London.

14   Department of Health (1996) *Primary Care: delivering the future*. HMSO, London.

15   Department of Health, Scottish Office Home and Health Department, Welsh Office (1996) *Choice and Opportunity: primary care: the future*. HMSO, London.

16   General Medical Council (1993) *Tomorrow's Doctors: recommendations on undergraduate medical education*. GMC, London.

17   Department of Health (1997) *The New NHS: modern, dependable*. Cm 3807. HMSO, London.

18   Department of Health (1998) *Our Healthier Nation: a contract for health*. A Consultation Paper. Cm 3852. HMSO, London.

19   Department of Health (1998) *Chief Medical Officer's Project to Strengthen the Public Health Function in England. A Report of Emerging Findings*. HMSO, London.

CHAPTER TWENTY-TWO

Public health and clinical practice

Nicholas Hicks

Introduction

This chapter places clinical practice in the context of a broader view of public health and then considers:

- **the contribution of clinical practice as a determinant of the public's health**, arguing that in developed countries clinical practice is a significant determinant of health
- **the contribution of public health to clinical practice**, suggesting that public health skills, values and sciences can be used to enhance both the organisation and delivery of healthcare for individual patients as well as for the population as a whole
- **the contribution of clinicians to the practice of public health**, describing how those with experience and expertise in clinical medicine can contribute to improving the effectiveness and quality of public health practice.

Clinical practice and public health in context

Throughout the world the organisation and funding of health services are matters of great concern and importance to the public and their governments. The importance that people attach to health services is reflected in the high investment countries make in spending between 5% and 14% of their national wealth on healthcare.

It is sometimes argued that an interest in health services distracts public health practitioners from more effective ways of working. But this is to misunderstand the multisectoral nature of public health practice. The goal of public health practice is to maintain and improve the health of populations. The practice of public health involves identifying the determinants of health and effective means of influencing them, and then applying that knowledge in practice. Over the decades many determinants of health have been identified. Many have nothing to do with clinical practice or health services and include the absence of war, the availability of clean water, the provision of safe food, adequate housing and education.

To be effective a public health practitioner must influence at least one determinant of health. But the power and expertise to influence the non-health service determinants of health usually lies with people who are not employed by health services and with people whose job titles do not include the term 'public health'. For example, politicians determine whether a country is at war or peace and have a significant influence on major determinants of health, such as the distribution of wealth in society and the quality of education available to the population. In local communities, senior officers of local authorities – including chief executives and directors of housing, social services and environmental health – have influence over important determinants of health. If the practice of public health requires influence over determinants of health, then those who seek to improve the public's health should seek appropriate positions in society so they can have the influence they desire. The precise role they seek will depend on the particular determinants of health they wish to influence. The implication is that real public health careers are not limited to those jobs traditionally viewed as 'public health', but include politics, local government, the civil service, education, housing, transport and many others. For public health practitioners working in the NHS it is important to know whether or not health services can be a significant determinant of health.

Clinical practice as a determinant of health

There is a widely held view that clinical practice has little influence on the health of the population. There are arguments to support this view, for example:

- there is little correlation between the amount a country spends on healthcare per head of population and age-adjusted death rates
- it is often hard to correlate variations in rates of use of common medical and surgical procedures (e.g. prostatectomy, cholecystectomy) with population morbidity for the relevant conditions[1]
- a significant proportion of healthcare (some suggest as much as 20 to 60%) may be less than appropriate[2]
- dramatic improvements in health have occurred before any plausible effective health services were available.[3]

Many of these and other similar arguments were advanced eloquently and influentially in the 1970s, not just in Britain but in the USA as well, by people such as McKeown, Illich and the McKinlays.[3–5] Indeed, the view that medical care and health services have little to do with improving the public's health has, for some, become dogma. But, perhaps, nearly a quarter of a century later, it is time to reconsider whether this view is as accurate as many appear to believe.

It is conceivable that health services might contribute to the health of the population by:

- reducing mortality and morbidity
- providing relief from distress in a way that McKeown refers to as the 'pastoral role' of medicine
- contributing more broadly to a sense of societal security and well being.

These possible contributions are considered below.

Clinical practice and reduction of morbidity and mortality

The health of both individuals and populations is influenced by many different factors. It is therefore difficult to measure directly the precise contribution to health of any single factor. If an action has a large and rapid effect on health, e.g. the outbreak of war or the contamination of drinking water, then it is easier to recognise and quantify its impact than it is for an action whose effect is smaller or slow to take effect, e.g. change in dietary habits. Similarly, some medical interventions have a large and immediate effect, e.g. setting a broken bone relieves pain and prevents disability. Such treatments are provided so frequently and so routinely that we are sometimes in danger of taking them for granted. For example, a broken leg no longer usually condemns people to a life of pain or disability, appendicitis and community-acquired pneumonia now only rarely threaten the lives of young adults and children, and commonly performed operations such as hip replacements, cataract removal and coronary artery bypass grafting relieve pain and restore life-enhancing function for many thousands of people each year.

But the impact of most clinical practice is not always dramatic or easily recognised. Indeed, many interventions whose effect on health is now acknowledged to be important, such as the use of aspirin to reduce mortality from coronary heart disease, have required the results of well-designed, adequately powered, randomised trials to demonstrate and quantify the magnitude of the links between intervention and outcome.[6]

Since the first randomised controlled trial (RCT) was published in 1948, the numbers of RCTs that have been performed has grown exponentially.[7] The Cochrane Database of Controlled Clinical Trials now contains the details of more than 200 000 randomised trials. Many of these document the effectiveness of both established and newly developed health service interventions. Each year, there are many millions of people who receive one or more clinical interventions. Even if the absolute benefit for each individual were small, aggregated across a population the net benefit might be significant.

Bunker and colleagues tried to quantify the impact of health services on population mortality and morbidity by using evidence from clinical trials, from routine healthcare statistics, from epidemiological studies and national censuses and surveys to estimate the achieved and potential contribution of clinical practice to changes in life expectancy and the numbers of years of avoided disability.[8,9] They conclude that:

> *three of the seven years' increase in life expectancy since 1950 can be attributed to medical care. Medical care is also estimated to provide, on average, five years of partial or complete relief from the poor quality of life associated with chronic disease.*

They recognise that their findings are estimates rather than precise measurements of the impact of clinical practice on health and that they had to make a number of unproven assumptions to reach their conclusions. Nevertheless, they believe that their estimates indicate the likely order of magnitude of the impact of health services on health. Putting its impact into perspective, a five-year difference in life expectancy is approximately the difference in life expectancy documented between top grade and unskilled workers in the Whitehall Study of British civil servants and the difference of life expectancy between 20-a-day smokers starting at age 20 years and those who have never smoked.[10]

Bunker also points out that, thanks to the results of clinical trials, we can be confident that clinical practice has a direct effect on health. Furthermore, the biological mechanisms underlying the impact of many clinical practices on health are well understood. By contrast, he observes that 'the association of many social factors with health is well known, but except for occupation, it is not known how they might act or whether they are proxies for some other yet-to-be identified factor.'

Support for the view that the impact of modern health services on a population's health can be comparable to that of other more widely recognised determinants of health can be derived from observation of local clinical practice. For example, the effectiveness of simple treatments such as aspirin, ACE inhibitors and beta-blockers given to survivors of acute myocardial infarct (heart attack) has been well documented in randomised trials.[11-15] In 1995 in Oxfordshire, the extent to which these interventions were used in survivors of heart attack was measured.[16] Assuming that the effects of these interventions are additive and that Oxfordshire residents are not dissimilar to the patients recruited to the trials, then one can surmise that in Oxfordshire about 60 premature deaths are being prevented or delayed among the 600 or so people who survive a heart attack each year. For comparison, 41 Oxfordshire residents were killed in road traffic accidents in 1995.[17]

Still more support for the view that health services have an impact on population health comes from the only RCT of the impact of different approaches to funding healthcare – The RAND Health Insurance Experiment. This study measured health service use and health status changes among people randomised to fee for service healthcare, or to fully pre-paid healthcare, or to care that required a co-payment at the time of use. Among the main conclusions of this study was that co-payment and fee for service medicine:

(a)   reduced the amount of care received by chronically sick people on low incomes, and
(b)   that their health was measurably worse as a consequence.[18]

Other observational data also confirm that loss of health insurance (which severely restricts access to healthcare) has substantial and sometimes devastating effects on the health of poor, sick populations.[19,20]

In summary, in recent decades three important things have happened: first, the range and effectiveness of medical treatment has improved; second, because of the huge increase in the numbers of randomised trials that have been performed, we now have a much better understanding of the link between clinical practice and health status; and third, the multiple patterns of health service provision in the USA have allowed health service researchers to measure the impact of different degrees of access to care. We can therefore be more confident that modern healthcare reduces both mortality and morbidity and that it is indeed a significant determinant of both the health of individuals and populations.

Social health: a dimension of public health/ the role of clinical practice

McKeown comments that[21]:

> When people are ill they want all that is possible done for them and small benefits are welcome when larger ones are not available. Moreover, inability to control the outcome of disease does not reduce the importance of the pastoral or samaritan role of the doctor. In some ways it increases it ... and, if I were ill ... I should like good medical attention, by which I mean clinical service which combines technical competence with humane care.

I suspect that these views accurately reflect the sentiments of the vast majority of the population.

The WHO defined health as 'a state of complete physical, mental, social well being and not merely the absence of disease and infirmity'. Although this broad definition is often considered to be unrealistically idealistic and makes health difficult to measure, most people would accept both that there are positive aspects of health as well as negative and that social health is an important dimension of the health of individuals and populations. It is generally accepted that health services can relieve some physical illness and mental illness, but the possibility that clinical practice might also contribute to a sense of personal and societal well being is rarely discussed.

Support for the idea that health services might contribute to societal well being comes in a monograph by Churchill, who argues that the purpose of health services is not limited to improving the physical and mental health of individuals or the population.[22] Indeed he asserts that the primary goals of health policy should be providing individuals with 'security', i.e. 'freedom to live without fear that their basic healthcare concerns will go unattended and freedom from financial impoverishment when seeking or receiving care', and providing the nation with a sense of 'solidarity', i.e. 'the sense of community that emerges from acknowledgement of shared benefits and burdens'. Whether or not these are the primary goals of health policy remains debatable. However, it is important to recognise that secure and confident access to (in McKeown's words) 'clinical service that is technically competent and humane' can contribute to both personal and social well being.

This analysis suggests that not only has the contribution of clinical practice to the physical and mental health of the population been underestimated, but its role as a determinant of positive societal health has also been understated.

The contribution of public health to clinical practice

The previous section suggests that modern clinical practice contributes significantly to the public's health. It is thus an important task for public health practitioners to seek to influence the delivery of healthcare to maximise the contribution of clinical practice to the public's health. There are several ways in which public health skills and values can be used to contribute to the practice of clinical medicine:

Shaping clinical services

The contribution of public health practitioners working in health authorities is described in Chapter 15 by Jewell. The shaping of local clinical practice requires public health practitioners to take an overview of local provision, to integrate epidemiological, social, economic and evaluative sciences with political wisdom and managerial competence, and to establish and run processes for the setting of priorities and the rationing of scarce resources for healthcare. It represents a major contribution of public health to clinical practice.

Clinical services delivered by public health practitioners

There is a long tradition of public health practitioners playing a direct role in the delivery of population-oriented clinical services. Such services include population screening programmes, child health preventive services including immunisation programmes, and communicable disease control services. Public health physicians may also give clinical advice to individual patients at ports and airports while acting as port health officers. Sometimes these public health clinical roles develop into specialities in their own right, often occupying a place between public health medicine and another medical speciality, e.g. consultants in communicable disease may have a background in public health, microbiology or infectious diseases.

Improving the quality of clinical decision making: a new role for public health medicine?

Some actions in clinical practice produce predictable and consistent effects in almost every patient. However, most medical interventions do not have such predictable consequences for individual patients. Instead they alter the probability of particular outcomes occurring. For example, about 80% of patients admitted to hospital with a heart attack would survive with little in the way of active treatment. The implication is that much of clinical practice revolves around the assessment of modification of risk. However, this is not the way that medicine has traditionally been taught.

Epidemiology, which is the basic science of public health, is also the basic science that underpins the measurement and manipulation of risk. It is the science which provides answers to clinical questions such as:

- how effective is this intervention?
- what is the prognosis of this disease?
- how safe is this treatment?
- what does this test result tell me about the chances of my patient having a particular illness?

The answers to such questions come from epidemiological studies whose results are described in vocabulary that is unfamiliar to many clinicians. The language of risk includes phrases such as odds ratio, relative risk reduction, absolute risk reduction, likelihood ratio, specificity, sensitivity, confounding, bias and intention-to-treat. Although unfamiliar to clinicians, this is the vocabulary and scientific basis of public health practice and of traditional aetiological epidemiology. The recognition that epidemiology can be used to improve the quality of clinical decision making, and hence the effectiveness of clinical practice both for individuals and for populations, offers new ways for public health physicians to work with clinicians and to influence clinical practice. Promoting the use of empirical evidence in clinical practice can be 'bottom-up' or 'top-down'.

A bottom-up approach is one which seeks to equip individual clinicians and other decision makers with the skills and resources to reflect accurately valid, relevant evidence in the decisions they take that affect the care of patients. In particular it requires that people should:

- be *motivated* to apply evidence in practice
- have the *necessary skills*, e.g. the ability to turn the problems they face into answerable questions, to find relevant information and to make sense of the information they retrieve
- have adequate and *timely access to relevant information*
- have their *work organised in such a way that they can apply their skills and make use of the information* available to them.

The bottom-up approach, although useful, has its limitations. The number and complexity of decisions that have to be taken in a modern healthcare system are too great to expect individuals to be able to obtain, interpret and integrate all the valid, relevant information for every decision that they take. This implies that, especially for common, clinically or financially significant decisions, it will often be necessary for much of the information retrieval, analysis and integration to have been done previously. This, in turn, implies that, for at least some sets of decisions, a top-down approach is also needed.

In a top-down approach, a limited number of clinical issues are selected as priorities. The relevant stakeholders are brought together to agree, in the light of knowledge of the evidence and the state of present practice, the content and nature of care that should be provided locally. This agreement may be summarised in the form of guidelines, which, if they are to have any impact, must be disseminated as part of a planned programme of implementation.

Taken together, these approaches begin to define how public health practitioners can work to influence the quality of decision making in clinical practice. They imply that useful tasks include:

- cultivating a *culture that values evidence*
- working to refocus both pre- and post-qualification *education* (cf. lifelong learning) as the education of many clinical and managerial staff (both senior and junior) has not equipped them to understand the strengths and weaknesses of different types of evidence or to make best use of new developments such as *information technology* and *systematic reviews*
- reviewing and contributing to the appropriate provision of *clinically relevant information* such as primary research data, *systematic reviews* and *evidence-linked clinical guidelines*
- ensuring the co-ordination of the work of the many groups whose work is aimed at improving the quality of care, e.g. education, clinical audit, R&D.

These tasks require leadership, well-developed technical skills and public health involvement in management, education and the assessment of the quality of care. They also imply close working between public health practitioners and clinicians, including public health participation in the management of provider institutions such as hospitals and primary care groups. Quality of care depends not only on the quality of the interaction between patient and professional, but also on the organisational environment in which care is delivered. In other words, patients and populations would be served best if there were mutually supportive and linked professional and organisational systems for maintaining and improving the quality of clinical practice.

The future: public health and clinical practice linked through clinical governance?

The Government's NHS White Paper and subsequent consultation document *A First Class Service*[23] reach similar conclusions about the importance of developing integrated organisational and professional approaches to continuously improving the quality of clinical practice. At the heart of these documents lies clinical governance, which has been defined as 'a system through which NHS organisations are accountable for continuously improving the quality of their services and safeguarding high standards of care by creating an environment in which excellence will flourish.'[24] In future, all NHS organisations will be expected to establish robust systems of clinical governance.

The concept of clinical governance is entirely consistent with, and indeed embodies much of, the public health approach to improving the quality of clinical practice described above. Writing prior to his appointment as CMO for England, Donaldson set out his views on how to ensure that clinical governance achieves its full potential. He emphasised the importance of leadership; a positive organisational culture in which blame is used only rarely; team-working; the provision of relevant clinical information; the strengthening of skills in accessing the appraising evidence; and the development of organisation-wide approaches to identifying and delivering opportunities for better clinical practice. These are all aspects and attributes of successful public health input to clinical practice.

It is intended that clinical governance will be as important as corporate and financial governance. NHS institutional boards will no longer be able to ignore their responsibilities for the quality of clinical care provided by their organisations. This will require the systematic and widespread application of many of the skills and values that public health practitioners possess. A political commitment to improving quality of care, to establishing effective clinical governance and to holding NHS institutions to account for the quality of care that they deliver, provides new opportunities for public health practitioners to apply their skills throughout the NHS.

In summary, this section has described how public health practitioners can contribute to clinical practice by shaping of health services, by involvement in the delivery of population-based clinical services, and by working with clinicians and managers to improve the quality of clinical decision making. In the near future, there will be considerable opportunities for public health practitioners to work closely with clinicians and managers, probably employed by provider institutions, to make a substantial contribution to the quality of everyday clinical practice.

Clinicians' contribution to the practice of public health

Previous sections have argued that clinical practice is a significant determinant of the public's health and that improving the quality of clinical care is an important and practical role for public health practitioners. The chapter would not be complete without acknowledging that clinicians also have an important contribution to make to the practice of public health.

Clinicians as advocates for health

Healthcare professionals, especially doctors and nurses, have a special and trusted status in most societies. They are also interested in promoting health and reducing the burden of disease. Collectively they are the repositories of huge amounts of health-related knowledge and expertise. This status and knowledge confers power and responsibility which, in turn, gives the professions the opportunity to act as powerful advocates for health in society. This advocacy role does not have to be limited to healthcare issues, and has in the past been extended to include advocacy about other broader determinants of health. For example, the Royal College of Physicians has campaigned vigorously against smoking and Professor Sir Douglas Black, a past President of the Royal College of Physicians, is best known for his Black Report,[25] which did much to highlight the importance of socio-economic inequalities as a determinant of health. Such public health advocacy, which gains much of its legitimacy from the involvement of its advocates in clinical practice, can be powerful. It is an important contribution of clinicians to public health. The professions should be encouraged to make more use of their special opportunities to act as advocates for health.

Shaping health services for populations

Not only do clinicians provide clinical care which in aggregate improves the health of populations, they also have a role contributing to the planning and management of clinical services. This may be by offering expert advice either as individuals or as a member of a professional body, e.g. a Royal College, the General Medical Council, or by accepting managerial responsibilities in relation to their local health services. The advent of clinical governance is likely to increase clinicians' responsibilities and opportunities in relation to public health and management.

   People who occupy dual roles that involve both clinical and managerial/public health responsibilities are important bridges between worlds that have often been too separate. The advantages that public health expertise can bring to clinical practice have been discussed already. It is my contention that the advantages that up-to-date clinical experience brings to the practice of public health include:

- first-hand contact with the public
- a practical knowledge of current clinical issues and controversies
- an opportunity to witness the delivery of clinical services and to develop a feel for those services that work well and those that do not
- a 'peer relationship' with other clinicians.

Involvement in clinical practice can serve as a very practical reminder that clinical decisions may not be as black and white as is sometimes suggested in journals and textbooks. Similarly, it serves as a reminder that information recorded in clinical data sets is often not as clear cut and precise as it sometimes claimed. Although none of these benefits are essential for the practice of public health, taken together they illustrate how those with first-hand experience of clinical practice can have a useful contribution to make to improving the quality of aspects of public health decision making in relation to the shaping of health services.

Clinicians thus have useful contributions to make to public health through the clinical services that they provide, by public health advocacy and by contributing to the shaping of health services.

Summary

This chapter has explored aspects of the relationship between public health and clinical practice. It has argued that modern health services can make an important contribution to the health of both individuals and populations. It is therefore an important public health task to work to ensure that clinical practice is delivered as effectively and efficiently as possible to meet the healthcare needs of the populations they serve. The chapter has also illustrated how public health practitioners working in the NHS can make a substantial contribution to the quality of clinical practice while noting that clinicians also have a useful contribution to make to the practice of public health.

References

1   Andersen TF and Mooncy G (eds) (1990) *The Challenges of Medical Practice Variations*. Macmillan Press, London.

2   Winslow CM, Kosecoff J, Chassin MR *et al.* (1988) The appropriateness of performing coronary artery bypass surgery. *JAMA*. **260**: 505–9.

3   McKeown T (1976) *The Role of Medicine: dream, mirage or nemesis?* Nuffield Provincial Trust, London.

4   Illich I (1976) *Medical Nemesis: the expropriation of health*. Random House, New York.

5   McKinlay JB and McKinlay SM (1977) The questionable effect of medical measures on the decline in mortality in the United States in the twentieth century. *Milbank Memorial Fund Quarterly/Health and Society*. **55**: 405–28.

6   ISIS-2 (Second International Study of Infarct Survival) Collaborative Group (1988) Randomised trial of intravenous streptokinase, oral aspirin, both or neither among 17 187 cases of suspected acute myocardial infarction: ISIS-2. *Lancet*. **ii**: 349–60.

7   Streptomycin in Tuberculosis Trials Committee (1948) Streptomycin treatment of pulmonary tuberculosis: a Medical Research Council investigation. *BMJ*. **2**: 769–82.

8   Bunker JP, Frazier HS and Mosteller F (1994) Improving health: measuring effects of medical care. *The Milbank Quarterly*. **72**: 225–58.

9   Bunker JP (1995) Medicine matters after all. *Journal of the Royal College of Physicians*. **29**: 105–12.

10   Marmot MG, Davey Smith G, Stansfeld S *et al.* (1991) Health inequalities among British civil servants: the Whitehall II study. *Lancet.* **337**: 1387–93.

11   Antiplatelet Trialists' Collaboration (APT) (1994) Collaborative overview of randomised trials of antiplatelet therapy- I: Prevention of death, myocardial infarction, and stroke by prolonged antiplatelet therapy in various categories. *BMJ.* **308**: 81–106.

12   Garg R and Yusuf S for the Collaborative Group on ACE Inhibitor Trials (1995) Overview of randomised trials of angiotensin-converting enzyme inhibitors on mortality and morbidity in patients with heart failure. *JAMA.* **273**: 1450–6.

13   Hall AS, Murray GD and Ball SG on behalf of the AIREX Study Investigators (1997) Follow-up study of patients randomly allocated ramipril or placebo for heart failure after acute myocardial infarction: AIRE Extension (AIREX) Study. *Lancet.* **349**: 1493–7.

14   Pfeffer MA, Braunwald E, Moye LA *et al.* (1992) Effect of captopril on mortality and morbidity in patients with left ventricular dysfunction after myocardian infarction. Results of the Survival and Ventricular Enlargement Trial (SAVE). *New England Journal of Medicine.* **327**: 669–77.

15   Yusuf S, Peto R, Lewis J *et al.* (1985) Beta blockade during and after mocardial infarction: an overview of the randomised trials. *Progress in Cardiovascular Diseases.* **27**: 335–71.

16   Dovey S, Hicks N, Lancaster T *et al.* on behalf of the Oxfordshire Myocardial Infarction Incidence Study (OXMIS) Group (1998) Secondary prevention after myocardial infarction: how completely are research findings adopted in practice? *European Journal of General Practice.* **4**: 6–10.

17   Office for National Statistics, Table VS3 (1996).

18   Brook RH, Ware JE, Davies-Avery *et al.* (1983) Does free care improve adults' health? Results from a randomized controlled trial. *New England Journal of Medicine.* **309**: 1426–34.

19   Lurie N, Ward NB, Shapiro MF *et al.* (1984) Termination from Medi-Cal: does it affect health? *New England Journal of Medicine.* **311**: 480–4.

20   Lurie N, Ward NB, Shapiro MF *et al.* (1986) Termination of Medi-Cal benefits: a follow-up study one year later. *New England Journal of Medicine.* **314**: 1266–8.

21   McKeown T (1979) *The Role of Medicine: dream, mirage or nemesis* (2e). Basil Blackwell, Oxford.

22   Churchill LR (1994) *Self-interest and Universal Healthcare: why well insured Americans should support coverage for everyone.* Harvard University Press, London.

23   Secretary of State for Health (1998) *A First Class Service: quality in the new NHS.* The Stationery Office, London.

24   Scally G and Donaldson LJ (1998) Clinical governance and the drive for quality improvement in the new NHS in England. *BMJ.* **317**: 61–5.

25   Department of Health and Social Security (1980) *Report of a Research Working Group: inequalities in health.* DHSS, London.

CHAPTER TWENTY-THREE

Public health nursing

Ron De Witt and Jackie Carnell

Introduction

Since the 1850s, successive governments have strived to address issues of public health and the 1997 newly elected Labour Government are no different in this respect. What is different, however, is the explicit manner in which this government aims to tackle public health issues, which has been characterised by the appointment of Tessa Jowell MP as the first-ever Public Health Minister. The role of the minister is to work across all government departments, with the sole intention of identifying those issues that impact upon the public's health and framing them within an overall policy framework. On the day of her appointment Tessa Jowell said:[1]

> We were elected on a manifesto commitment to tackle the root causes of inequality in health, caused by unemployment, caused by pollution, caused by bad housing. So my brief is to work across Government and across the Department of Health to ensure the causes are identified, that strategies are identified and acted on.

She went on to say: 'the needs of people don't conform neatly to departmental boundaries'.

A momentum of change is certainly gathering within the UK in relation to healthcare, with the recent publication of the government White Paper *The New NHS*,[2] which describes a new direction for the development and delivery of healthcare. A fundamental component of this new direction for the NHS is the increased emphasis on health needs, health improvement plans for the general population and the abolition of the internal market. It is the considered position of the authors that no one speciality or subdiscipline within nursing will be more affected by these changes, and have significant opportunities to lead the required changes, than the public health nurse.

This chapter will focus upon the difficulties encountered in promoting a public health nursing agenda, the opportunities that are now surfacing to place the public's health at the forefront of healthcare and will describe the positive contribution that public health nursing can make to developing these new ways of working.

Difficulties with the present approach to issues of public health

The premise of caring for defined populations, such as families and community groups, which is the unique feature of public health nursing, has traditionally been the responsibility of health visitors. Historically, their role has been to promote health and prevent ill health within these populations, as well as working with families to ensure that the debilitating effects of disability or illness are kept to a minimum. Family and community advocacy, as well as mobilising local services to meet the needs of the local population, were always part of their professional activities.

However, since the implementation of the Salmon Report in 1974,[3] which led to community nurses being employed by the NHS instead of local authorities, the public health dimension of their work has started to become clouded.

As many as 50% of the health visitors and district nurses became attached to general practices, with the remainder retaining their base in community clinics and their focus on the total community population. Their population became defined by those who were registered with that particular practice and the clear focus on the specific communities, within the geographical population, was lost.

The NHS internal market was introduced in 1990, and was characterised by GP fundholding and the emphasis on a primary care (GP) led NHS. By 1996 almost all health visitors were attached to general practice and 52% of the population were registered with fundholding practices. The work of the health visitor was now defined as a series of delegated tasks and activities, aimed at particular individuals, usually 0–5-year-olds, and only to those individuals who were registered with a specific practice. It is our belief that, although continuing to work in a community setting, their ability to focus upon populations, with prevention and promotion of health as their primary objectives, had been lost. In essence they were not being allowed to practise as public health nurses.

Responsibility for the health of school populations resided traditionally with the school nurse. However, during this period of change the School Health Service has fared no better, it became a service that didn't fit. A common question was 'If patients are registered with a GP, then why do we need a separate school service?' The role of the school nurse as a public health worker, providing a comprehensive service to the school population, was lost. Their work was broken down into screening and surveillance tasks, but the idea of providing a health-promoting service to the whole population of schoolchildren was swiftly forgotten.

But it is not only within primary and community care that the focus upon public health nursing has been diluted, elsewhere within the NHS the same story can be told. It is the view of the authors that a number of reasons lie behind the demise of the traditional public health nursing role.

Narrow, medical definition of public health

It is our belief that one of the principle issues is the narrow medical definition utilised to describe much of what falls under today's public health banner. This has resulted in a predominantly medical approach to the identification of health problems through the application of epidemiology, which are in turn addressed through medical interventions at ground level in terms of preventing and combating disease. This particular approach is not what the Acheson Committee[4] had in mind when they reported in 1988 that public health was concerned with more than sanitary hygiene and epidemic disease control. The committee considered that public health must involve not only 'efforts to preserve health by minimising and where possible removing injurious environmental, social and behavioural influences', but also 'in the provision of effective and efficient services to restore the sick to health and where this is impractical to reduce to a minimum suffering, disability and dependence'.

This preoccupation with medical intervention as the sole response to issues of public health, which runs counter to the views of the Acheson Committee, has resulted in an approach to public health which has left those who have a great deal to offer on the outside looking in, or at least with their wings clipped.

It is our view that a wider and more inclusive approach to the issue of public health should be acted upon if we are to rectify some of the current difficulties that plague the delivery of public health programmes. Such an approach should facilitate collective and collaborative action with the overall aim of improving the public's health. Robert Beaglehole and Ruth Bonita[5] capture the essence of such an approach in the preface to their book entitled *Public Health at the Cross-roads*, with the following statement: 'Public Health is the collective action taken by society to protect and promote the health of entire populations.'

Disconnection

The difficulties associated with the use of a narrow, medical definition have been further compounded by the methodologies utilised to define and deliver public health strategies. As a consequence we have a disconnection between health policy and actual activity on the ground. Four main reasons exist for this disconnection, these are:

- organisational structure
- working practices
- contracting process
- staff perceptions.

Organisational structure

In 1998 the NHS is 50 years old and since its inception it would appear that not a day has gone by when either the national press or one of the many NHS-related journals has not carried a headline predicting some crisis or other within the service. Loss of beds, closure of hospitals, increasing waiting lists and the unavailability of particular treatments are typical headlines in the press. As a consequence, we have also seen during this period successive governments and numerous committees and working groups seeking to reorganise the service in an attempt to address these perceived shortcomings. Such initiatives include the reforms of the 1990s, which focused primarily upon the structure of the NHS with the introduction of the internal market, the purchaser–provider split and GP fundholding.

It is our opinion that this focus upon ill health and organisational structure, which has characterised much of the reforms of the 1980s and 1990s, has ensured that unwittingly a disconnection has occurred between health policies and strategies and the delivery mechanisms for public health nursing on a day-to-day basis.

Those setting the public health agenda within health authorities have no line responsibility for, and little contact with, health professionals in the field, and as a consequence policy and strategy is:

- shaped with little or no interaction with those professionals on the ground who are aware of particular health needs
- formed into service contracts negotiated with trusts, GPs, voluntary bodies and private companies, which are in turn incorporated by these organisations into business plans and communicated to health workers. In this process of translation across the purchaser–provider divide, many of the essential features of policy are lost and modified.

Working practices

The issue of disconnection in terms of working practices is illustrated by the lack of co-ordination between the various professional staff who deliver the public health agenda in the clinical setting. As an example, health visitors, school nurses and occupational health all operate independently of each other, and at times in separate parts of the same organisations, without any reference to each other's function and contribution. We believe it is now both relevant and timely to question the operational independence of these groups, especially when they are all servicing the same public health agenda.

Contracting process

A further feature of the reforms of the 1990s is the focus on service contracts between purchasers and providers. Within some of these contracts patient services have been described in terms of the particular speciality provided, or even by procedure. Such an approach, while necessary to understand the range of services provided, has prevented an holistic approach to service delivery being taken in many instances, thereby facilitating the occurrence of further disconnection between health policy and activity. The contracting process has also promoted the concept of competition and worked against collaboration and partnership, which are the essential foundations upon which any public health agenda needs to be built.

This disconnection is further compounded by the way in which the public health agenda is determined and subsequently shaped, a process that excludes non-medical health professionals. They therefore face great difficulties in knowing how much emphasis to place on the different segments of the health policy, and indeed in feeling any sense of ownership of the health policy. Equally, few clinicians see the details of what is negotiated between the purchaser and provider.

One of the major problems has been the emphasis on contracting by stating the required number of tasks, contacts and activities, without any emphasis on what is supposed to be achieved in terms of health gain or health outcomes. This has worked counter to the traditional role of public health nurses and has made it impossible for them to respond to the health needs of individuals, families or communities, or even of practice populations as a whole. In other words, their practice has been prescribed for them by others.

Staff perceptions

Many public health opportunities are lost due to the narrow, medically orientated approach to issues of public health, thus leading to many healthcare professionals failing to recognise their own role in contributing to the public's health. For example, when we questioned health visitors, many believed that they spent only 10% of their time on public health issues. What do they do with the remainder of their time? Child development and child health was the reply. Is this not public health nursing?

Such feedback from discussions with healthcare professionals within the service is not uncommon. The vast majority do not see themselves playing any role in the delivery of the public health agenda. The primary reasons behind such a stance starts very early in the career of a healthcare professional. Examination of the pre-registration curricula of most healthcare professionals, contains little or no reference to their future role in public health delivery issues. This approach is compounded by the lack of any reference to the public health dimension in many of the current job descriptions for healthcare professionals.

Commonality between public health and nursing

As stated earlier in this chapter the appointment of the first public health minister emphasises the intention of this government to address issues of public health. But what do we mean by the term public health?

Donald Acheson, writing in *Public Health in England*,[4] stated that 'Public health is the science and art of preventing disease, prolonging life and promoting health through the organised efforts of society'. Professor Walter Holland,[6] writing in 1997, contended that public health's major function must be to:

- improve the surveillance of the health of the population centrally and locally
- encourage policies that promote and maintain health
- ensure that the means are available to evaluate existing health services.

Holland's review of public health illustrates that each of these elements has been constant in the medical speciality of public health over the past 130 years, albeit with different focus and emphasis at different times.

A further insight into public health can be gleaned from examining the final aspect of the Acheson Committee's consideration: 'the provision of effective and efficient services to restore the sick to health and where this is impracticable to reduce to a minimum suffering, disability and dependence'. Consider now, the descriptions utilised to describe nursing:

> *The unique function of the nurse is to assist the individual sick or well in the performance of those activities contributing to health, or its recovery, that he would perform unaided if he had the necessary strength, will or knowledge. And to do this in such a way as to help him gain independence as quickly as possible.*[7]

Roper[8] believes that there are core nursing activities required by patients whatever the setting: 'The nurse initiated part of nursing is helping patients to prevent, alleviate or solve or cope with the problem (actual or potential) related to their activities of living.' Benner[9] describes seven domains of nursing practice:

1   the helping role
2   the teaching/coaching function
3   the diagnostic/patient-monitoring function
4   effective management of rapidly changing situations
5   administering and monitoring therapeutic interventions and regimens
6   monitoring and ensuring the quality of healthcare practice
7   organisational and work-role competence.

These domains confirm that trying to identify what nursing is can be achieved in broad terms, but identification of specific nursing activities is not as easily defined.

The DoH has attempted to address this issue in its guidance on the nature of nursing in *The Challenge for Nursing and Midwifery in the 21st Century*[10]:

> *Nurses have ... always been close to patients offering care and comfort even when cure or relief has been unavailable. They have been educator and advisor to, helping people to help themselves. They have skills, human values and especially the ability to listen to people ... nurses have always had a special responsibility for trying to help those in need or at risk to maintain their independence and respect, particularly the frail and vulnerable.*

This document, having given an overview of what nursing is about, then describes what is constant in nursing:

The work of the nurse, whatever the setting, draws upon a tradition of caring, based around both skills and values and includes:

- *a co-ordinating function*
- *a teaching function, for carers, patients and professions*
- *developing and maintaining programmes of care*
- *technical expertise, exercised personally or through others*
- *concern for the ill but also for those currently well*
- *a special responsibility for the frail and vulnerable.*

Clearly there is a high level of commonality between these definitions of nursing practice and the broad-based approaches to issues of public health. Further evidence of the valuable contribution that nursing can make to the public health agenda can be found in the WHO view on how the role of the nurse will develop. It anticipates a shift to primary care from secondary care, with nurses becoming increasingly proactive in leadership and development.

The WHO (1985)[11] stressed that nurses will work increasingly within the community and participate in multidisciplinary working, and, where appropriate, provide leadership to such teams. Nurses will innovate and participate in planning and evaluation of care planning and become more active in providing health education. If this is so, the greatest opportunities are about to happen for the nurse whose work concentrates on the public's health.

The message that nursing must be based on the needs of patients/clients is confirmed in the 1993 DoH publication *New World, New Opportunities – Nursing in Primary Care:*[12]

Progress in primary healthcare will be made only if everyone with an involvement in, or influence on, primary healthcare thinks in terms, first, of the needs of patients, clients and communities, next to the skills required to meet those needs and then of the ways of harmonising the skills in order to fulfil primary health care a two-fold objective:

- *to improve individual and family health; and*
- *to improve health for total populations.*

In summary, therefore, the first half of this chapter has outlined the current service difficulties facing those who are attempting to introduce and develop a public health perspective into their nursing practice. This section has also outlined some of the numerous definitions of public health and attempted to highlight the high level of commonality between these public health definitions and the descriptions utilised to describe the nursing role. The remaining part of this chapter will now consider how this high level of commonality can be turned into opportunities for the nursing profession.

Public health nursing opportunities

Following the publication in 1984 of *Health for All by the Year 2000* by WHO[13] and *Public Health in England* by the DoH in 1988,[14] there was recognition of the importance of public health. However, real effort is now being made with the publication of the Green Paper on public health and the government's recent White Paper *The New NHS*.[2,15] Nurses have the most to contribute towards the new public health movement and the opportunities are clear.

Public health definitions that clearly link the delivery of a public health agenda to a role for which nurses are prepared is evident. Public health is a collective view of health needs and healthcare of the population which requires a collective approach, emphasising partnerships at all stages and levels of the public health process. This means partnerships with communities, clients and professionals if we are to effectively improve the public's health. We believe that to be effective, public health practitioners will require a firm sense of identity as 'public health nurses' based on a broad and inclusive approach to public health.

Such an approach should include medical care, health promotion, rehabilitation, and the underlying social economics and cultural determinants of health and disease; areas of expertise in which nurses abound. There is now tremendous potential for merging the efforts of medicine and nursing to tackle inequalities in the public's health. Nurses witness daily the effects of poverty and the wider environmental issues of health on individuals and families.

New directions in national health goals and targets will, hopefully, redirect resources towards achievement of public health goals. But it will require strong leadership and is most likely to be effective if motivated by a real desire to support public health and to strive for equality of opportunity for health, not cost containment. An important task, which public health nurses can contribute towards, is the balancing of effort devoted to controlling individual risk and dealing with programmes for underlying social and economic causes of ill health. This refocusing for nurses involves a move away from a predominant concern for individuals that has developed back to the population, social structure, and processes that generate health and disease.

Apart from a firm sense of direction, public health nursing requires a strong and clearly articulated theoretical foundation, based on a clear appreciation of the historical perspective of public health and a key goal of strengthening the partnership of the two processes of education and practice. Wherever the base, strong support and leadership of public health nursing education and training is essential to bridge the gap between academic and practical public health nursing and to ensure that students are socialised in the value of public health.

What then can be done to achieve a better balance in the nursing approach to the issue of public health? We believe that a number of responses can be utilised to strike a balance. The first step has to be an adaptation of a broad-based and inclusive approach to the issue of public health by all of the current categories of nurses. The need for such an approach is essential if the difficulties associated with the narrow definition of public health are to be avoided and if the valuable contribution that nurses can make to the delivery of public health programmes is to be recognised and utilised.

The science and art of public health nursing

Such an approach should be based upon the principles espoused by Acheson, who stated that, 'Public Health is "the science and art of preventing disease, prolonging life and promoting health through the organised efforts of society".'[4] Adopting a definition such as this one will enable the art or micro model of public health, as practised by public health nurses, to be given equal recognition to that of science or macro public health initiatives, which is the widely practised medical model of today.

Typical features of the science/macro/medical model include:

- the international, national and health authority mapping of epidemiological data and useage to advise on policies affecting health and the provision of health services to meet the needs identified
- the control of disease through immunisation and contact tracing of diseases such as TB
- the early detection of disease through screening procedures.

To take the micro public health agenda forward, front-line workers, whose *raison d'être* is practising the art of public health, are essential. And if these workers are not recognised, commissioned appropriately and allowed to practise as micro public health workers, progress will be severely hampered. Typical activities will include:

- the mapping of the health needs of local populations (community or practice populations) by the use of epidemiological data, collected by contact with individuals, families and local communities, and measuring it against the 'macro' figures
- using the information to work directly with other agencies to improve local services, or to empower and facilitate the efforts of individuals, families and communities to seek the improvement themselves
- working with individual parents to impact positively on their children's health, physically, socially and mentally
- facilitating early detection of deviation from 'normal' health by working with families in a shared assessment process
- minimising the effects of ill health by enabling families to cope with the least detriment to their lives
- all this to be done within a total population approach and with clearly defined priorities against which the objectives are set.

White Paper opportunities

In its White Paper, *The New NHS*,[2] the government made it clear that the service as a whole will be expected to strengthen the contribution made by nursing. Those activities described above, combined with the opportunities arising from this latest series of changes within the NHS, place the public health nurse in a unique position of opportunity. Implementation of the White Paper involves taking steps to strengthen staff involvement in service developments and in planning change. A key objective of the government is to enable all staff to maximise their contribution to health and healthcare.

Particular White Paper developments upon which a broad-based public health approach will be framed include:

- HIMPs
- PCGs
- health needs assessment.

Health Improvement Programmes

The HIMP is to be one of the key vehicles for taking forward the government's objective of improving the public's health. The HIMP will describe the health needs of the local population and what needs to be done to meet these needs. In essence, it is the local strategy for improving the public's health and healthcare delivery. The HIMP, which will be unique to each health authority area, will also describe standards and targets which all parties will need to achieve. Health authorities will not, however, draw up the details of the HIMP in splendid isolation. They are required to work with NHS trusts, PCGs, local authorities and healthcare professionals in defining the HIMP. By drawing in all of these partners, the HIMP will become the vehicle for translating the health, social and joint strategies within each area into practice.

This partnership responsibility with other bodies will mean, for example, that local authorities will have, in turn, a more clearly defined duty. The White Paper states that with regard to local authorities their duty will include to 'promote the economic, social and environmental well being of their areas'.

Primary care groups

PCGs, made up of all the GPs and community nurses in a particular area, will replace the thousands of existing commissioning and fundholder groups. This reduction in the number of commissioners, along with a much stronger community focus upon the needs of the population that falls within the catchment area of a particular PCG, will enable the public health nursing agenda to come more strongly to the fore. PCGs will serve populations of around 100 000 patients and take responsibility for commissioning services for their local community. They will also work closely with local authorities and, in particular, with social services.

The creation of PCGs will enable community nurses to focus upon the community sector as a whole, which was not the case previously with individual practices. PCGs will have freedom to make decisions about how they use their resources, consistent with the HIMP.

What will need to be avoided as we seek to establish the new arrangements is a sole focus upon organisational structures and boundaries. For these new arrangements to work, all health professionals and managers will also need to focus their attention upon the process of healthcare and the need for collaboration. PCGs offer a golden opportunity to work across the healthcare and social care spectrum, with all nurses maximising their influence upon the public's health. We must not allow previously held prejudices and organisational responsibilities to prevent the public receiving the health and social care they require. This need will be particularly important as health authorities and local authorities come together in new working arrangements.

As stated earlier, the process of defining the HIMPs will provide tremendous challenges and opportunities to identify and address issues of ill health, e.g. poor housing, within a common health and social policy approach. This process of integrated care, working across hospital, community, primary and social care traditional boundaries, will also present a number of specific challenges. These will include the need to reassess traditional boundaries between the health professions and the healthcare and social care professions. New roles will need to be established to ensure that the vision of integrated care is achievable. Nurses have a good track record in working in partnership with patients and carers. They will now need to consider how best they can enter into partnerships with other healthcare and social care professionals.

However, for this new approach to function as it should, time and effort will also need to be invested in determining the underlying health needs of the local population.

Health needs assessment

Under the new White Paper arrangements, health authorities will be required to carry out a number of tasks. These will include:

- assessing the health needs of the local population, drawing on the knowledge of other organisations and healthcare professionals
- drawing up a strategy for meeting these needs. As stated earlier this will take the form of an HIMP developed in partnership with all the local interests.

This particular focus will provide public health nurses with the opportunity to be involved in both the health needs assessment and the strategy-setting process to meet these needs. Nurses work within the settings that need to be analysed, holding key positions, ready to identify and collect valuable health information. The views of patients and clients are also essential components of health profiles. Nurses know from their experience of caring for people that health and clinical needs cannot easily be separated from patient-demand healthcare. Professional priorities need to be developed in tandem with the priorities of local people if public health is to be taken forward. Nurses are often closer to patients, clients and communities than other health workers, thus are often uniquely placed to gain insight into local views. A key aspect of public health practice is advocacy, and nurses must work constructively to influence policy and strategy as well as the mechanism of delivery. This is sometimes difficult as employees of health agencies. But it is important to find legitimate and constructive ways of making salient points.

In working with these communities it is vital that the many different defining attributes of a community are acknowledged if the true health needs of the population are to be identified. Gibson[16] defines these attributes as:

- social systems or networks
- organisational structure
- individual group or space
- boundaries
- movement in and out.

Public health nurses on the ground are more able to work with these different attributes and ensure that particular health needs are identified rather than lost to the system. This is particularly true of those patients suffering with mental illness. Whether they are able to be integrated into society is entirely dependent upon the community attributes defined earlier. Without an understanding of how communities operate and the potential subsets within them, particular health needs could, and would, be lost within the traditional macro approach to public health. Limited access and poor take-up of services are important contributory factors that perpetuate inequalities in healthcare, particularly in relation to minority ethnic groups and to the vulnerable in society, who suffer social exclusion. This may be due to language problems, poor understanding of healthcare services, or a failure to provide appropriate health services. The role of the public health nurse is fundamental in addressing problems of this nature. Attention should also be given to the need to find ways of involving the public within each of the communities in the decision-making process with regard to health policy. By developing this involvement and shared understanding of the local issues impacting on health and the causes of ill health, a real sense of ownership within the community is possible. Public health nurses are ideally placed to facilitate the development of such an approach.

Community attributes in action can be observed at this moment in time, up and down the country, by studying the debate around the formation of PCGs. These are intended to be based upon natural communities. As we write, many GPs are suggesting alternative, more appropriate PCG boundaries, based upon natural affiliations, to those suggested by health authorities. This is community attributes in action and it will continue to impact upon the public health agenda within the PCGs. Steps should therefore be taken to ensure that these community characteristics are reflected in all health needs assessment exercises undertaken within PCGs.

Leadership in public health

Opportunities would therefore appear to be abundant for re-establishing, and in some areas developing further, the public health nursing concept. But the mere existence of opportunities is not enough. Nurses need to demonstrate their competency to take on this new role. Public health nurses must take leadership roles in order to keep the public health vision alive, rather than waiting to be offered the responsibility, because there is a danger of public health nursing becoming everyone's business and no one's responsibility. Public health is nursing practice.

The basis upon which to build this case began back in 1994, when the Royal College of Nursing outlined some key activities for public health work in nursing[17]:

- assess the health needs of local populations through completion of health profiles
- support people to participate in the community to influence factors that affect their health
- build healthy alliances and a supportive infrastructure to provide information, resources and practical help for community initiatives
- increase health resources in communities by establishing local networks
- engage with the local statutory and voluntary groups to work towards health-related policies and actions
- increase uptake of health services by ensuring they are accessible, offered appropriately and effectively targeted.

The English National Board for Nursing, Midwifery and Health Visiting also contributed to the case for public health nursing in its publication *Creating Lifelong Learners*.[18] This places emphasis on the fact that nursing must be able to respond quickly and flexibly to patients, clients and family needs. The key characteristics of the role and function of nursing are listed below.[18]

- **Accountability** – expert practitioners should have the ability to exercise professional accountability and responsibility, reflected in the degree to which they use their professional skills, knowledge and expertise in changing environments, across professional boundaries and in unfamiliar situations.
- **Clinical skills** – expert practitioners should have specialist skills, knowledge and expertise in the practice area where they are working, including a deeper and broader understanding of client/patient health needs within the context of changing healthcare provision.
- **Use of research** – expert practitioners should have the ability to use research, enquiry and scholarship to plan, implement and evaluate concepts and strategies leading to improvements in patient care.
- **Teamwork** – expert practitioners should have skills in team working, including multiprofessional team working, in which the leadership role changes in response to changing client needs, team leadership and team-building skills to organise the delivery of care.

- **Innovation** – expert practitioners should have the ability to develop and use flexible and innovative approaches to practice that are appropriate to the needs of their client/patient or group, and are in line with the goals of the health service and the employing authority.
- **Health promotion** – expert practitioners should understand and use health promotion and preventative policies and strategies to achieve service targets.
- **Staff development** – expert practitioners should have the ability to facilitate and assess the professional development of staff for whom they are responsible, and to act as a role model of professional practice.
- **Resource management** – expert practitioners should have the ability to take informed decisions about the allocation of resources for the benefit of individual clients and the client group with whom they are working.
- **Quality of care** – expert practitioners should have the ability to evaluate quality of care delivered as an ongoing and cumulative process.
- **Management of change** – expert practitioners should have the ability to facilitate, manage and evaluate changes in practice to improve quality of care.

These qualities of expert practice should be evident in the leaders of public health nursing and, as such, pave the way for them to take on the mantle of driving forward the changes that are needed to carry out the latest challenge in improving the public's health.

The need to prepare nurses to take on the opportunities presented within the White Paper has been formally recognised by the NHS Executive with the publication in April 1998 of a consultation paper on a *Strategy for Nursing, Midwifery and Health Visiting*.[19] This strategy seeks to determine how best the nursing, midwifery and health visiting contribution can be strengthened and developed to enable the professions to respond to the opportunities and challenges arising from the government's policies for health and social care.

The consultation paper focuses in on three particular areas:

- improving health
- improving healthcare
- re-examining *A Vision for the Future*.[20]

Under each of these headings, nurses are asked to consider how best their roles can be supported and developed to meet the challenges of the future. The responses to the questions are to be used to inform the development of a strategy for nursing, midwifery and health visiting. It is anticipated that this strategy will be published in late 1998.

We are now at the critical stage of the evolution of the public health agenda. If the service chooses the narrow path, nursing will become marginalised. If, on the other hand, it chooses a broad, inclusive view of public health and translates this into practice, as suggested within this chapter, there are real prospects of nursing practice becoming the public health agenda. Connections are waiting to be made:

Where there is no vision, the people perish (Proverbs 29:18)

References

1   Jowell T (1997) *Health Care Today*. **50**: 24.

2   Department of Health (1997) *The New NHS: modern, dependable*. Cm 3807. HMSO, London.

3   Salmon Report (1974).

4   Acheson D (1988) *Public Health in England*. HMSO, London.

5   Beaglehole R and Bonita R (1997) *Public Health at the Cross-roads*. Cambridge University Press, Cambridge.

6   Holland W (1997) *Where Now for Public Health? The Art of the Possible*, Chapter 8. Nuffield Trust, London.

7   Henderson V (1969) *Basic Principles of Nursing Care*. International Council of Nursing, Geneva.

8   Roper N (1994) Definition of nursing. *British Journal of Nursing*. **3**(4): 355–7.

9   Benner P (1984) *From Novice to Expert: Excellence and Power in Clinical Nursing Practice*. Addison Wesley, Menlo Park, CA.

10 Department of Health (1993) *The Challenge for Nursing and Midwifery in the 21st Century*. Health Debate. DoH, London.

11 World Health Organisation (1985) *WHO Executive Board Emphasises Key Role of Nurses in Primary Care*. WHO Press, Geneva.

12 Department of Health (1993) *New World, New Opportunities: nursing in primary health care*. DoH, London.

13 World Health Organisation (1984), *Health for All by the Year 2000*. WHO, Geneva.

14 Department of Health (1988) *Public Health in England*. DoH, London.

15 DoH (1998) *Our Healthier Nation: a contract for health*. The Stationery Office, London.

16 Gibson C (1998) The concept of community: implications for community care. *Nursing Standard*. **12**(34): 40–3.

17 Royal College of Nursing (1994) *Public Health: nursing rises to the challenge*. RCN, London.

18 English National Board (1994) *Creating Lifelong Learners*. ENB, London.

19 National Health Service Executive (1998) *A Consultation on a Strategy for Nursing, Midwifery and Health Visiting*. Health Service Circula 1998/045. NHS Executive, London.

20 National Health Service Executive (1993) *A Vision for the Future*. NHS Executive, London.

CHAPTER TWENTY-FOUR

Public health scientists

Janet Baker

Who are public health scientists?

Public health scientists are defined in this chapter as those who have a knowledge base in statistics, epidemiology and the social sciences. In the UK they are currently at the centre of the debate facing public health as it tries to define the role and accreditation of 'public health specialists'.

Public health scientists believe that public health should be a 'broad church' which gains much of its strength from its multidisciplinary and multiprofessional base. Any attempt at a definition of public health should account for this richness. Public health scientists work in different parts of the NHS (trusts, primary healthcare teams, health authority and NHS Executive level), the local authority (e.g. environmental health, town planners, housing, social services), academic institutions, local government offices and voluntary organisations.

The report published by the CMO defined 'hands on' public health practitioners as those who 'spend a substantial part of their working practice furthering health by working with communities and groups. They need more specialised knowledge and skills in their respective fields. This group include public health nurses, health promotion specialists, health visitors, community development workers and environmental health officers.'[1]

The definition used for public health specialists (which includes public health scientists) is 'those who come from a variety of professional backgrounds and experience and need a core of knowledge, skills and experience. This core is in urgent need of definition so that generic public health specialists can be fully acknowledged for their contribution. This includes professions from backgrounds such as social sciences, statistics, environmental health, medicine, nursing, health promotion and dental public health. The knowledge, skills and experience needed include the ability to manage strategic change in organisations, to work in management teams and leadership of public health initiatives'.

Within health authorities in England there are disciplines other than public health medicine that are regularly contributing to public health activities.[2] The latest information available on staffing in health authority public health departments can be broken down as follows:

- 16% research or information officers and epidemiologists
- 4% as health promotion
- 48% public health physicians and trainees
- 6% pharmacists
- 5% medical advisers
- 8% nurses
- 3% consultants in dental public health
- 11% other job titles specific to public health.

As the audit reviewed public health departments, the numbers vary widely as some departments include health promotion. In addition, some look to other departments for their information support and comparisons therefore become very difficult. The importance of the survey was to show that there are a wide range of disciplines involved in public health programmes and that public health scientists are a significant proportion. If academic units and local authorities are included, the number of disciplines increases even further.

What is the contribution of different professions?

Public health needs sociologists, population-oriented doctors, clinicians, nurses, dentists, health promotion specialists, statisticians, economists, environmental health officers and others too. It needs all these specialists working together, to properly understand the true complexities of public health and to improve the public's health.

In the past there has been a tendency for public health in the NHS to be constantly pulled towards clinical services, which is only one (albeit important) aspect of public health.

To unite the public health function across all organisations, whilst properly exploiting its true intellectual and disciplinary diversity, is clearly never going to be easy, but the rewards for the public's health might well be formidable. The Government's approach to public health, which recognises the wider determinants of health and the wide expertise that is needed to deliver the strategy *Our Healthier Nation*, is enthusiastically welcomed.[3] It also recognises the need for the public health function to be strengthened.

As the profile of public health is raised, as a mainstream concern for health and local authorities through jointly developed health improvement programmes, it will be important for managers in health authorities and local authorities to have an understanding of the issues.

The contribution a public health scientist can make to public health is 'rigorous' science in the use of medical data, use of analytical techniques, statistical inference and interpretation. Active research experience also teaches the importance of organisation, motivation and collaboration.

At present there is no common definition for roles in public health and a wide variety of job titles are used and salary scales applied. Examples of the type of work done by public health scientists working in health authorities are summarised below[4]:

Health needs assessment

Scientists would contribute not only by looking at the numerical data available (epidemiological, use of facilities, etc.) to assess what is needed using various statistical techniques but also be in active discussion with 'communities', providers, users of services and others to identify their needs through focus groups or, more formally, a questionnaire.

Health strategy development/implementation

There are many examples of where scientists are involved in strategy development, either through providing information from literature reviews and critically appraising the evidence, analysis of epidemiological data, geographical mapping, or identifying the sociological implications of options. Where scientists take the lead is usually on health strategies which span many agencies, for example *Our Healthier Nation*, smoking, alcohol and general health promotion areas.

Service reviews

Examination of data sets, data collection, questionnaire design and analysis together with qualitative reviews of the service.

Epidemiology/information analysis (demographic or health service)

Analysis of trends in data sets to identify any significant changes, conversion of data into information to support health needs assessment, strategy and service reviews, and the production of the annual report of the DPH.

Research and development

Public health scientists are involved in a wide variety of research, e.g. the design of an accident information system which looks at data sets from different organisations; identifying the correlation between severity of accidents and the use of cycle helmets; providing statistical support to clinical trials; organising trials for smoking interventions; evaluation of interventions; health impact assessment of airports.

What are the main issues facing public health scientists?

The main issues that have been identified are the need to develop career pathways, education, training and development programmes, accreditation systems and equal opportunities for all to contribute. These are recognised in the CMO's project to strengthen the public health function and were first identified in a survey by Somervaille and Griffiths on the training and career development needs of public health professionals.[5]

Career progression for public health scientists

The pattern of the early career development of public health physicians and dentists has been established over many years. Employers are familiar with this pattern and feel they can make assumptions about the training and background of medically or dentally qualified persons. Some other groups, e.g. environmental health officers, have an established educational development pattern but for many public health practitioners following careers in the public health field there is no established pattern. This group enter organisations with degrees in virtually any subject and often progress by individual specialised training and study to higher degrees.

Employers and colleagues can experience problems in determining appropriate levels of responsibility, remuneration and professional development for them. The survey of public health departments in England identified a wide range of job titles and grades for staff with similar qualifications and doing essentially similar jobs.

Clear career paths in public health for all disciplines would help individuals to map out a path in developing a public health career. There needs to be a pro-active programme to ensure that people understand the contribution they can make to public health. There are some examples where public health scientists lead public health work on behalf of health authorities, local health authorities, the NHS Executive and the Regional Government Offices. Three examples follow.

Assistant Director of Public Health

The Assistant DPH is responsible for ensuring the production of health and social care strategies for major groups, such as people with mental illness, older people, people with disabilities and children. In addition, he/she oversees the production of a cross-agency health promotion strategy and ensures it links to other strategies.

Health science practitioner

A health science practitioner is responsible for identifying the health needs of disadvantaged groups. These may be centred on disability, deprivation, age, social exclusion, lack of permanent residence or ethnicity. Within the health authority the post-holder has lead responsibility for promoting the interests of black and minority ethnic communities. This includes designing, introducing and implementing a commissioning strategy for services for people in these groups. Ownership of the strategy was gained by a wide consultation with community groups, potential service users, providers and other agencies. Monitoring takes place through reviews and patient/care satisfaction surveys. Change has occurred and provider units have established equality groups and consultation networks. Interpreting services are in place. Practices have recognised the needs of people from minority ethnic groups and monitoring of ethnicity is improving.

Health of the Nation (*Our Healthier Nation*) co-ordinator

The co-ordinator is responsible for setting up healthier alliances, working with regeneration partnerships and putting public health on other agencies' agenda. Specific projects are a *Health for Youth* initiative, developing primary care services for young people through general practice, tackling HIV in prisons and community development work.

To date most public health scientists have experienced a career path that owes more to opportunism than planning. To assist in the development of people's careers, a framework for education, training and development and the development of an accreditation system (as outlined below) needs to be in place. The concepts detailed by creative career paths need to be addressed. It is essential that public health scientists visualise a personal career path without glass ceilings otherwise they are likely to leave the field of public health altogether.

A 'creative careers path review' covering all professions in the NHS has been undertaken. Further joint action is ongoing with the Equal Opportunities Unit to produce an action plan to take the recommendations forward. The recommendations made in the report include[6]:

- a more explicit understanding between the NHS and the individual about what each can reasonably expect of the other in relation to careers
- individuals should take more responsibility for shaping their own careers and the NHS should provide support and counselling
- a career development framework for everyone, and more positive action to identify and nurture the best talent within the NHS
- a clear assessment of the NHS's requirements now and in the future, matched by effective career counselling
- more emphasis on breadth and diversity of experience and retraining to meet new demands
- continued vigorous action to ensure that the NHS selects and retains good managers, regardless of their age, gender, race, disability, family circumstances or professional background
- increased flexibility in working patterns.

It is essential this framework includes public health scientists.

Education, training and professional development

The findings of the survey by Somervaille and Griffiths identified that although most staff are formally qualified in one relevant discipline, relatively few have formal public health qualifications. The survey also identified a widespread demand for appropriate training and career opportunities.[5]

Training and development needs to be valued and must be seen as being central to public health organisations and able to respond to the public health issues that face us today and in the future. Performance assessment should include the achievement of educational objectives for both the organisation and its employees.

Any consideration of training for public health needs to take account of the diversity of public health professionals and be underpinned by the principle of equity of opportunity for education, training, professional development and career advancement for all public health specialists.

Training programmes will need to be flexible, recognising the diversity of entry to the profession, as well as the potential tensions between generalist and specialist knowledge areas. Development of links between knowledge and practice will be important and encouragement of critical thinking, research and reflective practice are central. Training settings need to be diversified and secondments should be arranged so that practitioners are exposed to a wide range of organisations and the educational opportunities they offer.

Education and development needs are beginning to be considered both through the CMO's report and the Regional Offices. At least two regions have conducted surveys of educational and training needs and are developing strategies to take this work forward. Training programmes are being developed and funded through various mechanisms.

There are several excellent Masters courses available across the country and although varied in their content, they provide a fairly high level of public health education and allow professionals to acquire basic technical skills. However, there are fewer opportunities for Diploma or Certificate type studies which might appeal to a broader group of professionals wanting to share in some basic public health skills. Development here could also provide a useful induction level education for those thinking of entering the public health field. Options such as modular/stand alone courses and distance learning should be considered as ways of creating a more flexible approach. A work-based learning contract and modular courses, with transferable credits that can be put towards any level of academic achievement (diplomas, certificate, first degrees), is seen to have considerable educational potential. To focus on an MPH/MSc could perhaps be viewed as being too narrow.

Taught courses, even at Masters level, do not provide a complete training package. There is a need to ensure that trainers, mentors, placements and secondments are all part of a rounded public health training. Whilst this type of activity is already accepted as part of the public health physician training, it remains to be developed for all public health professionals, particularly public health scientists. The implementation of this training culture does of course have cost implications for employers, which might be minimised if such activity was truly integrated for all public health professionals and co-ordinated at a regional level.

Integral to the training/education toolkit is continuing professional development (CPD) and the Faculty of Public Health Medicine decided along with other Royal Colleges that in order to keep up to date and have credibility, its members should undertake CPD. CPD needs to be extended to include all public health professionals at this level of responsibility and be organised more effectively. Joint CPD should take place across all the agencies.

One way to integrate service and academic work may be to target research monies at joint projects of local relevance. This is happening in some areas already, e.g. the Public Health Resource Unit in Oxford has several projects underway which are benefiting from the 'coal face' knowledge of particular issues and the academic skills of analysis.

There is a specific requirement for a leadership development programme which should be integral to public health training. This is of vital importance for public health, in the role of trying to deliver change and influence other people's agendas. The two pilot leadership programmes in North Thames and West Midlands are welcomed, with participation in the programmes open to all those working in the public health field.

Measures needed to ensure a high standard of public health practice/development of a professional group

Standards need to be set to ensure that individual scientists acquire the technical expertise and skills necessary to execute the public health function. For example, the Faculty of Public Health Medicine sets the standard for public health physicians by examining both technical competencies and practical skills. Training programmes, and the staff involved, need to be accredited to a high standard and have sufficient resources to carry out their role. Ideally, there should be one professional or organisational body which formally monitors standards.

However, in the long term, excellence in public health practice will only be achieved if high-quality graduates are attracted to the profession. A high standard of recruits will only be sustained if trainees are secure in the knowledge that there is a commitment to help them obtain suitable jobs at the end of their training programme.

One of the issues that has been continually debated over the last few years by public health scientists and practitioners is whether a new professional group should be established. However, if we are looking to identify a new profession, we need to think through the very important characteristics of a profession:

- there is a body of knowledge or skill held as a common profession
- there is an educational process based on this body of knowledge for which the professional group as a whole has a recognised responsibility
- there is a standard of qualification for admission to the professional group based on character, training and proven competence
- there is a standard of conduct on courtesy, honour and ethics which guides the practitioner in relationships with clients, colleagues and the public
- there is a formal recognition of status by colleagues and by the State as a basis of good standing
- the organisation of the professional group is devoted to its common advancement and its social duty rather than the maintenance of an economic policy; the needs of clients are placed above those of the practitioner or his or her employer of the moment.

These issues are currently being debated and taken forward by the Multidisciplinary Public Health Forum (MDPHF), a national grouping of public health professionals, in conjunction with other organisations, primarily the Faculty of Public Health Medicine and the Royal Institute for Public Health and Hygiene. Recently, a tripartite agreement was signed by the three organisations with the aim of drawing up and administering a framework of accreditation which would define the skills and knowledge necessary for professionals working in public health. The overall project is expected to take three years.

The Faculty of Public Health Medicine has also voted to increase its membership to include a diplomate category of membership, which, for the first time, will give public health scientists the opportunity to obtain, by examination, a diploma in public health and become members of the Faculty.

The MDPHF sees professional accreditation as vital to ensure that the public health function is carried out effectively and that the population of the UK is served by properly trained and competent public health professionals.

A feasibility study has been commissioned by the NHS Executive to establish whether standards can be developed for public health practitioners, which will include scientists, and what systems should be in place, including costs, benefits and timescale.

Competencies

In attempting to identify competencies for public health practitioners, it is important to link this with the essential public health functions and the competencies professionals and teams will require to deliver the new health strategy *Our Healthier Nation*. However, a definition of the core knowledge, skills and experience required is essential if the contribution of public health practitioners is to be recognised.

The diversity of disciplinary competencies within multidisciplinary public health is its major strength, and training programmes should not be designed to produce uniform generalists. While this diversity also makes it difficult to identify generic competencies, it is essential that all team members have opportunities to develop the skills and competencies identified below:

- to have basic understanding of the core disciplines which contribute to multidisciplinary public health practice, together with an understanding of how other organisations are structured and function
- to be able to communicate and to work across agencies
- to be able to manage and implement change
- to be able to engage the public in policy development
- to be able to engage the public in health needs assessment
- to be able to look at the health impact assessment of public policy
- to develop a broad understanding of key current public health and health policy issues and debates, e.g. inequalities in health, developing and implementing health strategies.

In addition, some members of the team will be employed for their specialist skills in any of these disciplines and will be expected to develop these to a high level. Technical excellence is central to the public health function. It is also important when looking at competencies to define the values and attitudes that should be held:

- the application of scientific rigour to whatever we do
- an understanding of the importance of being person-, team- and organisation-oriented
- being able to justify what we do as we are paid by public monies.

The competencies and the need for certain qualifications will vary according to the job function. The feasibility study commissioned through the NHS Executive should identify possible areas where standards could be developed.

What about the future?

The future is very bright for public health scientists. For the first time we have a health strategy that recognises the wider implications of health and the need for many professional groups to be involved in implementing the strategy. The CMO's project to strengthen the public health function in England recognises the issues facing public health scientists and the short-term action proposed will address the following capability and capacity issues.

- career structure and pathways
- remuneration
- workforce planning
- education and training
- recruitment and retention
- continuing professional development and lifelong learning
- leadership.

It also recognises the need to look at the competencies required and, in the medium term, to establish an accreditation system for public health scientists. Public health scientists would like to see this followed through by a national training programme developed for public health scientists across all government departments, which gives them a background knowledge of the wider public health agenda, equips them to pass the examination for the diploma in public health (examined by the Faculty of Public Health Medicine or equivalent professional organisation) and provides them with the core skills identified in this chapter.

Standards should be developed for public health scientists and public health practitioners more widely. These standards will not only affect any training programmes developed but will assist in CPD and identifying appropriate remuneration scales for different occupations.

Workforce planning should be integrated across all disciplines and should recognise the contribution that public health scientists can make to the delivery of the public health agenda. This will require a joint approach between Postgraduate Deans, Regional Education and Development Groups and Education Consortia.

Scientists should be encouraged and helped to continue their professional development through CPD and opportunities such as learning sets, secondments and mentoring should be more widely available. In terms of careers, public health scientists should expect a career development framework and more positive action to identify and nurture talent, with no artificial glass ceilings to limit their ability.

The leadership programmes in North Thames and West Midlands, following evaluation, will need to continue or an alternative be offered in order that leadership skills are developed more widely. Over the next two years less than 50 people will be trained in leadership skills – this is just the tip of the iceberg.

The public health profession needs to ensure that it is multidisciplinary and is inclusive of public health nurses, physicians and other practitioners. It also needs to establish links outside the traditional boundaries of the NHS and be flexible in its own approach in looking to take up the opportunities on offer.

References

1   Department of Health (1998) *Chief Medical Officer's Project to Strengthen the Public Health Function in England: a report of emerging findings.* DoH, London.

2   Smith DC and Davies L (1997) Who contributes to the public health function? *Journal of Public Health Medicine.* **19**(4): 451–6.

3   Department of Health (1998) *Our Healthier Nation.* The Stationery Office, London

4   Cornish Y (1998) *Professional Development in Public Health for Public Health Practitioners from Non-Medical Disciplines: developing a strategic framework for the West Midlands.* South East Institute of Public Health.

5   Somervaille L and Griffiths R (1995) *The Training and Career Development Needs of Public Health Professionals.* Report of postal survey and discussion workshops. Institute of Public and Environmental Health, University of Birmingham.

6   Caines K and Hammond V (1996) *Creative Career Paths in the NHS: the agenda for action.* NHS Women's Unit, DoH.

CHAPTER TWENTY-FIVE

The socially constructed dilemmas of academic public health

John Gabbay

How best to underpin the new era?

Academic public health has two major characteristics. The first it has in common with all academic disciplines, indeed with all human knowledge: it is a social construction. In other words, it takes its shape and content from the organised human activity that produces it. So, for example, what we know about the relationship of ill health to poverty owes as much to the way the research community is organised within society as it does to any underlying natural truths about disease aetiology. The second characteristic, which is peculiarly poignant in academic public health, is that it is beset by a series of irresolvable opposing demands.

Many of the problems of public health practice are caused by its unusual nature as an activity, that has on the one hand been spectacularly successful in improving the population's health, and yet on the other hand has often been fragmented, directionless and marginalised. Similarly, the academic discipline provides some of our most important insights into the nature of health and disease and yet somehow seems to be continually in disarray. The recent literature, for example, has many discussions about the intellectual bankruptcy of epidemiology and the need for a new paradigm. Yet it is that very discipline which has been elucidating the links between unemployment and ill health, smoking and cancer, fat and heart disease, HIV and AIDS, health outcome and health technology, and between fetal growth and just about every conceivable adult ailment!

Perhaps as an academic discipline we demand too much of our rare skills while covering too wide an area. And now the new public health coupled with the new emphasis on NHS research and development, which rely so much on those public health academic skills, stretch them even further across both biomedical and non-medical aspects of public health. Do these new developments provide just another twist in a long history of impossible demands to be met while struggling at the margins of the medical profession, or are they an opportunity to establish a new and even more successful academic infrastructure?

The academic base for public health is necessarily eclectic and broad-ranging, but strongly dependent on epidemiology. The nature of that epidemiology has changed over the past century. Mervyn Susser has described a transition from the era of sanitary statistics, rooted in miasma theory, through an era of infectious disease epidemiology, rooted in the germ theory, to the recent post-war era of chronic disease epidemiology.[1,2] This recent phase is, he argues, rooted in the 'black box' paradigm, in which the mechanisms of the underlying disease are invisible to the investigator.

The recent phase also marks for Susser the final transition from an 'epidemiology of substance' dealing with real problems which need to be solved for public health reasons, to an 'epidemiology of technique, at risk of existing for its own sake regardless of subject matter'.[3] Some sectors of epidemiology seem obsessed with discovering ever more minor and often misleading exposure–disease relationships. Wing asserts that all major associations, such as smoking and cancer, have now been elucidated, so that most papers reporting the association of exposure and disease – and they are legion – have a relative risk of 3 or less.[4] Usually such a result cannot be taken scientifically as a reliable indication of real risk, since it is dubious whether the inevitable biases, confounders and measurement difficulties can be excluded as the reason for the apparent association. Certainly, relative risks of that order cannot be acted upon until amply confirmed by further studies, and are therefore of no use to public health practitioners. They are, however, a great source of copy for journalists, who have a field day reporting claims that vasectomy can cause prostate cancer, yoghurt can cause ovarian cancer, or women who don't eat enough olive oil are at greater risk of breast cancer.[5] All of which does little to help the credibility of public health professionals and a lot to worry and confuse the public. Here, then, is one of the dilemmas for academic public health: should we pursue risk-association epidemiology in the hope of finding new and real risks that can be used to improve the people's health (thereby using precious academic resources in a pursuit of diminishing returns)? Or is it time to abandon an exhausted research paradigm and focus on new types of questions (thereby perhaps missing major new causal factors that have as yet eluded us)?

The current paradigm has been accused not only of the exhaustion of useful work on risk-factor exposure, but also of focusing on the wrong part of the chain of causality, and hence missing the point that the most important public health questions are social and political, rather than biomedical. As Wing writes:

> ...any questions of context, such as where the exposures have come from, why some individuals but not others were exposed, or what other changes occurred in order to produce the exposures, have been eliminated from the realm of scientific interest.

He notes the ludicrousness of studying, for example, the relationship of race to disease without ever studying racism, or the role of radiation exposure in causing cancer without ever studying the processes of the military–industrial complex that produce the radiation. Thus, he remarks, epidemiologists have investigated smoking as the cause of lung cancer in terms of individual behaviour, whereas it would be perfectly respectable within another paradigm to focus the scientific effort on the tobacco agribusiness, cigarette marketing and the social rewards of smoking. This might matter less were it not that the endeavours of epidemiologically-based public health have done little to prevent global tobacco consumption from exacerbating the health inequalities between rich and poor, north and south.

Susser remains foremost among those who have diagnosed the increasing emptiness of academic epidemiology. He prescribes a shift to a new paradigm in which we do not try to discover universal laws about the causes of diseases, but develop an ecological approach based in the biological sciences. The new approach, which he calls eco-epidemiology, would accept the complexity of systems that interact at many levels – molecular, cellular, physiological, social, climactic – to produce any given phenomenon. It is difficult to discern exactly what Susser's new paradigm of eco-epidemiology would look like, but he is clear that by investigating in depth those many levels of interaction for any given problem, we would gain deeper insight and better control over it than we do with our current paradigm. Naturally such a multi-level biomedical approach to any one complex phenomenon would limit the generalisability of our findings, but Susser asserts that it would nevertheless give us much more useful knowledge for improving the public health than the relatively fruitless pursuit of our current paradigm. Indeed, he insists, if we persist with the latter into the next era of public health we risk terminal stagnation and the disappearance of epidemiology as the scientific basis of practice.

However, Susser's analysis is ingenuous in two respects. First, despite his extensive use of Kuhn's analysis of scientific endeavour, he fails to apply Kuhn's key concept that the emergence of a new paradigm depends upon social and economic factors way beyond the internal logic of the science and beyond the control of the scientists.[6] New paradigms are not simply invented by clever people: they emerge from a complex web of external factors affecting the scientific community. They are social constructs. Therefore we cannot design a new paradigm of epidemiology simply by analysing the problem and writing a prescription which the scientific community then goes away and swallows whole. Second, it may be a mistake to expect a new paradigm based chiefly on the biomedical sciences to usher in a new era of preventive public health, since, as we have already seen, the most intransigent public health problems are social and economic. Thus any successful new paradigm for academic public health will need to depend much more heavily on the social sciences than Susser admits.

Whether or not there is a need for a dominant paradigm based on any particular theoretical approach,[7,8] the idea of a multi-level approach to epidemiology is certainly attractive. There is otherwise a danger that academia will degenerate into a kind of scorn exchange between micro-epidemiologists pursuing the biological mechanisms of disease and macro-epidemiologists searching for the social causes, and between clinical epidemiologists focusing on the pathogenic factors in individuals and public health epidemiologists focusing on the disease determinants of communities.[9–11] Already there are methodological arguments of the deaf between triallists ('if it's not a randomised controlled trial why waste your time?') and those who use observational data,[12] between the individual approach ('aggregate community studies will miss individual associations') and the ecological approach[13]; and of course between the quantifiers ('if you can't measure it don't study it') and the proponents of qualitative studies.[14] There is increasing respect for the latter of each of those contrary views – observational, ecological and qualitative methods – but it is the former of each pair that most strongly shape the prevailing paradigm of academic public health. And yet many of the key problems of the new public health seem to defy solution by micro-epidemiological, individualistic, trials-based, biomedical, quantitative clinical epidemiology.

This leads us to another of the dilemmas for a new academic public health in its struggle for respect and recognition among the other medical sciences. Should it try and rely on a new biomedical paradigm, which would have the advantage of helping epidemiology hold its own in the face of molecular biology and the new genetics? Or should it consciously draw much more than it does on social and behavioural sciences, thus risking being dismissed as a 'soft' science by the medical elite, which holds so much sway over the public health research world? The former would push us towards elucidating the molecular and cellular mechanisms whereby diseases are caused, and therefore has much to commend it. It is one thing to know, for example, that at a population level, babies born a certain size are more likely to develop heart disease in later life. It is quite another to understand the hormonal and molecular mechanisms which result in that happening, so that we can intervene to prevent the consequences. There is a tremendous intellectual challenge in doing so, and an honourable tradition of success from such an approach. Hence the medical research community has good incentive to regard 'wet epidemiology' (i.e. epidemiological studies which involve, for example, the analysis of blood samples) as its strongest suit. And yet the wider public health research community would see this as medical hegemony that flies in the face of the obvious: that the main causes of public ill health are not biochemical but social, economic and political.

One enormous difference between the bioscientists' and social scientists' approach to science is the way in which they deal with the question of values, which again leaves the public health academic caught in a dilemma. Biomedical scientists try to strip away all cultural, ethical or political values from the objects of their investigation. If they find that the mean weight of a given population is 85.2kg, then that is a simple value-neutral fact; the interest will come from using that fact, say, in formulating and testing hypotheses about the dietary determinants of body mass. For the social scientist such facts and hypotheses are frankly boring. They would be much more interested in why anyone would care about people's weight in the first place, how and why some people are able to exert better control over their diet, or why agribusiness is politically empowered to influence dietary research. These questions would be openly driven by the investigator's values – such as a political conviction that the distribution of food is unjust. For the public health practitioner, the political ends are almost second nature; they drive the work. After all, we do the job because we want to right wrongs – be it to reduce health inequalities, bring wayward doctors to heel or fight for clean air. Yet the bioscientist sees such subjective prejudices as a danger – they may colour one's interpretation of the facts and so lead to false conclusions. Rothman, a leading epidemiological investigator and theoretician, has stated that position very clearly: 'The time for a scientist to be a political and social mover is after hours. Otherwise the conduct of science to achieve political ends will corrupt both endeavours.'[15] But, like it or not, the public health academics *do* make ethical and political choices consciously or otherwise, when they decide what to study, how to study it, which factors to take into account, how to interpret the results, or where and how to disseminate the results. As Neutra illustrates nicely in a thought experiment, if we found an environmental risk factor that is equally associated with Alzheimer's disease or hangnail, we would not simply toss a coin in deciding which to investigate.[16] At every stage from choosing our research programmes to implementing (or, more likely, *not* implementing) the results, public health science is inherently value-laden. Which brings us back, of course, to Wing's critique of an epidemiology that studies the effects of race on disease without ever mentioning racism. Treating race as a value-free risk factor does not, as its proponents would suggest, make an epidemiological study more scientific. On the contrary, the unconscious decision to exclude racism from the discourse is an inherent political bias that shapes the science. So what are the public health academics to do? Openly admit the values that drive their research and shape the results, hence risking the scorn of bioscientific peers? Or choose suitably 'value-free' research topics and methods that enable them to cling to the notion that they are doing real science – hence risking a betrayal of the very values that drive them?

There are those who say that many British public health academics who are not engaged in aetiological research have made the wrong political decision in pursuing health services research as opposed to the wider public health. Such academics have followed their NHS colleagues, the argument goes, away from the true public health.[17] They have abandoned health promotion centred on local communities, local government, environmental, social and political issues. Instead – and perhaps because that is where research funding has been easiest to acquire – they have allowed their research agenda to be drawn into supporting the bureaucracy of health services commissioning, the chimera of clinical audit, or the evangelism of evidence-based medicine, clinical effectiveness and now clinical governance. The critics lament the fact that even though clinical medicine is only a minor determinant of public health, scarce research skills have been deployed in evaluating local clinical services, running clinical trials, studying the cost-effectiveness of clinical interventions and undertaking systematic reviews. In short, academics are accused of ditching public health epidemiology in favour of clinical epidemiology. Indeed the argument goes even further among those who take the global view that the greatest burden of ill health is in the developing world, and is due to the macro-economic forces that cause poverty, unemployment, food shortage, preventable disease and war.[18] Given that the greatest public health problems lie in those directions, how can British academic public health physicians justify the disproportionate time they spend on local health problems, let alone health services research? Surely to achieve the greatest good they should direct their attention to the wider global determinants of health?

The answer to such charges can be made at several levels, but two points will suffice here. The first is that the involvement of public health academics in health services research may yet yield rich rewards for the public health. Health services soak up a very great deal of the spending intended by policy makers to improve health, and throughout the world that expenditure is threatening to grow out of hand. By helping to establish which are the most cost-effective interventions, public health academics can do a great deal to target those vast resources more efficiently and effectively, if not to begin to contain them. There may be doubts about the impact of the NHS R&D programme in tackling these problems over the 1990s but no question that this heralds a significant and long-overdue movement to improve the knowledge base so as to bring about more clinically effective practice.[19,20] There is now the potential for channelling the tidal wave of health technologies that has threatened to deluge health services. A major sea change is under way and it is doubtful whether it could be achieved if public health academics refuse to help to lead that programme. And why should they refuse, given that most are doctors who chose to go into public health because they were frustrated with the limitations of treating individual patients and desperate to make wider use of their clinical knowledge to improve health?

This leads to the second point in response to the charge that public health has misdirected its attentions, which is that the academics have naturally followed the paths set for them by the structures in which they work. Any research paradigm is the product of the circumstances that spawned it. It should therefore come as no surprise that public health research is focused around a medical paradigm, despite all academic departments professing to rely on non-medical scientific expertise in multidisciplinary research teams. Nearly all these teams exist within medical schools. They are headed by medical men (almost none are women despite the high numbers of women in public health) who are paid as medics not as academics, and who think with a medical mindset. They support a profession run by public health physicians, which works almost exclusively in the NHS, and whose professional body is a faculty of the medical royal colleges. Their value as research groups is judged by a Research Assessment Exercise alongside the medical disciplines of psychiatry and general practice, and the majority of their funding comes from a medically dominated NHS R&D programme, the Medical Research Council, and medical charities. Is it not entirely predictable that most public health academics would focus more easily on health service matters than on the wider public health? Or that they would fall into line with the NHS R&D programme's reliance on evidence from randomised clinical trials at the expense of research into political, organisational and behavioural factors that affect healthcare delivery? Of course it is, because public health departments that adopted a non-medical paradigm would find it very hard to survive in the competitive world of research. Here then is yet another dilemma. Should academic public health stay in its comfortable medical home doing well at what it best knows how to do? Or should it set out to seek its fortune elsewhere in the academic domain, wandering in a wilderness comforted only by an inner glow of logical and ideological soundness?

No-one but the bravest of zealous pioneers would choose the latter option without first seeing a substantial change in the infrastructure of both the professional and academic environments. Take first the professional environment. Public health doctors in the UK have been tearing themselves apart over the question of how best to accommodate the wide range of professions who contribute to the public health movement. The question is still unresolved, and there remains a plethora of public health umbrella organisations, none of which has a strong voice in public policy making. Each has a different view of the kind of evidence upon which policy-making should best be based – a different research tradition.[21] (Compare, for example, the professional journals of health promotion specialists, environmental health officers, communicable disease specialists, and health economists.) Each lives in quite different cultures (compare the worlds of local authorities, health commissioning agencies, hospital and community trusts, government departments, nongovernmental organisations, voluntary bodies, and research organisations). And none has a career structure that will match that of the public health physicians (compare the status and prospects of a high-powered graduate health promotion officer from the local authority with those of a specialist registrar in the health authority working, perhaps, on the same 'healthy alliance' project). Although each of the many groups has a substantial role in the new public health movement, it is difficult to know whether Babel, Balkanisation or Brownian motion give the best metaphor for the lack of cohesion. In such a condition, public health professions are not likely to produce a viable alternative to the medically dominated academic model. They require a strong cohesive professional voice, which has the power and influence to demand – and secure funding for – an academic base that meets their needs.

There can be no doubt that some aspects of public health practice require a new non-medical paradigm. For that to emerge, the structure of research departments, careers and funding will need to alter radically the power relations between the different academic disciplines. Yet in the academic world of the UK, what do we find? Academic public health departments exist mainly within medical schools, judged for their contribution to community-based *clinical* subjects and funded mainly by clinically dominated organisations. And within those confines they are becoming increasingly successful. It is therefore not enough to complain about medical hegemony in academic public health – not only does that ignore the successes of the medical model, but also it unrealistically expects a paradigm shift in the science underpinning public health without major shifts in the underlying structures. There will not be a non-medical paradigm until there is non-medical academic leadership, and that cannot realistically happen in medical schools, or in the face of medically inclined funding sources. At the very least, there should be clearly identified funding streams for strong academic departments outside medical schools to deal with some of the wider aspects of public health. Perhaps that would help to resolve one of the most fundamental dilemmas of academic public health – the fact that it is still organised in a way that encourages the use of medical methods to solve the non-medical as well as the biomedical problems of public health.

References

1   Susser M and Susser E (1996) Choosing a future for epidemiology. I Eras and paradigms,
     II From black boxes to Chinese boxes and eco-epidemiology. *American Journal of Public
     Health.* **86**: 668–77.

2   Susser M (1998) Does risk factor epidemiology put epidemiology at risk? Peering into the
     future. *Journal of Epidemiology and Community Health.* **52**: 608–11.

3   Susser M (1989) Epidemiology today: a thought-tormented world. *International Journal of
     Epidemiology.* **18**: 481–8.

4   Wing S (1994) Limits of epidemiology. *Medicine and Global Survival.* **1**: 74–86.

5   Taubes G (1995) Epidemiology faces its limits. *Science.* **269**: 164–9.

6   Kuhn T (1970) *The Structure of Scientific Revolutions* (2e). University of Chicago Press,
     Chicago.

7   Savitz DA (1997) The alternative to epidemiologic theory: whatever works *Epidemiology.*
     8: 210–12.

8   Krieger N and Zierler S (1997) The need for epidemiologic theory. *Epidemiology.* **8**: 212–14.

9   Mackenbach JP (1995) Public health epidemiology. *Journal of Epidemiology and Community
     Health.* **49**: 333–4.

10   Shy CM (1997) The failure of academic epidemiology: witness for the prosecution. *American
     Journal of Epidemiology.* **145**: 479–86.

11   Poole C and Rothman KJ (1998) Our conscientious objection to the epidemiology wars.
     Journal of Epidemiology and Community Health. **52**: 613–14.

12   Black N (1996) Why we need observational studies to evaluate the effectiveness of
     healthcare. *BMJ.* **312**: 1215–18.

13   Susser M (1994) The logic in ecological: I The logic of analysis. II The logic of design.
     American Journal of Public Health. **84**: 825–35.

14   Speller V, Learmonth A and Harrison D (1997) The search for effective health promotion.
     BMJ. **315**: 361–3.

15   Rothman KJ and Poole C (1985) Science and policy making (editorial). *American Journal of
     Public Health.* **75**: 340–1.

16   Neutra RR (1996) Epidemiology differs from public health practice. *Epidemiology.* **7**: 558–9.

17   Editorial (1994) Population health looking upstream. *Lancet.* **343**: 429–30.

18   Beaglehole R and Bonita R (1997) *Public Health at the Crossroads.* Cambridge University
     Press, Cambridge.

19   Peckham M (1991) Research and development for the NHS. *Lancet.* **338**: 367–71.

20   Baker MR (1998) Taking the strategy forward. In: MR Baker and S Kirk (eds) *Research and
     Development for the NHS: evidence, evaluation and effectiveness* (2e). Radcliffe Medical Press, Oxford.

21   McPherson K (1998) Wider 'causal thinking in the health sciences'. *Journal of Epidemiology
     and Community Health.* **52**: 612–13.

PART 3

Facing the future

CHAPTER TWENTY-SIX

Futures I

Walter Holland and Susie Stewart

Introduction

Previous chapters have dealt with a number of current concerns. We have recently reviewed the development of public health in the UK in the past 100 years.[1] There have been dramatic improvements in health, in the health services, in the environment and in quality of life over this period. But much remains similar. Many of the problems that bedevilled us in the past still do so, perhaps in a less serious way or in a somewhat different form. New problems have also emerged. A striking finding has been that we have not learnt sufficiently from past events or experience.

In this chapter, we will consider briefly the major problems of the past and then describe what we see as an ideal future for public health. There are, of course, many constraints to overcome along the way. But unless we strive for an ideal, it is unlikely that any constructive change will be achieved.

Major problems of the past

The main issues that have been, and remain, important in public health can be considered under a series of headings

Issues affecting health

Housing

This first claimed attention in the mid-1800s and has been a constant concern over the years.

Nutrition

One of the major influences on the health of a population is how it feeds itself. In the past undernutrition was the main problem, including vitamin deficiencies such as rickets. Improvements have been made, but now we see the problems of obesity.

Morbidity and mortality

Although there has been a dramatic decline in mortality from infectious disease, associated with the development of effective immunising agents and antibiotics, TB is still responsible for several hundred deaths per year. The dread of some diseases, such as diphtheria, measles and whooping cough, has been replaced by others, such as HIV infection, chlamydia and legionella. There has been a sharp decline of mortality in children and pregnant women. But we now have the continuing problems of cancer, cardiovascular disease and stroke, and an increase in disability associated with an increasingly ageing population.

The environment

There has been substantial improvement in air quality but, in spite of this, concerns with the pollution from increasing road traffic remain. Although the past hazards of inadequate sanitation and sewerage and polluted water supplies have largely disappeared, new ones have appeared; for example, lead and other heavy metals in paint, petrol or oil; the use of pesticides in farming; and the content of some animal feeds in the food chain.

The cons of progress

Not all the changes that have occurred this century have been good for health. Among relatively new or continuing problems is the increase in cigarette smoking, particularly in the young. Improved transport systems and changes in society have led to curtailment of the amount of exercise taken and this is associated with coronary heart disease, stroke and arthritis. Abortion and fertility are issues of ethical and public health concern. Although immunisation against measles and whooping cough has led to some reduction in mental illness, nonetheless these illnesses are a continuing concern. Violence, including child abuse, shows no evidence of disappearing. But, above all, deprivation stands out as a factor of major impact on health throughout the whole period. There has been an indisputable improvement in the standards of life and in state provision for those in greatest need. But even with these changes in welfare, inequalities in levels of health between the various social groupings have remained to the detriment of the more deprived, and are unacceptable at the end of the twentieth century.

Organisational issues

For public health, organisation concerns have always been important. Perhaps the most central of these has been the relationship of public health to clinical practice, both in hospitals and general practice. We have discussed the major issues surrounding this relationship elsewhere, so there is no need to rehearse them again here. In addition to relations with clinical practice, difficulties with other professional groups such as social workers and environmental health officers (sanitary engineers) have also been common. The failure to recognise changes in attitudes, educational standards and relationships between different professional groups has bedevilled the speciality in its ability to develop multidisciplinary working.

In order to perform effectively, public health needs to be able to communicate openly and honestly, to review progress, and to evaluate health service, environmental, behavioural and other issues. The conflicts between public health and political and other administrations have been frequent – and the freedom to speak and report frankly has sometimes been curtailed.

Another serious concern has been how to allocate limited resources within the context of exploding demand for healthcare. Those concerned with populations must have a key place in discussions on how priorities are best decided and implemented, and this has not always been the case.

Education, research, manpower

Another difficulty that has bedevilled public health over the years has been a search for its sense of identity, as illustrated by its changing names – social medicine, community medicine, preventive medicine.[2] This confusion has not helped in the development of a coherent method or content of both undergraduate and postgraduate education for those involved in practice. This confusion has also played a part in the variable attraction of the subject in the recruitment of both medically and non-medically qualified individuals. Research and its findings have also often been neglected – too often the subjects tackled have either been of a trivial nature, or have underestimated the complexity of interacting factors or been dismissed as unnecessary; for example, 'common sense tells us that a particular action is a waste of time, so no research is needed'. All these factors have influenced recruitment to the subject and thus its confidence and its standing.

Having briefly reviewed some of the major issues let us now consider an ideal structure for public health in the future which might enable the speciality to be more effective and influential in tackling the issues that have been described. We envisage this ideal to be achievable by 2025.

The ideal for public health

Governance

Central government will continue to be accountable to Parliament. We will not speculate on methods of election or the presence or not of two chambers. There is a central Public Health Department with a Secretary of State, a Minister for Health Gain and a CMO. Within the Department of Public Health there is a division concerned with the provision of clinical services, with a minister at its head who would be of equivalent rank to the Minister for Health Gain. The provision and function of clinical services, as a NHS paid from general taxation, continues. The budget for the Department of Public Health contains a large component for the provision of health services – as in the past. The managerial, operational control of health services is exercised, as in 1999, by the NHS Executive (Figure 26.1).

There is an elected regional government. Within each Region there is a public health authority, with a specific component concerned with the provision of clinical services. The authority contains both elected and appointed members. The officers of the authority

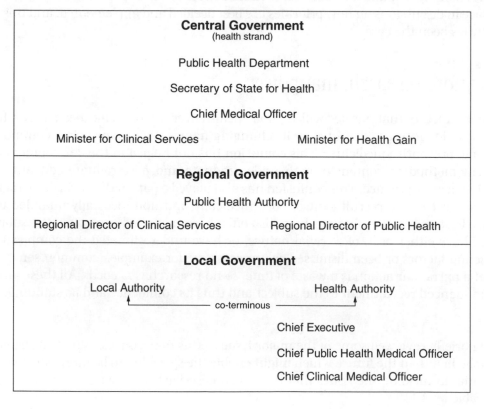

Figure 26.1:   Ideal public health structure in 2025

include a Regional DPH and a Director of Clinical Services, as well as other appropriate individuals. The Director of Clinical Services is accountable to the Regional DPH. The geographical distribution, and number, of Regions is similar to the present situation – that is, there are eight Regions in England and Wales – although the boundaries differ slightly.

Below Regions are elected local authorities, similar to the unitary authorities of the present, responsible for environment, housing, education and transport. Within each local authority there is a co-terminous health authority, with a Chief Executive, Chief Public Health Medical Officer and a medical Director of Clinical Services. The health authority consists of individuals who have either been elected to the local authority or who have been specifically nominated by the elected members of the local authority, as well as a number of appointed members. In addition there is, in each area, a number of hospitals with their own Boards.

It thus follows that the past lack of democratic governance at regional and local level has been remedied. The co-terminosity of health and local authorities facilitates the co-ordination and integration of policies to improve health for defined populations. The division of posts between public health and clinical services recognises the division of responsibilities and confirms that clinical services are only one part of the health service equation, albeit an important one. The explicit organisation also recognises that there is an earmarked, ring-fenced budget for public health, of which clinical services are one component. The budget for health continues to be met from general taxation, but the involvement of elected members at local and regional level ensures that health resources can be used for non-health administered services, such as traffic-calming measures in housing estates with large numbers of small children to reduce the risk of traffic accidents, the provision of health education in local schools or counselling services for family planning.

Functions and responsibilities of public health

In order to fulfil their role, public health practitioners at all levels are:

- forthright in the advocacy of programmes that improve health, and in a position to state clearly and openly the dangers of some actions – clinical, environmental or political
- able to influence the size of budget for public health activities; they can thus ensure that long-term public health action which will improve levels of health are considered on a separate dimension from short-term healthcare-delivery issues which always used to take precedence
- able to assume a clearly identifiable role in helping to guide the policies not only in the field of health, but also in schools, environmental agencies, welfare agencies, housing departments and every sphere of activity that has an influence on health.

As the prime responsibility of public health is to promote health and prevent and control disease, the Chief Public Health Medical Officer at both regional and local levels has responsibility for public health information services. Public health has key needs in the collection, analysis and dissemination of accurate information, and is thus responsible for the design and implementation of its information requirements – demographic, social, environmental, and measures of health and clinical service utilisation and outcome. This is based on records of individuals, not events.

The major types of problem with which public health deals are:

- outbreaks of disease caused by infective or toxic agents; for example, smallpox, typhoid, BSE, radiation
- problems arising from social and environmental issues, such as inadequate housing, unemployment, poverty, abortion, fluoridation of water
- behavioural concerns, such as smoking, excessive consumption of alcohol, drug-taking and insufficient exercise
- health service issues, including assessment of healthcare needs and outcomes and the effectiveness and efficiency of particular services.

Public health practitioners, although employed by health authorities, have specially secured positions, as MOHs had before 1974. They are thus able to inform the public responsibly on public health matters, and can fight actively the promotion of products such as cigarettes, which have a well-proven effect on health. They can guide other authorities in the implementation of simple public health measures, such as fluoridation of public water supplies, which provide enormous benefits, particularly in more deprived sectors of the population.

Each health authority has the duty to publish an Annual Report of Public Health. This report highlights any particular problem that has arisen in the local area in the past year, reports on progress of action taken on issues that have been of concern in the past and periodically reviews issues of concern or interest; such as, for example, the prevention of mental illness, progress in the elimination of unsafe workplaces and the problems of homelessness.

Staffing of Public Health Departments

Public Health Departments at each level – central, regional, local – are led by a Chief Public Health Medical Officer or DPH. All departments are multidisciplinary. The major academic disciplines represented are epidemiology, medical statistics and some aspects of the social sciences, including economics. They have all been trained in interdisciplinary work. Some of the medically qualified members of the team have specific skills in the handling of outbreaks of disease, and the law has been clarified so that they have full responsibility and the necessary powers to act appropriately in the investigation and control of outbreaks. There are both formal and informal links to the microbiological and toxicological laboratories at all levels, so that their facilities and expertise can be used to best effect. The senior staff in a department are all rewarded as consultants and supported by both staff in training as well as appropriate numbers of technical and clerical individuals.

Education, training and research

In medical schools, education in public health now begins in the first pre-clinical year, with basic courses on epidemiology, medical statistics and social sciences. Each of these subjects counts in the necessary tests each student has to pass. As students progress in their medical training, the knowledge from the three basic sciences is integrated in order for them to have a reasonable appreciation of the application of public health to the improvement and maintenance of health. During the basic 5-year course each student will have had an attachment of at least 1 month to a public health department to experience the practical, service aspects of the subject. Some students, who opt for a longer medical training – for example, BMedSci or PhD – will have had the opportunity for much greater involvement in public health and its component disciplines and will have undertaken a small research project (or in the case of a PhD a bigger project) in, for example, mounting a survey of healthcare needs, evaluating the effectiveness of a programme of health education in schools or developing techniques for health surveillance.

Those medical practitioners opting to follow a career in public health pursue a career pathway similar to that introduced in the late 1990s after the changes introduced by the then CMO, Sir Kenneth Calman; that is, after house officer posts they do general professional training followed by specialist training. Specialist training is done at one of the Regional Institutes which is within a university with a medical faculty. Non-medically qualified aspirants to posts in public health – for example, nurses, statisticians, social scientists – are expected to have at least a Master's degree in their basic subject. They will then have had about 3–6 months' education in the biological sciences as applied to medicine. They then join their medical colleagues for further education and training in epidemiology, medical statistics and the social sciences as applied to public health. This 1-year theoretical course in the sciences of public health for all disciplines includes specific training in interdisciplinary work. After this year, trainees are involved in service or academic activities for a defined training period of at least 3 years. This training period involves increasing responsibility and development of specific expertise. As with other disciplines, public health now consists of an increasing number of sub-specialities – information, health promotion, disease control and so on.

Research and academic departments are much more integrated with service authorities. Most academics hold joint appointments between academic and service authorities. The relationship between the two is much more constructive than in the past. As public health must be involved in appropriate studies, whether epidemiological, sociological, psychological or statistical, to enable hypotheses to be tested and solutions implemented for the control of ill health, the need and ability to interact between service and academic practitioners has become easier and much more active than in the past. Since the academic units exist at regional level, they provide the academic support so essential for individuals at local level. The regional departments are also adequately staffed so that they are able to provide the necessary service support, so often needed at local level, for example, in the investigation and control of an outbreak, without influencing their educational and research function.

Tasks at local, regional and central level

Public health is not concerned only with the control of disease and improvement of health. The factors that contribute to these affect all our lives. Thus public health is involved with communities at all levels. Public health professionals work with representatives of the people in their communities to find out what are their concerns, and also to inform and help them to improve their own conditions and influence their personal behaviour in order to maintain and improve their health. In addition, they work with and guide those responsible for the planning and provision of those activities which affect the health of the population; for example, housing, water and sewerage, education, social services, employment, transport and clinical services.

Although public health practitioners are employed by the relevant authorities, thus enabling them to have access to and responsibility for health information systems, formal links exist to the authorities responsible for the activities referred to above. Thus the number of individuals employed at a local health authority is greater than it was in the 1990s, and the method of appointment again includes representatives of the local/regional authority.

Research in the previous 10 years has begun to tackle the different ways in which individuals, the media, politicians and authorities perceive the risks of particular behaviours, environments or actions. Epidemiological research has also progressed in disentangling the relative contributions of, for example, drinking, smoking and air pollution on the development of coronary heart disease. As a result of this research the ways in which public health practitioners are able to communicate with the media, pressure groups and the public has improved. Educational programmes now incorporate ways of risk communication to various groups. Individuals practising public health are now selected for different positions in the speciality not only on the basis of their factual knowledge, but also on their diplomatic, political and communication skills. Research in the field is far more closely linked to practical questions, so that not only can the factors responsible for particular problems of ill health be investigated, but also evaluated possible solutions found.

An important change in the relationships and tasks of public health practitioners since the 1990s concerns their links to the other clinical disciplines. In many areas of the country, commissioning of health services is done by groups of GPs serving populations of about 100 000 people. These commissioning groups are assisted in this task by public health practitioners who provide guidance in the assessment of the healthcare needs of the population, evaluation of the health services provided, and in the determination of priorities and options for preventive or health promoting, curative and rehabilitative services. These public health practitioners, usually 1–2 consultants 1–2 trainees and associated technical staff, also have responsibility for participation in the appropriate local authority body concerned with education, housing, environment, etc., so as to ensure that a coherent policy to improve health is developed.

Public health practitioners are similarly involved in hospitals. Their roles within these institutions are, first, in cross-infection control and surveillance and in participating in the evaluation of the services provided within the hospital. They have a crucial role in co-ordinating, but not directing, the activities of GPs, community staff and hospital staff.

Public health departments at each level have a major role in the assessment and monitoring of the services and policies that are planned and provided for the maintenance and improvement of health of the population in their area. As they are responsible for monitoring, a clear separation exists between those working with general practice, with hospitals and with those in the 'main' headquarters. Obviously, co-operation between the three groups is crucial, and all are accountable to the DPH.

It is important to emphasise that the executive, managerial roles of public health are far more distinct than in the past. Public health practitioners have executive, managerial roles for the design, maintenance, adequacy and quality of the information system. They have power, and authority, in the investigation and control of outbreaks of disease. However, their other tasks are investigative, advisory and participatory. They are responsible for the assessment of the healthcare needs of populations, the evaluation of such services, the regular reporting on the health status of their population, the investigation of the factors that lead to ill health and the methods of coping with these.

The results of these tasks are then communicated to those responsible for the delivery of individual services in hospitals and the community (e.g. GPs, nurses, physiotherapists), and to those involved in developing and managing policies and services in housing, education, nutrition, welfare, environment, etc. The public health practitioners have a duty to guide and participate in the deliberations of health authorities and local authorities, both in their discussions on currently provided services as well as priority setting in the planning of new activities. As we have emphasised above, these tasks involve working with individuals and groups within the community, as well as with the bodies responsible for the provision of services.

The tasks and roles of public health are now far wider than 25 years ago. Thus the number involved in public health is much greater. The GP commissioning group serves a population of about 100 000. There are usually between five and seven such groups within the area of a health authority. Within each health authority there are usually two or three hospitals. Each Public Health Department therefore, has at least 15 consultant-grade practitioners and an appropriate number of other staff and trainees. The speciality of public health is thus strengthened and capable of performing its tasks. Recruitment is no longer a problem, since it is evident that public health performs an important and interesting role.

Conclusion

Public health has learnt from the lessons of history, so that now, in 2025, it has regained its powerful, effective voice. It has learnt that the most effective method by which to influence decisions in all aspects of life, and thus in the improvement of health status, is to be responsible for the investigation of the factors that lead to ill health, the determination of methods to improve health, the surveillance of health and the factors that influence it. It guides and participates with those responsible for the delivery of services to individuals and communities in the application of findings and knowledge. It does not attempt to direct, or manage, clinical or other individual services. It has achieved its goal of being able to communicate with the media and public openly and frankly on policies that influence health and has learnt how to transmit effectively knowledge on absolute and relative risks. It has learnt to value and co-operate with the academic disciplines central to the speciality and has developed strong educational programmes and a high profile so that it can recruit individuals of the highest calibre.

Public health has finally come of age.

References

1   Holland WW and Stewart S (1998) *Public Health, the Vision and the Challenge.* Nuffield Trust, London

2   Holland WW (1994) Changing names. *Scandinavian Journal of Social Medicine.* **22**: 1–6.

CHAPTER TWENTY-SEVEN

Futures II

Kenneth Calman

Introduction

Predicting the future can be difficult. Perhaps the only sensible way forward, therefore, is to try to set out those areas which might see developments, recognising that in many instances new ways of thinking and new initiatives will come from unanticipated sources. For the purposes of this chapter, public health will be interpreted widely and will reflect all those disciplines which might have a role in improving the health of people. This must also be the objective of research, to change the health of the population for the better. This inevitably raises issues about the value base that is used in achieving that goal, and the purpose of improving health. Is it for the many, or the few? Is it an end in itself, or one method of improving quality of life? The answer to these questions will set the framework for research and help to evaluate any new developments designed to improve health. It will certainly raise questions about costs and effectiveness of their implementation.

At the end of the day, it is ideas and new ways of thinking that are important. The culture of curiosity and the spirit of enquiry need to be at the heart of professional education. They should not be seen as add-on extras which take up time, space and money. The ability to create new frameworks and concepts and change the way in which health and healthcare are delivered should be in the job description of every professional. Without research there will be no change at all.

Possible future developments can be divided into several categories, the first of which is one of general issues, such as the importance of fully utilising the current knowledge base and the techniques for horizon scanning and identifying promising new ways forward. The second category reflects methodologies that might be developed. Finally, there is a series of specific areas related to those factors that determine health. Each of these will now be discussed in turn.

Some general issues

The improvement in the health of the population might be achieved by a variety of routes and mechanisms, many of which are not dependent on new knowledge, but on using existing information more effectively. There is much to be gained by putting into practice what we already know about improving health. Such developments might include the following.

- Improving the organisation of public health to deliver better health programmes. Many different professional groups are involved in health, as are many organisations, both statutory and non-statutory. Greater collaboration between health authorities and local authorities would be part of this. Clarification of the messages and actions, agreement on these by all parties and working together would begin to reduce confusion in the public's mind about health issues. Improving the health of the public requires an interdisciplinary approach, utilising a wide range of sectors.
- Involving the public in the process is critical and in itself gives ownership of the problem and thus a greater chance of success. The communication to the public about matters relating to health can be improved.
- Issues around risk, its understanding and management, are crucial. Skills of advocacy and public presentation of complex issues are all part of the role of the public health practitioner. Such individuals do not come from any particular professional group, but involve all disciplines: scientists (biomedical, behavioural and social), health professionals, managers and politicians who have an interest in health matters.
- The use of legislation and enforcement to change health is an important component. This has been done successfully in the introduction of seat belts, drink and driving limits, regulations on air and water quality, and many others. Such regulations generally limit individual freedom, but are done for the good of the population as a whole. The public need to take a full part in this process and recognise the value and the limitations of the outcome.
- Part of this process is about education, for professionals and the public. Understanding of science, and the process of discovery, is not well developed with policy makers and the public. There is much to be done in areas such as risk and its management. It will require individuals with leadership skills who are able to help in this process and so assist in changing perceptions and attitudes of both public and professionals.
- Clarity about what a good outcome means will also be needed. How will it be measured, and how will we know if we have achieved the outcome required? Such questions need active public involvement so that the benefits of any changes can be recognised at the start of the process.
- A number of different organisations now encourage the process of horizon scanning, sometimes called foresight initiatives, intelligence or surveillance. In essence, a process is set up which sets out to identify new developments at the earliest possible moment in order that they can be assessed and, when appropriate, introduced. This

must be an active, not a passive, process and depends on building networks on topics which link to those people who are at the leading edge of change in the subject. This network must be broad enough to anticipate developments in a range of fields. Examples of this might include the identification of new screening techniques, or of new infective agents, or the re-emergence of old diseases such as TB.

- The importance of values has been emphasised already. These are relevant as new developments will question our ethical principles. Moral issues are crucial to an understanding of the decisions to be made in improving the public's health. Patient rights and the common good may be in conflict and decision makers need to recognise this. Human rights issues, the problems of confidentiality and the definition of a 'person' are just a few of the examples that might be chosen to highlight ethical issues. Genetic engineering and the possibility of human cloning are fundamental issues that raise many difficult questions. These will not be the last, and as science progresses, so such issues will continue to arise. New developments to improve the health of the public will certainly not be without a re-consideration of basic values.

New methodologies

One of the most difficult aspects of research is to develop tools or methods that can be used to answer public health questions. In some instances the question posed may be straightforward, but the technique for answering it not available. The converse is also true, that a validated research method can be used to answer questions that are not particularly useful, simply because the method is available. For example, there are limits to the value of epidemiological techniques, they cannot define causation. On the other hand, the polymerase chain reaction (PCR) for measuring small quantities of DNA (deoxyribonucleic acid) opened up a whole new field for research. Molecular techniques and the new genetics have revolutionised the way we can redefine problems and begin to answer new and old questions. The development of computers, geographical information systems and other information technologies has allowed new questions to be answered. Newer techniques in the social sciences are helping us to understand behaviour, perception and attitudes. A final illustration is the definition of the link between the environment and health. Many substances and conditions in the environment are likely to affect health. However, making the definitive link and quantifying the effects can be very difficult. Consider the problem of road traffic and air pollution. Clearly, there are potential harmful effects but the quantification of the impact is more difficult. We need new, and more refined, methods of health-impact assessment. How do you assess the effect of investing in improving air quality on health, and would it be better value for money than reducing the lead content of water? How do you measure the impact of sustainability and reduction of energy use on human health? Questions like this require new methodologies.

The implication of this discussion is that future issues in public health are likely to be linked as much to the development of new methods of enquiry as to the questions themselves. For this reason horizon scanning needs to include a search for new techniques which might assist in improving our understanding of better health.

Some specific areas for development

It is possible to set out those factors that determine health, which can then be used to consider what new developments might occur in each. The factors include:

- biological factors, such as ageing and genetic influences
- social and economic factors, such as education, housing, employment, income and poverty, and cultural aspects
- the environment, including the quality of the air, water and soil, transport, climate changes; this topic also includes infection
- lifestyle issues, such as diet, smoking cigarettes, drug abuse, alcohol and physical fitness
- health services, and the way they are delivered and accessed; this topic includes developments in medicine, diagnostic techniques, and rehabilitation.

This section considers such issues from two different directions. The first is the definition of some of the major issues ahead, and the second, new methods that might be available to improve health. It should be noted again that this is a difficult exercise and it is just as likely that new problems and solutions will come from unexpected places.

Biological factors and the understanding of disease

This is likely to be one of the most exciting areas in public health. The human genome project is one of the most important research developments for the future. The development of cloning may have significant consequences for improving health. The new genetics allow not only the possibility of new treatments, such as in genetic engineering, but, perhaps more importantly, for our understanding of disease. The reclassification of disease with the introduction of more specific therapies will be particularly relevant.

One of the most interesting areas of biology is in an understanding of the process of ageing. Why does it occur, and can it be slowed down? These again are fundamental questions which, once research methods are developed, may change the way in which we think. Another issue is an understanding of the way in which the brain functions at a molecular level. An understanding of memory, of the patterns of behaviour, of mental health problems and of learning would allow significant shifts in improving health.

As a final illustration of the way in which research in the basic sciences might assist in improving health, the topic of maternal–fetal interactions can be used. For many years it has been known that such interactions as smoking, alcohol, drugs and diet have an effect on fetal growth and development. More recent work shows that the impact can be very long-lasting and can influence disease in adult life, such as heart disease and hypertension. The consequences of this are profound, and as the knowledge builds up so it will become possible to intervene more specifically. The ethical and social consequences of this are unknown.

Social and economic factors

The brief list given in the introductory section outlined some of the significant problems. Social and economic factors are closely linked to the level of health. Educational attainment is related to health, as is employment status and poverty. This latter is one of the most significant predictors of health, worldwide. Poverty is not only about a lack of material factors but is about the personal, social and psychological consequences. Changing these will not be easy and is part of the political process in any country. Yet all the evidence suggests that these factors are major determinants of health. The research agenda must identify new methods of intervention which can reduce inequities and inequalities. There are no simple solutions.

Reference was made above to new research on ageing. From a social point of view, ageing and the care of the elderly presents a major challenge in all countries. It is linked closely with service development, and with issues of quality of life and disability. It returns to the question raised at the beginning of the chapter, the purpose of health. Is it valuable to live a long life if the end part is associated with disability and suffering? The purpose must be to limit the period of time in which there is significant morbidity (sometimes known as the compression of morbidity). This is a major public health problem. It is partly about access and availability of care, but is also about health promotion, lifestyle improvement, disability management and a whole range of social issues. Amongst these are the problems of isolation and loneliness. Those with an interest in improving the health of the public need to take this range of issues seriously.

A further major public health issue, now increasingly recognised as such, is violence. This can range from the effects of war through to the problems in a domestic setting. The consequences are huge and lives are affected in a most profound way. The action required is likely to be of a societal or community nature. Research is needed urgently into the causes and possible methods of intervention. In the domestic setting it is closely associated with the role of women. In almost all societies women are disadvantaged, yet they are the principal carers and decision makers in relation to health. As a subset of this, the education of women is crucial, as are equal opportunities for their development and role in society.

Lifestyles

Many health problems have their origin in poor lifestyles, and some of these have already been mentioned. The key difficulty is in changing behaviour. For example, the vast majority of the population know that smoking cigarettes has serious health consequences.

Yet over 20% continue to smoke. Why? It must be that the value to them of continuing is greater than the wish to change. This 'value-based' concept emphasises the need for research into behaviour and attitudes. We need to understand more clearly issues about motivation and perception, and new directions in this area are likely to come from psychology and sociology. New models of behaviour are required. What is not in doubt is the impact of lifestyle on health.

As part of a study, lifestyle, ethnic health and gender issues are important. The differing patterns of disease and risk factors must mean that such topics must be considered at all stages in programmes to improve public health. Health for all is not an empty slogan, and in research terms such matters are of profound importance.

Environment and communicable disease

Much is already known about the link between environment and health, although, as has been mentioned, much still remains to be done. Some of the key issues that will face us all over the next decade will be related to environmental problems, including climate change, air quality and food safety. The effects can already be predicted to some extent. More traditional areas, such as the quality of housing, remain critical and link directly to poverty and the quality of the whole environment. With such subjects, although we will need more research, our existing knowledge could allow us to change the environment for the better. For example, issues of air quality and health are increasingly recognised. Much could, and is, being done to improve the atmosphere.

Infectious disease is still with us, and over the past 20 years the re-emergence of old infections (e.g. TB and malaria) and the emergence of new ones (e.g. HIV, transmissible spongiform encephalopathies and Ebola) have presented us with some serious problems. The need for surveillance at country, regional and global levels is obvious. This should be coupled with a strategy for active control of the problem and a strong research base.

Immunisation programmes are amongst the most cost-effective healthcare measures available. The elimination of smallpox in the world set the standard and there is a real possibility of eliminating polio and measles. New technologies and new knowledge are opening up avenues for different approaches for vaccine development. Infections that have proved difficult to control with vaccines may now be within reach, including HIV, meningitis and malaria. Such initiatives demonstrate how developments in one area of knowledge can be of benefit in others.

The role of health services

The health service can contribute greatly to improving health and quality of life. This can occur through two main mechanisms, and it is likely that there will be considerable developments in both over the next decade.

The first of these is in the development of clinical practice, with the use of new methods of diagnosis and treatment. Diagnostic techniques have been revolutionised over the past two decades, with innovations in both imaging and laboratory-based methods. Scanning techniques have completely changed the accuracy of diagnosis and allowed new methods of intervention with direct vision of the problem and the outcome. This, together with developments in minimally invasive surgery, is likely to alter disease management.

New, and very powerful, drugs for the treatment and control of disease have appeared over the past few years. It is likely that they will continue to be discovered, often, as has been said before, from unlikely sources. These will all require adequate evaluation and assessment before widespread introduction. With them they bring problems of side-effects and resistance. A particular concern for the next decade will be drug-resistant micro-organisms, already a major problem in some places. The role of the pharmacist is likely to develop further as their special skills are used to improve patient care.

Finally, there are likely to be new developments in rehabilitation and palliation. If one of the goals of improving health is to change quality of life, then this must be an area for new thinking and ideas in physiotherapy, dietetics, occupational therapy and nursing. As examples of this the work in stroke units or in rehabilitation after cancer surgery show how much can be achieved using existing knowledge.

The second area to consider is that of improving the management of health services. This would include access to services, better ways of providing them and a more effective assessment of need for the population as a whole. Changes that have already occurred have been dramatic, with the greater use of outpatient facilities, concentration of specialist equipment, the use of guidelines and protocols. Evidence-based medicine, a new name for a well-recognised process, is now embedded in health service culture. However, care must be taken not to interpret the phrase too narrowly, and qualitative as well as quantitative data will still be required. The public dimension to changing and improving health services is clear, and there will be increasing involvement of patients in the process, something to be welcomed. Patient choice, and the responsibility that goes with it, will become the norm.

Linking clinical practice and service delivery is screening for early disease. It is already possible to screen for a variety of diseases and to intervene, thus changing the natural history of the illness. While some programmes are successfully established, others need a greater input of quality and evaluation. Over the next decade new methods of screening are likely to become available (genetic screening would be one of these), which will change the way in which particular diseases are managed. This is likely to be one of the most exciting areas of health service development, linking high technology with improved patient care.

The health service, if it is to become more effective, will have to link with a wider range of partners, including the local authorities, the voluntary sector and a wide range of community-based projects whose aim is to improve health and quality of life. This is likely to be one of the most exciting and challenging areas of health service improvement.

Just as in medical science, there needs to be a culture of creativity and challenge to existing ideas and concepts in all of the areas described. There is as much need in health services for experiment and rigorous evaluation as there is in the laboratory setting.

Some conclusions

This chapter has tried to point out the remarkable changes that have already occurred to improve the health of the population. A wide range of disciplines has been involved. Much change could still occur if we were to make full use of existing knowledge. In addition, research in a wide variety of areas is likely to demonstrate that even more will be possible in the future. It is a good time to be involved in improving the health of the public.

CHAPTER TWENTY-EIGHT

Futures III

Lord Hunt of King's Heath

Experience as a councillor in both Oxford and Birmingham and a long-standing interest in local government provide me with a perspective on the key role that local authorities have, and will continue to have, in promoting the public's health.

In Birmingham, over the past 15 years, the local authority has shown powerfully how it can lead its people out of the depths of depression, resulting from the destruction of so much of its traditional industries in the early 1980s. New industries, new investment and new confidence have been brought to the city, the catalyst for which was undoubtedly the City Council.

This is not the first time it has happened. It was one of Birmingham's greatest leaders who encapsulated for me what it is that local government can offer to the health of our country. In 1873, Joseph Chamberlain was elected Mayor of Birmingham. In a speech at the time, he appealed for the help of his council colleagues in a radical programme of improvement: 'The town', he promised, 'shall not with God's help, know itself'. Chamberlain was as good as his word. He organised the purchase of the two gas companies and water works, so that these undertakings could be modernised and expanded under municipal control. He appointed an MOH, and established a Drainage Board to supervise the scientific disposal of sewage and refuse. He extended the paving and lighting of streets, opened six public parks, saw the beginning of the public transport service and himself laid the foundation stone of the Council House which was to become the hub of this vast municipal enterprise. The impact on the city was enormous and it had an equally major impact on the health of the people living in Birmingham. It was one of the most visible signs of the inter-relationship between local government and the health of the people.

We are now embarking on a similar journey in which local government is reconnected with health in a profound way. Much of the division that has characterised the relationship between the NHS and local government over so many years, a division that goes back to the beginnings of the NHS when Nye Bevan fought (and won) for most of the NHS to be run by government-appointed organisations as opposed to local government, must now be put away. Bevan wanted a minister accountable to Parliament to control the entire running of health. As he said, 'When a bedpan drops in a ward in St Thomas' Hospital, its echo should respond in the Palace of Westminster.' Over the 50 years of the NHS, Bevan has perhaps been taken a little too literally – a few too many bedpans dropped and rather too much echo at Westminster!

But times change and we are embarking on massive constitutional change in this country:

- devolution in Scotland and Wales
- the new Northern Ireland Assembly
- prospect of voting reform
- reform of the House of Lords
- elected Mayor and Assembly for London
- prospect of legislation in the next session over elected mayors and cabinet systems of governance in other local authorities.

Local government is facing up to a massive change agenda, including the introduction of:

- best value
- new financial framework
- new ethical framework
- democratic renewal
- a whole mass of White Papers and legislation on local government legislation including education, transport and social services.

The health service faces an equally daunting agenda in:

- replacement of the internal market
- massive development of primary care
- major modernisation of our hospitals
- tackling chronic health problems.

Who of us could be certain what the governing institutions of our country will look like in 10 years time? Who can be certain what local government and the NHS will look like? It is a time of great fluidity and the time is ripe for us to take advantage of that flexibility to put the NHS/local government relationships on a new footing, putting behind us previous failures in relationships, which have led to:

- gaps in services
- inadequate support for people discharged from hospital
- unacceptably poor health for thousands of people.

The time is ripe for us to put aside our divisions and differences in:

- culture
- funding
- decision-making process
- accountabilities
- medical and social care models.

The scale of the health problems are so daunting that unless differences are put aside there is little or no chance of tackling the gross inequalities in health in our country, inequalities demonstrated by the following figures.

- Amongst men of working age, mortality is nearly three times greater for social class V compared with social class I. Over the past 10 years, mortality rates among young men (15–44 years) have not reduced, while those in other age groups have fallen markedly. In parts of Birmingham and Coventry, male healthy life expectancy is below retirement age.
- The poorer you are, the less healthy you are likely to be. If the whole population had experienced the same death rates as those of non-manual groups, there would have been 550 fewer stillbirths and 80 fewer deaths in the first year of life in 1994; 600 fewer deaths in children and 13 500 fewer deaths in men aged 20–64 in 1991–93.
- A baby boy born today into social classes I and II can expect to live 5 years longer than a baby born in social class IV or V.
- Children in social class V are five times as likely to suffer accidental death than children in social class I.

These figures show what Tessa Jowell, Minister for Public Health, has called 'persistent and damaging inequalities in health between different occupational and ethnic groups, between geographical areas and between men and women'. The Government's Green Paper *Our Healthier Nation* points out that poor health has complex causes. Some are fixed, for example ageing or genetic factors. Some are to do with how we all live our lives (diet, physical activity, sexual behaviour, smoking, alcohol and drugs). Social and economic issues play a part too (poverty, unemployment and social exclusion), as does our environment (air, water quality, and housing). But access to good services, like education, transport, social services and the NHS itself, are also important. Tackling these issues involves a range of linked programmes, including measures on welfare to work, crime, housing and education, as well as on health itself.

This is not easy. At the national level, getting different Whitehall departments to work together has proved to be very difficult indeed. We all know the Whitehall tradition of strong departments where traditionally ministers have earned their reputations by defending departmental interests. The results have been conflicting policies which have often cut across each other when implemented at local level. Examples of this include:

- government rules in relation to housing associations, which stopped investment in housing for people discharged from the NHS
- funding policies, which over the years have squeezed local government allocations in order to give more to the NHS, have backfired, as social services departments have been unable to give sufficient support to people we want to discharge from hospital, so NHS beds get blocked
- the well-intentioned initiative to halve the time taken between the arrest and sentencing for persistent young offenders – sorting this out involves three government departments, to say nothing of the numerous agencies and quangos who will also have a role.

This departmental jungle has then been replicated at local level within local government departments and between local authorities and other local agencies. This has to end. In attempting to give everyone a stake in society, the damage done by poor housing, ill health, poor education, the lack of decent transport, and above all the lack of work, must be tackled. The problems are linked. Poor education means a poor job. A poor job often leads to poor housing. Poor housing contributes to poor health. Poor housing and poor health make it harder to bring up a family.

The establishment of the Social Exclusion Unit within the Cabinet Office, chaired by the Prime Minister, is a most powerful and visible sign of government recognition that to begin to tackle these issues, joined-up policies are needed.

Consider the focus on four of the biggest problems:

- poor housing estates
- problems of children expelled from school who are truant
- street homelessness
- young, single men with no jobs, little education and no skills.

To address these problems policies have got to be pulled together between the many different departments and agencies at national and local level. HAZs are so interesting because they aim to do just that. They are designed to overcome the well-recognised barriers between health and local authorities, and this is crucial to tackling intractable health problems in some of the most deprived areas.

The HAZs that have been agreed make impressive reading, as shown by the following three examples.

- In the South Yorkshire coalfield communities, a heart health programme will be implemented and rehabilitation services will be redeveloped to better support the casualties of the coal and steel industries.
- In the East End of London, recognising that you are healthier if you have a job, the HAZ will target improving job opportunities for disadvantaged young people, particularly from ethnic minorities, working in partnership with the local authorities, New Deal agencies, local employers (including trusts) and voluntary groups.
- In Tyne and Wear there will be a new partnership approach to improving the health of elderly people; with a new system for assessing high risk, improved access to public transport, improved special provision housing, and a programme to improve home insulation and reduce hypothermia.

There are many other opportunities for collaboration:

- across the whole health and social care interface
- in the strong involvement of local authorities in the development of HIPs by each health authority, to agree a programme to improve health and healthcare with widespread local ownership
- around the table in each PCG, so that when GPs make crucial decisions about the commissioning of services, they have the benefit of a direct local authority input

- in the much larger number of chairs and non-executives with a local government background who have recently been appointed to the boards of NHS trusts and health authorities.

Local authorities are around the NHS table as never before. But with greater influence comes greater responsibility, and the NHS has never needed more help from local government in supporting the modernising of the health service. One of the biggest problems the health service faces is the failure of the public to support NHS plans to change the way hospital services are provided. The plans come about because of the training requirements of doctors, safety standards and the need to centralise highly specialist services. A recent report published by the British Medical Association, Royal College of Physicians and the Royal College of Surgeons argued that the growing complexity of medicine means that specialist treatments can no longer be provided safely in small local hospitals, where consultants work alone without the back-up of a full medical team. The report says that there should be no single-handed consultants in any of the main medical or surgical sub-specialities and there must be a big increase in the number of consultants to provide services of the necessary high quality. It acknowledges that the average-sized District General Hospital, serving populations of 250 000–350 000 will remain the backbone of the NHS for some time. But although these can provide most hospital services, it will not be possible for each locality to have its own acute hospital and A&E unit. Hospital closures are not intended and those hospitals no longer able to provide acute services will be valuable in providing outpatient services and rehabilitation. This provides a model by which the NHS can be brought up to the standards of the twenty-first century, with major new hospitals built and supported by an increasingly strong primary care system.

It is not always going to be easy to persuade the public of the case for change. Experience in Birmingham is a case in point, where continuous disagreement over at least 20 years has meant that every major plan for change has hit the buffer of public, political and media opposition. That opposition has resulted in the failure to invest in the capital infrastructure. This paralysis led towards the setting up of an Independent Panel to enquire into the future of the city's health service. I was asked to chair the Independent Panel and our members included the Bishop of Birmingham; the former leader of the Conservative group on the City Council; the Labour chair of Social Services Committee; the Liberal Democrat Lord Mayor Elect; and people from our many ethnic communities, business and the voluntary sector. During our work, we held public hearings – Select Committee-style – where various NHS organisations were subject to robust questioning about their proposals. What the process did more than anything else was to focus on the needs of the city as a whole, rather than any individual organisation, and for the first time in 30 years we had a real sense of constructing a city-wide coalition to support change. It is that engagement with the citizenry which should be at the heart of NHS/local government relationships.

Local authorities will need to get involved in these debates increasingly in a sustained and serious way. In a sense, this is surely a visible sign of the leadership role of local authorities, in promoting the aspirations of local people. Leadership is truly at the heart of local government, but local authorities cannot act alone. NHS/local government partnership is vital and it has to be a solid partnership. It cannot be left to chance, and failure to engage cannot be tolerated. The public would not forgive us; nor should they if we don't get our act together and start to knock heads together to ensure that services are properly co-ordinated and the links between good environment, good housing and good health are fully exploited.

In spelling out the potential of partnership, the potential problems must not be ignored. Don't let us kid ourselves that this is at all easy. As David Hunter of Leeds University has said, 'These are complex management issues... People working across boundaries cannot afford to become too immersed in a single corporate ideology, cultural framework or set of values ... empathizing with multiple cultures will be essential'. Collaboration is fine in theory but it is difficult to achieve. More exhortations to work together will not be enough A complicated process of moving staff and organisations forward cannot be underestimated. There are still differences in style, approach and accountabilities, which will have to be confronted. Collaborative working might well be tested by legal constraints on delegation of powers. And there will always be a need to have mechanisms in place that can resolve disputes between partners, without undermining the partnership.

But at the end of the day, it always comes back to a question of leadership. This is a message that goes particularly for councillors and non-executive directors on NHS boards. In the complicated area of collaborative working, they are going to have to let go and to accept some risks, and above all to give strong support to the people in the field leading change.

In conclusion, the potential NHS/local government relationship is very good and can achieve much for the public. Nye Bevan, founder of the NHS said, 'The Service must always be changing, growing and improving'. Let that be our watchword, too.

CHAPTER TWENTY-NINE

Postscript/signposts

Siân Griffiths and David J Hunter

The Government's health policy remains an important area of unfinished business. As we go to press, a clutch of important initiatives are in the pipeline, including a report on how the public health function can be strengthened, and perhaps most important of all, the White Paper setting out the new health strategy which will bring together in a single document the Government's various initiatives which have in common a public health dimension.

If the Government's health policy has a distinctive focus then it lies in the attempt to bring about a fundamental shift in respect of how health and healthcare are viewed. Running through virtually all the changes underway in health and in other policy areas is a determination to narrow the health gap between rich and poor and improve the health of local communities. The lynchpin of all the various initiatives is the Health Improvement Programme (HIMP). It will provide the strategic direction for the NHS, local government and other partners. Whether the mechanism for delivering the HIMP is a HAZ or a less elaborate form of partnership, there will be a critical role for public health in its widest sense in delivering on the new agenda. Indeed, in its absence HIMPs cannot succeed.

The Government's unfolding health policy puts public health centre stage in clinical governance, clinical effectiveness and improving the public's health. It is the last of these which constitutes probably the biggest and most complex challenge because no single profession or organisation can do it all. But if health has entered the mainstream and is now everybody's business, it will be essential to ensure that those charged with making it happen both possess the requisite skills and are present in sufficient strength. This has been the main focus of the review of the public health function led by the previous CMO of England and now under the guidance of his successor. The review has identified the need for greater cohesion amongst public health practitioners at national and local levels, identifying six areas for action:

- with the public and within communities
- between local government and health authorities

- within primary care and thus the healthcare system
- developing research and development
- enhancing the capacity of practitioners
- creating a central focus for leadership.

Competent practitioners and greater capacity will be required to make sure that the emerging policies make sense for communities at all levels and in all the various settings and sectors which are relevant to health.

Managing for health demands managers with a range of skills quite different from those required to run institutions like hospitals. Fitness for purpose is vital because without proper attention given to the implementation of the changes they will fail. A false dichotomy has emerged between public health specialists and health service management. But the boundaries between them are shifting dramatically. In order to implement the Government's agenda for health, managers are needed who understand the contribution of population-based approaches to health.

Perhaps more than at any other time in their history, and as the contributions to this book have amply demonstrated, those doing public health are change agents and catalysts working to implement a health policy which has at its centre managing for health. But the shift remains a fragile one and could easily collapse in the face of familiar pressures from the healthcare system, notably, the drive to cut waiting lists, the reconfiguration of acute inpatient services and the need to balance the books. The commitment to joint working and creative partnerships could similarly be threatened by failure to understand the cultural differences between the healthcare, local government and voluntary sectors, and the need to take time to build trust. Those practising public health must, as guardians of the public's health, do all they can to prevent such outcomes.

Index

abortion 272
Abrams Committee 161–2, 165
    annual public health reports 175
accidents, road-traffic 59
accountability
    managerial 163–4
    nurses 247
    professional 164
Acheson Report 29, 31, 136, 218
    annual reports 171, 172, 173, 174, 175,
        218
    health authorities 160, 163, 166,
        167, 170
    nurses 237, 240, 243
    policy context 16
advertising, tobacco 18, 97, 98, 99, 102
Advisory Committee on Genetics Testing 133
advocacy role
    clinicians 232
    nurses 246
ageing 6, 121–5
    efficiency of services 125–7
    future 129, 285
    minimising the need for care 127–8
    understanding 284
    see also elderly people
Agenda 21: 4, 198, 204, 207
Agriculture Act (1947) 49
air quality 60, 69, 286
alarm system, Newcastle 74
alcohol
    fetal alcohol syndrome 128
    occupational health 120
American Medical Association (AMA) 89
Amsterdam Treaty 18, 53
annual public health reports 7, 29, 164, 170,
        171–2
    Acheson Report 171, 172, 173, 174,
        175, 218
    future 276
    issues 172–4
    options for change 174–7
    scientists, public health 252

anticipatory care in general practice
    Castlefields case study 186
    primary 180–1
    secondary 181
    tertiary 181–2
    see also health promotion
Article 129 (now 152), Maastricht Treaty 18, 53
Ashkenazy population, Tay Sachs disease 134
Assistant Directors of Public Health 254
Association of British Insurers 132
asthma 182, 195–6
Australia, smoking 99, 101

Beattie, A 205
beef export ban 18
benefits scheme 39
Bevan, Aneurin ix, 289–90, 294
Beveridge Report 160
Bexley, housing 74, 75
biological issues, future development 284–5
Birmingham
    housing 74
    local authority 289, 293
Black Report 34, 35, 36, 217, 232
Blair Government *see* Labour Government
bottom-up approach, clinical decision making
        229
botulism 50
brain, molecular functioning of 284
Brazil, food 51
BRCA1 and BRCA2 genes 134
breast cancer 134, 181
Brent, multidisciplinary work 150
Brundtland, Dr Gro Harlem 17
BSE crisis 12, 18, 47
Butler, Josephine 24
butter 53–4

Calderdale, housing 75
California, smoking 99, 101, 103
Calman, Sir Kenneth 4, 16, 201, 277
Campbell, Sir Colin 133
Canada, genetics 131

cancer
   breast 134, 181
   cervical 181
   colorectal 134
   lung 138
   ovarian 134
career development opportunities
   multidisciplinary public health 153–4
   scientists, public health 255–6, 259
career progression, public health scientists 253–5
Castlefields, Runcorn 185–6
   anticipatory care 186
   clinical governance and clinical resource
      management 187
   community development 187
   health needs assessment 186
   interagency working 186–7
Central Europe 200
Centre for Communicable Disease Surveillance and
      Control 107
certification powers 29–31
cervical cytology 181
Chadwick, E 23, 24
Chamberlain, Joseph 289
Chartered Institute of Environmental Health
      198, 201
Choice and Opportunity: Primary Care: The Future
      219
Chief Environmental Health Officers 163
Chief Executives 164
Chief Medical Officer (CMO) 170
children 6, 113–14
   abuse 272
   definition of public health 107
   domestic violence witnessed by 88
   food 52, 54
   future 112–13
   health problems suffered by 109
   informed consent and genetics 132
   mortality rates 121
   parenting 110
   parents as primary healthcare providers 109
   political power 108, 109–10
   poverty 110
   prevention of health problems 110
   public health needs 107
   responsibility for public health 110–11
   vulnerability 108
cholera 23
cigarette smoking *see* smoking

class *see* socio-economic factors
climate change 60
clinical decision making 229–30
clinical governance 13, 185
   Castlefields case study 187
   future 220, 230–1, 232
clinical practice 223–4, 233
   clinicians' contribution to public health
      practice 231–3
   as determinant of health 224–8
   future 287
   public health's contribution to 228–31
clinical resource management 185
clinical services 228
cloning 132, 284
Clothier Committee 133
Cochrane, Professor Archie 216
Cogwheel Report 216
colorectal cancer 134
commercial sector
   health promotion 210
   interagency working 183
Committee on Medical Aspects of Food Policy 47
Common Agricultural Policy (CAP) 52–4
Communicable Disease Control 163, 167, 218
communicable diseases
   and climate change 60
   future developments 286
   policy context 16
communications
   future 278, 282
   multidisciplinary public health 151–2
community alarm system, Newcastle 74
community clinics 165
community development 184
   Castlefields case study 187
   health promotion 206, 210–12
Community Development Programme 43
community health services 160
community medicine 214–16
   specialists 215–16
community nurses 8
   health promotion 209
   inequalities in public health 43
   Salmon Report 236
   see also nurses, public health
community paediatricians 111
community perspectives in interdisciplinary
      approach 147–8
community physicians 27–8, 160, 217

community psychiatric nurses 186
compartmentalisation 14
computers *see* information technology
confidentiality issues, genetics 132
consent and genetics 132
Conservative Government
    benefit scheme 39
    Director of Public Health, corporate role
        175
    food 52
    inequalities in public health 34, 36
    market-style reforms of NHS 12
Consultants in Communicable Disease Control
        218
continuing care 148
continuing professional development (CPD), public
        health scientists 256, 259
contracting process 238–9
contract staff 117
coronary heart disease 48, 50
Coronary Prevention Group 48
corporate tax as occupational health incentive
        118
counselling
    genetics 134
    health promotion 205
crime viii, 69
Croydon, housing 74
cytochrome P-450 138

danger from traffic 59
decision making, clinical 229–30
dementia 124, 129
demographic changes 121
    see also ageing
Department of Health (DoH)
    genetics 133
    health promotion 207, 209
    inequalities in public health 37
    local government perspective 196
    nursing, public health 240–1
    policy context 12, 13
        Health for All 14
        health promotion 207
Department of the Environment, Transport and
        the Regions 60, 76, 196
deprivation *see* poverty
designer foods 48
determinism, genetic 132, 136
diabetes mellitus 138, 182

diagnostic techniques 287
diet *see* food
Diploma in Occupational Medicine 118
directors of finance 149
Directors of Public Health (DPH)
    Acheson Report 218
    annual reports *see* annual public health reports
    future 168, 170
    health authorities 159
    role and responsibilities 161, 162
    tensions 163, 164, 166–7
Directors of Social Services 163
disabilities, people with
    access to work 119
    ageing population 123–4, 126–7, 128,
        129
    housing 70, 74
Disabled Facilities Grants 70, 74, 75
discrimination, genetic 132
disease, understanding of 284–5
District Health Authorities 27
district nurses 236
Doll, Sir Richard 215
domestic violence 5, 85, 87
    definition 86
    extent 87
    future developments 285
    Glasgow initiatives 90–2
        health service audits 91, 92
        protocols 91, 92
        training programmes 91, 92
    health effects 87
        on child witnesses 88
        emotional and mental health 88
        physical 87–8
    implications for health service 88–9
    nature of 86–7
    service delivery, attempts to improve 89–90
drugs, future developments 287
Duncan, William Henry 4, 5, 23–6, 29,
        32, 214
    commemoration in annual report 171

Eastern Europe 200
eco-epidemiology 263
E. coli 12, 200
economic issues
    ageing population 124–5, 126, 129
    annual public health reports 174
    clinical resource management 185

food 49–52
  Common Agricultural Policy 53
funding of healthcare, impact on public health
    226
future 275
health promotion 211
housing 70
local government perspective 194, 196
multidisciplinary work 149, 150, 154–5
national expenditure on healthcare 223
smoking 97, 99, 102
education 6
  as enhancer of intelligence 128
  health 128
    see also health promotion
  of health professionals
    future 277–8, 282
    genetics 134
    multidisciplinary public health 153–4
    nurses, public health 242
    public health medicine 215, 273
    scientists, public health 255–6
  interagency working 183
  opportunities 188
  and psycho-social health viii
  smoking 96–9
Education (Provision of Meals) Act (1906) 49
elderly people 70, 74
  see also ageing
Emergency Medical Services 160
employers' liability insurance 118
employment
  changing patterns 116–17
  and inequalities in public health 38, 39
  see also occupational health
England, smoking 95, 99, 101
English National Board for Nursing, Midwifery and
    Health Visiting 247
Environmental Health Commission 198, 199,
    200, 201
Environmental Health Officers 199, 200–1
  career progression 253
  health promotion 209
environmental health services
  historical perspective 215
  interagency working 183
environmental issues 8, 198–201, 272
  ageing population 126–7
  communicable diseases 163
  food 51

future 221, 283, 286
genetics 136, 137
policy context 12
smoking 102, 103
sustainability 4
transport 60
epidemiology 4, 8–9, 229, 261–7
  genetics 131–2, 135
  'lay' 148–9
  limitations 283
  nurses, public health 237
  scientists, public health 252
  social medicine 215
ethical issues 283
  genetics 132–3, 134
ethnicity and smoking 96
eugenics 137
European Agency for Health and Safety at
    Work 18
European Medicines Evaluation Agency 18
European Union
  Directive on the Legal Protection of
      Biotechnological Inventions 132
  food 52–4
  health promotion 211
  policy context 18–19
'evaluation bypass' 166
evidence-based medicine 166, 287
evolutionary mechanisms 136
Ewles, L 205
exercise 50, 61, 272
  and ageing 128

Faculty of Community Medicine (later Faculty of
    Public Health Medicine) 216
Faculty of Occupational Medicine 118, 120
Faculty of Public Health Medicine 218
  continuing professional development 256
  membership 153, 219–20, 257–8
  standards 257
family health services authorities 162
fear of traffic 59
fertility 272
fetal alcohol syndrome 128
fetus 284–5
  uterine environment and later health
      127–8
films, portrayal of smoking in 103
finance directors 149
financial issues see economic issues

Finland
    primary care perspective 181
    smoking 99
fish 51
food 5, 47–8, 54–5, 272
    BSE 12, 18, 47
    E. coli 12, 200
    European and global contexts 52–4
    future 221
    social history 48–9
Food Act (1875) 49
food poisoning 50
Food Safety Act (1990) 48
Food Standards Agency 16, 167
Four Counties Public Health Network 152
Fresh, Thomas 25–6
fruits 51–2, 54
Fulham, housing 75
fundholding GPs 236
future of public health 9, 219–21, 280–1, 288
    biological factors and understanding disease
        284–5
    children 112–13
    education, training and research 277–8
    environment and communicable disease 286
    functions and responsibilities of public health
        275–6
    general issues 282–3
    governance 274–5
        clinical 220, 230–1, 232
    health authorities 168–70
    health promotion 211–12
    health services, role 286–7
    lifestyles 285–6
    local authorities 289–94
    multidisciplinary approach 155–7
    new methodology 283–4
    scientists, public health 259–60
    social and economic factors 285
    staffing of Public Health Departments 276–7
    tasks at local, regional and central level 278–9

gender issues
    ageing and disability 127
    life expectancy 123
General Medical Council 164, 219
general practitioner contract 180, 181, 208
general practitioners (GPs)
    ageing population 126
    budget control 162
    future 279
    historical perspective 215
    inequalities in public health 42, 43
    occupational health 118
    smoking advice 97, 100
    tensions 165
Gene Therapy Advisory Committee 133
genetic disease vs. genetic susceptibility 134–5
genetic engineering 284
genetics 6, 131, 138
    epidemiology 131–2
    ethical, legal and social framework 132–3
    future 220, 283, 284
    policy considerations 133–6
    preventive action, scope for 136–8
    thrifty genes 128
genotypic prevention of disease 137
geographical information systems 283
Germany, food 53
'Ghost Acres' phenomenon 51
Glasgow, domestic violence initiatives 90
    Health Gain Commissioning Team 90–2
    policy framework 90
Glasgow Women's Health Policy 90
global context of public health 17
    food 52–4
global warming 60
Godber, Sir George 216
Greece, food 53
Griffiths, Roy 160
Griffiths Report 163
group home development 74

haemochromatosis, hereditary 134
Hammersmith, housing 75
Harrow, multidisciplinary work 150
Hawthorn effect 120
Head Start programmes 183
Health Action Zones (HAZs)
    health promotion 211, 295
    housing 73
    inequalities in public health 40, 42
    local government perspective 194, 292
    policy context 15
Health and Morals of Apprentices' Act (1802)
    115
Health and Safety at Work Act (1974) 115
health authorities
    annual public health reports 173, 177
    future 220, 275

Health of the Nation 219
  health promotion 209, 211
  inequalities in public health 40–3
  multidisciplinary public health 145–6, 150,
      151, 156
  occupational health 118
  policy context 14
  public health practice 7, 159
    future 168–70
    history 159–62
    tensions 163–8
  smoking 101
  staffing in public health departments 251
Health Education Authority 209, 211
Health Education Council 204
Health for All 4, 28, 218, 219
  health promotion 204, 207
  policy context 13, 14, 36, 207
  Regional Health Promotion Unit 29
Health Improvement Programmes (HIMPs)
  annual public health reports 177
  future 168–9, 220
  Guidance 1
  health authorities 166
  health promotion 211–12
  housing 73, 76
  importance 295
  inequalities in public health 40
  local government perspective 194
  multidisciplinary public health 156
  nursing, public health 244, 245
  policy context 15
health insurance 132, 226
health needs assessment 180, 218, 220, 252
  Castlefields case study 186
  nursing, public health 245–6
Health of the Nation 219
  co-ordinators 254
  health promotion 166, 207
  heart disease targets 48
  inequalities in public health 36–7, 307
  obesity targets 50
  policy context 13–15, 16, 207
Health of Towns Association 24, 31
Health Promoting Hospitals 209
health promotion 8, 203
  Bevan on ix
  children and young people 110
  current issues and dilemmas 210–11
  future 211–12

  genetics 136–8
  history and theory 203–6, 215
  local government perspective 193–4, 195
  nurses, public health 248
  occupational health 118, 119–20
  policy context 12, 206–8, 210
  responsibility for 209–10
  and service provision, tensions between 166
  see also anticipatory care in general practice;
      education, health
Health Promotion Committees 208
Health Promotion Units 211
Health Service Practitioners 254
Health Services Research (HSR) 125, 126
health technology assessment 125, 261–7
health visitors 8
  community development 184
  perceptions of public health 239
  role 180, 236
  working practices 238
Healthy City Initiative 204, 218
  Glasgow 90
  Liverpool 4, 31
Healthy Living Centres 15, 183, 211
Healthy Schools Initiative 183
heart attacks 226
heart disease 48, 50
hierarchies, professional 151
high-rise accommodation 69, 74
Hillingdon, housing 75
Holland, Professor Walter 240
Holme, Dr Samuel 24
homelessness 67, 71, 73, 74, 80
Home Repair Assistance grant 70
homicide 87
horizon scanning 282–3, 284
hospitals
  central planning 217
  future 279, 293
  history 215
housing 5, 66–7, 271
  action needed 75–8
  conditions inside the home 67–8, 81–2
  conditions outside the home 68–9, 82
  costs, links with poverty and poor housing 83
  exclusion from public health, reasons for 72–3
  good-practice examples 73–5
  hazards 84
  homelessness 67, 80
  interagency working 182

Liverpool 24
  services related to 69–70
    co-ordination 71–2
Housing Action Trust 74
housing associations 70, 71, 74
Human Fertilisation and Embryology Act (1990) 133
Human Fertilisation and Embryology Authority 133
Human Genetics Advisory Commission 132
Human Genetics Advisory Committee 133
human genome project 284
Hunter Report 216

illiteracy 188
immunisation 180, 286
Independent Inquiry into Inequalities in Health vi, viii, 38
independent living schemes 71
individual relationships and multidisciplinary public health 152–3
industrial emissions 115–16
industry 183, 210
inequalities in public health 34–6, 43, 193, 291
  children 114
  policy context vi–vii, viii, 11, 36–7
    Black Report 34, 35, 36, 232
    Blair Government 37–43
    Health of the Nation 36–7, 207
    Our Healthier Nation 16
inequalities in transport 61
infant mortality rates 121
information analysis 252
information services, public health 276
information technology
  environmental health perspectives 200
  future 283
  social exclusion 188
informed consent and genetics 132
innovativeness, public health nurses 248
innumeracy 188
Inspectors of Nuisances 27
insurance
  employers' liability 118
  life 132
  medical 132, 226
intelligence 128
interagency working *see* multidisciplinary public health

internal market
  clinicians and public health doctors, tensions between 165
  health promotion 207–8
  nurses, public health 236
international context of public health 17
  food 52–4

Jenkins, Patrick 36
Joint Approach to Social Policy (JASP) 39
Joint Care Planning Teams 216–17
Joint Commission on Hospital Accreditation 89
Jones, Agnes 24
Jowell, Tessa 235, 291

Karelia, Finland, primary care perspective 181
Kirklees, housing 75

Labour Government
  agenda for public health 172
  focus on public health 235
  inequalities in public health 34, 37–8
    role of health service 40–3
    social exclusion 38–40
  local authorities 194
  policy context 11, 12–13, 15, 16
'lay' epidemiology 148–9
leadership
  development programmes 256, 260
  local authorities' role 293–4
  and multidisciplinary public health 152
  nursing, public health 247–8
legal issues
  future 282
  genetics 132–3
  health promotion 205
  occupational health 118
leisure department 183
Levy, Barry 3
liability insurance, employers' 118
life expectancy 121–3
  clinical practice as determinant of 226
  and homelessness 67
  and quality of life vii
  socio-economic factors 35
life insurance and genetic discrimination 132
lighting levels, workplace 120
Liverpool 4, 23–6
  City Health Plan 177
  new beginnings 29–32

New Public Health 28
rise and fall and renaissance of public health
    26–8
Liverpool Health of Towns Association 24
Liverpool Sanitary Act (1846) 24
Local Agenda 21: 198
local authorities 7–8, 192–7
    annual public health reports 177
    community medicine 214–15
    environmental health 200
    future 275, 289–94
    and health authorities, tensions between 163
    health promotion 209
    housing 70, 76
    inequalities in public health 42
    interagency working 182–3
    Medical Officers of Health 27
    nursing, public health 244
    occupational health 117
    policy context
        Health of the Nation 14–15
        health promotion 12
Local Environmental Health Action Plan 4
Local Government Association 61, 196
Local Transport Plans 61
London Food Commission 48
lone parents 39
'low-fat' foods 48
lung cancer 138

Maastricht Treaty, Article 129 (now 152) 18, 53
Massachusetts
    life expectancy 123
    smoking 99, 101
managers and professionals, tensions between
    163–5
maternal–fetal interactions 284–5
McCormick, Professor James 180
measles 272, 286
media
    epidemiology 262
    health promotion 210
medical insurance 132, 226
Medical Officers of Environmental Health 160
Medical Officers of Health (MOH) 2, 26–7,
    159–60, 163, 214–15
    annual reports 7, 29, 173
    Duncan, William Henry 4, 5, 23–6, 29, 32,
        214
        commemoration in annual report 171

health promotion 203
Mental Health Schemes 182
mental illnesses, people with
    housing 70
    informed consent and genetics 132
Mersey Health Region 28–32
metabolism 138
minimally invasive surgery 287
Minister for Public Health
    annual public health reports 175, 176
    appointment 1, 12–13, 172, 220
    health promotion 209
    policy context 15, 16
    role 235
Ministry of Agriculture, Fisheries and Food
        (MAFF) 49
Ministry of Food 49
Ministry of Health (MOH) 160
Ministry of Health Act (1919) 166
Minnesota 99
moral issues 283
    genetics 132–3, 134
morbidity 272
    reduction through clinical practice 225–7
Morris, Professor JN (Jerry) 215
mortality 121, 122, 272
    inequalities 291
    reduction through clinical practice 225–7
multidisciplinary public health 6–7, 75, 143, 219
    benefits 146–50
    challenges 273
    development 150–5
    different ways of working 145–6
    future 155–7, 287, 294
    King's Fund research project 144–5
    nurses, public health 247
    primary care perspective 155–6, 182–3
        Castlefields case study 186–7
    tensions 166–7
Multidisciplinary Public Health Forum (MDPHF)
        219, 257, 258

National Environmental Action Plan 4
National Environmental Health Action Plans
        (NEHAPs) 199
National Health Service (NHS)
    ageing population 126
    community medicine departments 216
    community nurses 236
    domestic violence 89–90

future 293, 294
genetics 133, 135
Health of the Nation 15
health promotion 207–8, 211
history 160, 162, 215
inequalities in public health 37, 40–3
and local authorities, relationship between
     192, 193, 194
multidisciplinary public health 143, 156
   King's Fund research project 144
occupational health 116, 117, 119, 120
reorganisations 217–19, 238
resource allocation 217
scientists, public health 255
National Health Service Act (1977) 166
National Health Service and Community Care Act
     (1991) 207–8
National Health Service: A Service with Ambitions
     219
National Health Service Executive
   annual public health reports, lack of 173–4
   health promotion 209
National Health Service Reorganisation: England
     215
National Lottery 211
natural selection 136
needs assessment
   health 218, 220, 252
      nursing, public health 245–6
      primary care 180, 186
   housing 71
Netherlands, life expectancy 123
Newcastle, housing 74, 75
New Commitment to Regeneration Programme
     196–7
New Contract for Welfare 38
Newlands, James 25–6
New NHS: Modern, Dependable 220
   annual public health reports 171
   health authorities 168
   health promotion 208
   inequalities in public health 40
   multidisciplinary public health 155
   nurses, public health 235, 242, 244–6
New Public Health 28, 31
NHS Direct vi
nicotine replacement therapy (NRT) 97, 98, 100,
     102–3
Nightingale, Florence 24
noise pollution 60, 69

'non-fat fats' 48
non-insulin dependent diabetes 138
non-smoking clubs 97, 99
North Downs Community Trust 147–8
Northern Ireland, policy context 13, 15
Norway, smoking 99
No Smoking Day 101
nurses, public health 8, 235
   commonalities between public health and
        nursing 239–41
   and housing 74
   inequalities in public health 43
   opportunities 242–8
   present approach to public health, difficulties
        with 236–9
   see also community nurses
nutrition *see* food

obesity 50
occupational health 6, 115–17, 120
   health promotion 210
   Our Healthier Nation 117–20
   smoking restrictions 98, 102, 120
   working practices 238
occupational psychologists 119
Office of National Statistics 167
older people *see* ageing; elderly people
opportunistic screening 181
organisational concerns 273, 282
Ottawa Charter for Health Promotion 4, 28, 204
Our Healthier Nation vi, 220, 251, 291
   annual public health reports 176, 177
   co-ordinators 254
   education sector 6
   health promotion 166, 169–70, 208
   inequalities in public health 38, 40
   local government perspective 196
   multidisciplinary public health 156–7
   occupational health 117–20
   policy context 13, 15–16
   targets vii
outsourcing 117
ovarian cancer 134
Oxfordshire, multidisciplinary work 148

paediatricians 109, 111, 113–14
palliation 287
parenting 110
parents as primary healthcare providers 109
part-time staff, occupational health 117

patenting of genetic material 132
Patient's Charter 219
Peckham, Professor Michael 185
personalities and multidisciplinary public health
      152–3
pesticides 51
pharmacists 287
phenotypic prevention of disease 137–8
physical activity 50, 61, 272
      and ageing 128
PKU neonatal screening programme 134
planning departments 183
policies, public health vi–vii, viii, 11–17, 295
      and clinical practice, disconnection between
            237–9
      European Union 18–19
      genetics 133–6
      health promotion 12, 206–8, 210
      housing 73, 75–7
      inequalities in public health 36–7
      international context 17
      transport 61
polio 286
political imperatives and multidisciplinary public
            health 155
political power, children and young people 108,
            109–10
Polkinghorne, Reverend Dr John 133
pollution
      and housing 69
      occupational health 115–16
      traffic 60
polymerase chain reaction (PCR) 283
population
      size
            and organisation of public health 29
            and responsibility of primary care groups
                  168
      structure 121, 122
Portugal, food 53
poverty 5, 272, 291
      children 110
      and diet 49, 52
      future developments 285
      and housing 70, 83
      and occupational health 116
pragmatism and multidisciplinary public health
            155
pregnant women
      domestic violence 88

maternal–fetal interactions 284–5
      smoking 95, 97, 101
      uterine environment and later health
            127–8
Prevention and Health 207
prevention of health problems *see* health
            promotion
primary anticipatory care in general practice
            180–1
primary care 7, 179, 188–9
      anticipatory care
            primary 180–1
            secondary 181
            tertiary 181–2
      budgets 162
      Castlefields case study 185–7
      children 112
      clinical governance and clinical resource
            management 185
      community development 184
      future 168–70, 220
      health needs assessment 180
      Health of the Nation 14
      health promotion 208, 209
      history 215
      housing 71–2
      inequalities in public health 42–3
      multidisciplinary public health 155–6, 182–3
      nursing, public health 244–5, 246
      social exclusion 187–8
      see also general practitioners
Primary Care: Delivering the Future 219
Priority and Planning Guidance 40
privacy issues, genetics 132
professionals, public health
      challenges 4
      contribution to practice of public health 231
            advocacy role 232
            shaping health services for populations
                  232–3
      and managers, tensions between 163–5
promotion of health *see* health promotion
psychologists, occupational 119
psycho-social health viii
public health, definitions 3
Public Health Act (1848) 24, 159
      environmental health 199
      food context 48
Public Health Commissions/Forums 177
Public Health Common Data Set 173

Public Health Laboratory Service 160
purchaser–provider separation 12

qualitative vs. quantitative work 154
quality of life vii, 3

randomised controlled trials (RCTs) 211, 225, 226
Rathbone, Eleanor 24
recruitment of employees 116
regional development agencies (RDAs) 19
Regional Health Authorities (RHAs) 29, 173
Regional Health Promotion Unit 29
regionalisation 19
Registered Social Landlords 70, 71
rehabilitation 287
relationships and multidisciplinary public health 152–3
research
    community 8–9
    efficiency of services 125, 126
    funding, local government perspective 194
    future 277–8, 281
    genetics 135, 138
    health technology assessment 262, 265, 266–7
    into housing 77
    into public health medicine 215, 273
    scientists, public health 253
    use by public health nurses 247
resource allocation 217, 273
Resource Allocation Working Party (RAWP) 217
resource constraints
    health promotion 210
    multidisciplinary public health 154–5
resource management, clinical 185
    Castlefields case study 187
    nursing, public health 248
reviews of services 252
Rotherham, transport 62–4
Royal College of Nursing 247
Royal College of Physicians 101, 232
Royal Institute for Public Health and Hygiene 257
Runcorn see Castlefields, Runcorn

salmonellosis 50
Salmon Report 236
Sardinia, thalassaemia screening 134
scanning techniques 287
schizophrenia 138

School Health Service 236
school nurses 236, 238
schools
    food 49, 54
    health promotion 210
    interagency working 183
    nurses, public health 236, 238
    smoking 96–9
scientists, public health 8, 250–1
    career progression 253–5
    competencies 258–9
    contribution of different professions 251–3
    education, training and professional development 255–6
    future 259–60
    issues facing 253
    standards 257–8
Scotland
    policy context 13, 14, 15
    smoking 102
Scottish Inter-Collegiate Guideline Network (SIGN) 182
Scottish Needs Assessment Programme Report 85, 86
Scott Samuel, Alex 206
screening
    breast cancer 181
    cervical cytology 181
    future developments 287
    genetic 134, 287
    opportunistic 181
seat-belt legislation 207
secondary anticipatory care in general practice 181
secondments, housing 75
Second World War 49, 160
security issues, housing 69, 70
Seebohm committee 27
self-employment, occupational health 117, 118
Semple, Andrew 27, 28
settings approach to public health 31
Shaw, George Bernard 2
Sheffield
    multidisciplinary work 150
    transport 62–4
sheltered accommodation 71
shopping 50–1
SIGN guideline development 181–2
Simnett, I 205
Single Regeneration 211

smallpox 286
Smokebusters 99
Smokers Advice Clinics 97, 100
smoking 5–6, 95–6, 97–8, 103, 220–1
    future developments 285–6
    harm reduction strategies 98, 102–3
    reducing adult prevalence 97–8, 100
        through access restrictions 102
        through demand reduction 100–2
    reducing teenage prevalence 96, 97, 99–100
        through access restrictions 99
        through education 96–9
    Royal College of Physicians' campaign against
        101, 232
    tobacco advertising and sponsorship ban 18,
        97, 99
    tobacco control white paper 16
    trends 272
    workplace bans and restrictions 98, 102, 120
smuggling, tobacco 102, 103
social care managers 186
social exclusion
    inequalities in public health 38–40
    nursing, public health 246
    primary care perspective 187–8
    and psycho-social health viii
Social Exclusion Unit (SEU) 196, 292
    inequalities in public health 38, 39, 40
social health 227–8
social interaction 60
social medicine 215
social paediatricians 111
social science 264
social services 162
    historical perspective 215
    nursing, public health 244
    Seebohm committee 27
Social Services Mental Health Organisation 182
Society of Health Promotion Education and
        Promotion Specialists (SHEPS) 204
socio-economic factors
    children and young people 110
    food 52
    future developments 285
    housing 70
    inequalities in public health 34–6, 291
    smoking 95–6
    transport 61
South Bristol Health Park 151
sponsorship, tobacco 18, 97, 98, 99, 102

status issues, multidisciplinary public health 154
Stott-Davis consultation model for GPs 180
strategy development 252
Strategy for Nursing, Midwifery and Health Visiting
    248
stress and transport 59
suicide and attempted suicide 88
support services, housing 71
susceptibility, genetic 135, 137
sustainable development 198, 201, 221

taxation
    as occupational health incentive 118
    tobacco 102, 103
Tay Sachs disease, screening 134
team work 247
    see also multidisciplinary public health
technology
    health 261–7
    information 188, 200, 283
teenagers 6, 113–14
    definition of public health 107
    future 112–13
        primary care groups 112
    health problems suffered by 109
    parenting 110
    parents as primary healthcare providers 109
    political power 108, 109–10
    poverty 110
    prevention of health problems 110
    public health needs 107
    responsibility for public health 110–11
    smoking 95, 96, 97, 99–100
        access restrictions 99
        reduction through education 96–9
    vulnerability 108
telephone 'quit lines' 101–2
temporary staff, occupational health 117
tensions in health authorities
    clinicians and public health doctors 165
    doctors and multidisciplinary public health
        166–7
    general manager and professional 163–5
    health and health services 166
    local government and health authority 163
    strategic and operational 165–6
tertiary anticipatory care in general practice
    181–2
testing, genetic 134
thalassaemia screening 134

thrifty genes 128
time issues 154
tobacco smoking *see* smoking
top-down approach, clinical decision making 230
training
    child public health 112
    Environmental Health Officers 199, 200–1
    future 277–8
    multidisciplinary public health 153–4
    nurses, public health 242
    scientists, public health 255–6, 259
    Tomorrow's Doctors (GMC) 219
transport 5, 59
    accidents 59
    air quality 60
    challenge 62
    environmental damage 60
    food 51
    inequalities 61
    interagency working 183
    physical activity 61
    policy context 17, 61, 65
    Sheffield and Rotherham transport challenge
        62
      future 64
      public consultation outcomes 63–4
      Transport and Health Group 62–3
    social interaction 60
    stress, fear and danger 59
Transport and Health Group, Sheffield and
        Rotherham 62–3, 64
Treaty of Amsterdam 18, 53
tribalism culture 151
trust and multidisciplinary public health 153
Tudor-Hart, Julian 180, 189

United Nations (UN) 17
    Agenda 21: 4, 198, 204, 207
    Convention on the Rights of the Child 108
    Declaration on the Elimination of Violence
        Against Women 86
United States of America
    ageing population 123, 125, 129
    challenges to public health 3
    definition of public health 3
    domestic violence 89
    food poisoning, costs 50

    genetics 134
    Head Start programmes 183
    smoking 99, 100, 101, 103
user perspectives in multidisciplinary approach
        148–9
uterine environment and later health 127–8

vaccination 180, 286
vascular disease 128, 129
vegetables 51–2, 54
Vermont, smoking 99
'victim blaming' 211
Vienna Declaration 86
violence 272, 285
    see also domestic violence
voluntary organisations
    health promotion 210
    housing 71
    interagency working 183

waiting lists 219
Wales 13, 14, 15
Waltham Forest, housing 74
wardens, sheltered accommodation 71
waste-disposal sites 116
welfare rights workers 183, 186
Welsh Health Planning Forum 13–14
West Germany, food 53
wheelchair-accessible housing 74
whooping cough 272
Wilkinson, Kitty 24
Working for Patients reforms 161
Working Together for a Healthier Scotland 85
workplaces *see* occupational health
World Health Organisation (WHO) 17
    Alma Ata declaration 28, 203
    definitions
      health 227
      public health 167
    Health for All see Health for All
    health improvement targets, European 204
    nursing, public health 241
    Ottawa Charter 4, 28, 204
World War II 49, 160

young people *see* children; teenagers
youth services 183, 186–7